Virginia Mason Medical Center:
The First 100 Years

Volume 1

D1738311

Virginia Mason Medical Center:
The First 100 Years

Volume 1

John Kirkpatrick, MD

Katherine Galagan, MD

Editors

Cover design by Marcia Friedman, Friedman Peterson Design

Top photo: VMMC founders and staff, 1929, L to R, back row:
Drs. John M. Blackford, J. Tate Mason Sr., Maurice Dwyer, George A.
Dowling, Frederick Pilcher (intern), J.T. Dowling, R. Brittain, Minor C.
Lile, Harrison Wesson (intern). Front row: Drs. Aubrey Carter (intern),
Pius A. Rohrer, Noble Dick, Mr. Lewis Dare, Drs. Al Ballé, Joel W. Baker,
Lester J. Palmer, Minor Payne (intern), John N. Wilkinson. Not pictured:
Dr. Louis H. Edmunds. (PH 0125, Virginia Mason Historical Archives)
Bottom photo, left: Unidentified radiation oncology staff positioning patient
on linear accelerator, 1976 (PH 1000, VMHA).
Bottom photo, right upper: Nurse Marge McQuillan and Dr. Richard Dion
with newborn twins, circa 1960 (PH 1309, VMHA).
Bottom photo, right lower: Dr. Nanette Robinson (R) receiving award from
Dr. Donna Smith (L), 2019 (PH 9068, VMHA).

ISBN: 9798602454390

Printed in the United States of America

DEDICATION

History is memory,
and therefore we remember all those,
past and present,
who have given their best efforts, time and passion
to make Virginia Mason
a medical center of excellence

AUTHORS AND CONTRIBUTORS

Gillian Abshire, RN, MSN

Director, Graduate Medical Education

Barry Aaronson, MD, FACP, SFHM

Hospitalist, & Section Head (1999 - 2003), Hospital Medicine

Chief Medical Informatics Officer, Virginia Mason Medical Center

John Adams, MBChB, FRANZCP

Past Clinical Fellow (1983), Section of Psychiatry & Psychology

Ruth Anderson, MT(ASCP), MBA

Emerita Senior Vice President

George M. Auld, CPA

Emeritus Director of Finance

Kasra R. Badiozamani, MD

Retired Staff Physician, & Section Head (2014–19), Radiation Oncology

Oneil Bains, MD

Staff Physician, and Section Head (2013–present), Sleep Medicine

David Beaudry, MD

Emeritus Physician, Section of Ophthalmology

C. Craig Blackmore, MD, MPH

Staff Radiologist, Department of Radiology

Director, Center for Health Care Improvement Science

Jeffrey Carlin, MD

Staff Physician, & Section Head (2007 – 2017), Rheumatology

Director, Arthritis Clinical Research Unit (2015 – present)

Roy J. Correa, Jr., MD, FACS

Emeritus Physician, & Section Head (1974 – 1980), Urology & Renal Transplantation

Sally Cramer, RN

Retired, Clinic Nurse (1986 – 2018)

Cyrus Cryst, MD, FASN

Staff Physician (1992), & Section Head (2008–present), Nephrology

Medical Director, Renal and Pancreas Transplant Service (2008 – 2013)

Ellie David, writer

William DePaso, MD, FAASM

Emeritus Physician, & Section Head (2001 - 2013), Sleep Medicine

F. Richard Dion, MD

Emeritus Physician, & Section Head (1962 - approx. 1980), Pediatrics

Albert B. Einstein, MD, FACP

Former Staff Physician & Medical Director of the VM Cancer Center,

Section of Hematology / Oncology (1976 - 1993)

Farrokh Farrokhi, MD

Staff Physician, & Section Head (2014–present), Neurosurgery

Peggy Flanagan, LICSW

Former Social Worker, Section of Psychiatry & Psychology (1975-2001)

Paul Fredlund, MD

Emeritus Physician, Section of Endocrinology

Medical Director, Graduate Medical Education (1976 – 1979)

Medical Director, Continuing Medical Education (1995 – 1999)

Ken Freeman

Vice President, Enterprise Business Development

Melvin I. Freeman, MD, FACS

Emeritus Physician, & Section Head (1969–1995), Ophthalmology

Medical Director, Continuing Medical Education (1984 –1995)

Affiliate Clinical Investigator, Benaroya Research Institute (1995-present)

Andrew Friedman, MD

Staff Physician, & Section Head (2002–present), Physical Medicine & Rehabilitation

Katherine A. Galagan, MD

Emerita Physician, Department Chief (2001–2009) & Director of Clinical Laboratories (2001-2013); Pathology and Clinical Laboratories

Harry Geggel, MD

Staff Physician, & Section Head (2003 – 2018), Ophthalmology

Tony Gerbino, MD

Staff Physician (2001-present), Sections of Pulmonary, Critical Care, and Hyperbaric Medicine

Former Section Head (2006 -2017), Pulmonary Medicine

Ingrid Gerbino, MD, FACP

Chief, Department of Primary Care (2016 - present)

Robert P. Gibbons, MD, FACS

Emeritus Physician, & Section Head (1980 - 1995), Urology & Renal Transplantation

Michael Gluck, MD, AGAF, FASGE

Emeritus Physician, & Chief of Medicine (2013–2017), Gastroenterology

Craig Goodrich

Senior Vice-President/Chief Financial Officer

Debbie Gordon

Executive Assistant to Jeanne Jachim

Thomas Green, MD, FAAOS

Emeritus Physician, & Section Head (1979–2013), Orthopaedic Surgery

Mark D. Hafermann, MD, FACR

Emeritus Physician, & Section Head (1983 - 1993), Radiation Oncology

Emeritus Medical Director, Virginia Mason Cancer Center (1993 – 1998)

Charles J. Hammer, Jr, MD, FAAD

Emeritus Physician, & Section Head (1968 – 1994), Dermatology

Neil B. Hampson, MD, FACP, FCCP, FUHM

Emeritus Physician, & Section Head (1999 - 2006), Pulmonary, Critical Care & Hyperbaric Medicine

Medical Director, Center for Hyperbaric Medicine (1989 – 2010)

Affiliate Clinical Researcher, Benaroya Research Institute (2010–present)

Scott Hansen, MD

Section Head, Hospital Psychiatry Consultative Service

Daniel Hanson, MD, FHM

Staff Physician, & Section Head (2003 - 2008), Hospital Medicine

Director of Quality & Safety (2010 – 2013), Hospital Medicine

James Holm, MD, FACP, FACEP, FUHM

Section Head & Medical Director, Hyperbaric Medicine (2010 - present)

John R. Holmes, MD, FACC

Emeritus Physician, & Section Head (1994 - 2006), Cardiology

Jeanne E. Jachim

Vice-President, VMMC and President, Virginia Mason Foundation

G. Ted Johnson, MD

Emeritus Physician, Section of Emergency Medicine

Medical Director, SENSE program (1983-96) & Patient Education (1993-96)

Steve Juergens, MD

Former Staff Physician, Director (1990–2003), Chemical Dependency
Program; & Section Head (2000 – 2003), Psychiatry & Psychology

Gary Kaplan, MD, FACP

Chief Executive Officer, VMMC (2000 - present)

Julie R. Katz, RN

Administrative Director, Research & Academics

Rita Kelly, RN, retired

Reiley Kidd, MD

Emeritus Physician, & Department Chief (1988 – 1995): Radiology

John Kirkpatrick, MD, FACP

Emeritus Physician, Co-Founder & Section Head, Lewis & John Dare
Center (2000 – 2013)

General Internist, Section of General Internal Medicine (1976 – 2000)

Cynthia Kirtland, M.Div.

Supervisor, Spiritual Care and Support

Steven Kirtland, MD

Staff Physician, & Section Head (2017 – present), Pulmonary Medicine

Current Chief of Staff, VM Hospital (2009 - present)

Brian Knowles

Executive Director, Bailey-Boushay House

Kathleen Kobashi, MD, FACS

Staff Physician, & Section Head (2007-present), Urology & Renal
Transplantation

Richard Kozarek, MD, FASGE, FACG, AGAF

Executive Director, Digestive Disease Institute

Gastroenterologist, Section of Therapeutic Endoscopy

Dawna Kramer, MD

Emerita Physician, Department of Radiology

Joyce Lammert, MD, PhD, FAAAI, FACP

Medical Director of Physician & APP Recruitment, Development & Services

Former Executive Medical Director, Hospital (2013 - 2019)

Former Chief of Medicine (2007 - 2013)

Nancy Lencioni, ARNP, retired

Lisa Lotus, Former VMMC Archivist (2008 - 2012)

Donald E. Low, MD, FACS, FRCS(C)

Section Head (1991 - 2019), Thoracic Surgery & Thoracic Oncology

Director, Digestive Disease Institute Esophageal Center of Excellence

President, Ryan Hill Research Foundation

James MacLean, MD

Emeritus Physician, & Section Head (1982 – 1997), Neurology

Stephen J. Melson, MD

Emeritus Physician, & Section Head (1988–2000), Psychiatry & Psych.

Linda Mihalov, MD, FACOG

Staff Physician, & Section Head (approx. 2007 - present); Gynecology, Gynecologic Oncology, & Urogynecology

Diane K. Miller, MBA

Emerita Vice President & Executive Director of The Virginia Mason Institute (2008 – 2016)

Liz Woody Moehrke, CGRN, retired; Section of Gastroenterology

Neeta Moonka, MD

Physician Advisor, Supply Chain

Michael Mulroy, MD

Emeritus Physician, Department of Anesthesiology

Craig Murakami, MD, FACS

Staff Physician, & Section Head (2001 - 2008), Otolaryngology

Medical Director, Cosmetic Services

Dottie Nelson, PT

Retired, Physical therapist (1969), & Director (1975-1993), Physical Medicine & Rehabilitation

Maxine Nelson, MSW

Former Social Worker, Section of Psychiatry & Psychology (1987 - 1998)

Gerald (Jerry) Nepom, MD, PhD

Member and Director, Immunology and Diabetes Programs, Virginia Mason Research Center (1985 - 1994)

Director, Benaroya Research Institute at Virginia Mason (1994-2015)

Director, Immune Tolerance Network (2010–present)

Sandy Novak, MBA

Retired, Administrative Director (1978- 2007)

Ulrike Ochs, MD, FAAD

Staff Physician, and Section Head (2002 - 2014), Dermatology

Don Olson, BA, MHA

Emeritus Hospital Administrator

Brian D. Owens, MD

Emeritus Physician, Department of Anesthesiology

Former Director, Graduate Medical Education & Designated Institutional Official (2003 – 2016)

Keith Paige, MD, FACS

Former Staff Physician, & Section Head (2005 – 2014), Plastic & Reconstructive Surgery

Daniel L. Paull, MD, FACS

Emeritus Physician, & Section Head (1997–2008), Cardiothoracic Surgery

Stephanie Perry, MA, SFHM

Director of Hospital Medical Services

Pat Pethigal, RN, BSN

Retired, Administrative Director, GI Services

Huong T. Pham, MD

Staff Physician, & Section Head ('09-14; '19 – present), Radiation Oncology

William Poppy

Senior Vice President, Information Technology & Payer Contracting

Catherine Potts, MD, FACP

Staff Physician, & Former Chief (2010-2016), Dept. of Primary Care

Former Section Head (1994 - 2010), Bellevue Regional Medical Center

Astrid Pujari, MD

Medical Director, Integrative Medicine

Patrick A. Ragen, MD, MS

Emeritus Physician, Section of Hematology / Oncology

Lawrence Rainey, PhD

Emeritus Psychologist, Section of Psychiatry & Psychology

Edmond J. Raker, MD, FACS

Emeritus Physician, & Section Head (1988 – 2016), Vascular Surgery

David M. Robinson, MD, FAAAAI

Staff Physician, Section of Asthma, Allergy & Immunology

Affiliate Clinical Investigator, Benaroya Research Center

Michael Rona

President Emeritus

Austin Ross

Emeritus Executive Administrator

Robert Rudolph, MD, FACP

Emeritus Physician & Section Head (1993–97), Hematology/Oncology

John A. Ryan, Jr, MD, FACS

Emeritus Chief of Surgery (1991 – 2001); Section of General Surgery (1977 - 2012)

Edward K. Rynearson, MD

Emeritus Physician & Section Head (1972-88), Psychiatry & Psychology

Current locums associate, Loss and Separation Program

Margot Schwartz, MD, MPH

Staff Physician, & Section Head (2013 - 2015), Infectious Disease

James Schlenker, MD, FACS

Staff Physician, & Section Head (2014–present), Plastic & Reconstructive Surgery

James Simmons, MD

Emeritus Physician, & Section Head (1974–89), General Internal Medicine

Associate Program Director of Internal Medicine Residency (1993-98)

Donald Smith, MD, FACOG

Former Staff Obstetrician/Gynecologist (1972 – 1980)

Arden Snyder, PhD

Emeritus Psychologist, Section of Psychiatry & Psychology

Richard Soderstrom, MD, FACOG

Former Staff Obstetrician / Gynecologist (1965 – 1984)

Wyndam Strodtbeck, MD

Chief, Department of Anesthesiology (2018 - present)

Bill Thurman, MFA, MSW

Former Social Worker, Section of Psychiatry & Psychology (1975 - 2013)

Taylor Ubben

Retired, Supervisor, Medical Photography

Paul Weiden, MD, FACP

Former Staff Physician, Section of Hematology/Oncology (1981 - 2001)
Former Medical Director, VM Cancer Clinical Research Unit
(1995 - 2001)

Michael Weinstein, MD, MRM, FAAPMR, FAHA

Emeritus Physician (1986 – 2001), Physical Medicine & Rehabilitation

Patti Wilbur, RN

Retired Staff Nurse, & Director (2002–2015), Gastroenterology

Robert Wilburn, MD

Emeritus Physician, & Section Head (app.1980 - 2008), Nephrology
Emeritus Medical Director, Renal & Pancreas Transplant Service

David Wilma, author and historian

Roger Woolf, PharmD

Director of Pharmacy (1992 – present)

Julianna Yu, MD, FACEP

Staff Physician, and Section Head (2008 - 2017), Emergency Medicine

David Zehring, MD

Former Staff Physician, Plastic and Reconstructive Surgery

Art Zoloth, PharmD

Former Director of Pharmacy (1970 – 1992)

CONTENTS

FOREWORD: An Analogy to the Past

This collection of medical staff memories contains vivid stories of individual and group accomplishments that pushed Virginia Mason Medical Center along a path of extraordinary professional competence. Thinking about these accomplishments led me to reflect on what specific actions contributed to these results.

To start the story, I remember arriving at Virginia Mason in July of 1955, 35 years after the founding of the organization. I remember not being very impressed with the old brick building, and equally unimpressed that entering required climbing a few steps and ducking through a modest-height door. The main entrance used to be at the Seneca Street corner, and patients on stretchers had to be carried up the steps.

Once inside, I sought out Don Faber, the hospital administrator, who was sharing a 10 foot-square office with his secretary. About then I was thinking I might have been wrong to accept this administrative fellowship, particularly after turning down an offer to join the staff of a large new hospital in the San Francisco Bay area. Fortunately, my next encounter was meeting with John Dare, the administrative executive who would be my preceptor. John was the key to my accepting the position; at the time he was President of the Association of Western Hospitals and very well respected in the field. We had a good meeting. Things were finally improving.

It wasn't long before I sensed the value of a joint hospital clinic organization. The medical staff members were cohesive, and the typical friction often found between physicians and the hospital executive team was minimized. Personal relationships were constantly strengthened through social events. A typical event would be a dinner hosted by Tom Carlile. MD, and his wife, Berta, or others. John Dare might be entertaining on a piano. Cocktails were numerous and the dinner was informal and friendly.

This is not to suggest that all was quiet and calm. There were questions about how to expand the property that led to multiple meetings with the city and community neighbors; lay board members of the hospital were often key to the property acquisitions. There were also difficult decisions to make such as whether to develop a satellite clinic system. This issue was fiercely contested by some physicians who felt that the best course was to focus on specialty medicine at the downtown site rather than expand into primary care.

The decision to create the Virginia Mason Health Plan got off to a rocky start, and after several years and a subsequent sale to Aetna Insurance Company, it ceased to exist. But the single most difficult question was whether and how to create a single not-for-profit organization, buy out the partners and redefine the decision-making structure. This was finally accomplished under Roger Lindeman and his leadership team, along with lawyers and the medical staff study group chaired by Jim MacLean.

I recall that ultimately only one partner voted against the proposal. That partner was neurosurgeon Ed Reifel, who humorously noted that he really supported the proposal, but voted "no" because he couldn't believe that any group of physicians could ever approve anything unanimously.

Reflecting on the history in these pages led me to reflect on why Virginia Mason Medical Center is so different. There are numerous special attributes that make the difference.

A lot had to do with how new physician associates were selected. There was an intense review of the need for the addition, with early definition of the type of educational background needed. Thorough interviews and reference checking followed.

Selected physicians were thoroughly briefed on the culture and expectations of the organization, and there was a constant focus on providing care for the whole person in an integrated care model.

In the early period of employment there was an emphasis on performance excellence, which was evaluated by a well-defined peer review process. There was further emphasis on the importance of team work with other staff and employees, which came to be known as Team Medicine.

Physicians were encouraged to participate in local, regional and national associations, which helped harvest outstanding technical developments that could then be used at home or shared with others outside the organization. This provided constant improvement to practices and organizational innovation.

Recognizing and rewarding individual accomplishments was another regular practice. Emeritus members were not abandoned and regular briefings of members were constant.

Finally, the essential piece of Virginia Mason's innovative practice was the absolute inclusion of physicians in decision-making processes.

This book, a collection of histories of the clinical staff's origins and accomplishments, is entertaining and complete and reflects each author's belief that recording the past is important. It is a rare gem and worth actively reviewing. Special commendation goes to Drs. John Kirkpatrick and Katherine Galagan, who encouraged submissions, edited and carried them through to publication.

Today's world is very different than the world in which the events and accomplishments detailed in this book unfolded, but innovation and creativity are constant and accelerating. The future is bright for Virginia Mason because of the cultural building blocks of excellence and "team medicine" that formed its foundation.

Austin Ross
Emeritus Executive Administrator (1955 - 1991)
Author of *The First 75 Years, Virginia Mason Medical Center, 1920-1995*
Seattle, WA
November 25, 2019

EDITORS' PREFACE

I remember reading the impressively detailed history of The Mason Clinic's Department of Radiology written by Reiley Kidd, MD, and first published in the *Bulletin* in 1995. It was written on the occasion of the Medical Center's 75th anniversary, and covered the years from 1920 to 1995. Reiley's personal interest in genealogy made his work informative, interesting and very complete. After reading this comprehensive volume, I immediately thought how great it would be to have similar information about each section of the Medical Center: the people who worked there, their major accomplishments, the changes they experienced and some reminiscences of their time at Virginia Mason.

With the impending Centennial of our medical center, it seemed a good time to record the history before it was lost, so I asked 34 of my emeritus colleagues if they would participate in such a project and 25 answered affirmatively. That was in 2015. To my great and good fortune, about a year later I sat next to Katherine Galagan at an annual breakfast for retired physicians. After she heard what I was up to, Katherine generously offered to help with editing. She had previously edited and published several books for the College of American Pathologists leading to a Lifetime Achievement Award from the CAP, and she had done other books for relatives and friends. Little did she know how our project would grow, with another 50 or more writers signing on. Some of their writings exceed 60 pages, with one over 90 pages long. Needless to say, the amount of time she has donated over the past three years has been enormous and I am indebted to her for this monumental effort.

Virginia Mason has commissioned author David Wilma to research a history covering the first 100 years of Virginia Mason Medical Center, which will be an overview of the highpoints of Virginia Mason since its founding in 1920. This follows the 50-year history written by former Virginia Mason intern Allen Nourse, MD, and the 75-year history written by administrator extraordinaire Austin Ross. Our book, meanwhile, focuses more on the back story of the individuals who worked here, where they came from, what talents they brought and their achievements locally, regionally, nationally and, in some cases, internationally. We've also included their research findings, breakthroughs and numerous "firsts".

Their contributions to medicine and Virginia Mason were enormous, the care given to patients was excellent and the teaching was superb, drawing outstanding medical students to Virginia Mason's training programs in anesthesia, surgery, radiology, medicine and, for a time, pathology. All of this led to "first class patient care" as Virginia Mason became the premier referral center in the Northwest. You'll read about the camaraderie and, in the opinion of several of the authors, the "special sauce" that has made Virginia Mason such a unique place.

The book is in two volumes, with the first focusing on the sections within the Departments of Medicine, Primary Care, and Hospital Services, followed by numerous chapters on various important support services within the medical center, including graduate medical education, administration, the Bailey-Boushay House and many more. The second volume contains the histories of the Departments of Surgery, Anesthesiology, Pathology and Radiology, as well as short chapters on the history of Benaroya Research Institute, the Pharmacy and Medical Photography.

This history has limitations, however, and they must be acknowledged. First, the focus is on the physicians who served in the sections. There is simply not enough time or space to acknowledge the thousands of others who have given their best work to the Medical Center – the nurses, administrators, medical assistants, technologists and technicians, physician assistants, managers, housekeepers, dieticians, mechanics and so many others who are the heart and soul of Virginia Mason. To all of them go our heartfelt thanks for making the advances and accomplishments described in these chapters possible.

In addition, these chapters have been written within the boundaries of the memories of each writer, which are understandably incomplete. As much as possible we have tried to verify the facts through the considerable efforts of VM Archivist Jeni Spamer and VM Library and Archives Technician Lisaann Cohn. Their help was invaluable and we extend our deep gratitude to them for all the effort they have expended on behalf of this project. We realize, however, that there may be errors and omissions and for that we apologize.

We would also be remiss in not thanking the many authors involved. Some have taken time from retirement to write these pages, and others have fit the writing and reviewing into already overloaded work-days. Almost all of the current section heads and department chiefs have reviewed these chapters and added invaluable comments and corrections. To all of these physicians, writers, and reviewers, past and present, we offer our profound thanks. These volumes would not exist without your efforts.

We also would like to extend our thanks to the Historical Society, our archivist Jeni, and previous archivists, for their past and present efforts to preserve the history of Virginia Mason and bring it to life. They have laid a groundwork from which these volumes have sprung, and some members have served as authors and reviewers as well.

Finally, we must acknowledge our spouses, Cori and Joe, for their patience, timely and helpful suggestions, critical questions, keen editing and incredible tolerance for the many hours we have spent deeply engrossed in this project. Thank you for your wonderful love and support - we couldn't ask for better partners in life!

For all of its limitations, these volumes capture a time past and present that is unique and memorable. We hope you enjoy this trip through Virginia Mason's storied past, written by those who lived it!

John Kirkpatrick, MD
Katherine Galagan, MD
Seattle, WA
November 22, 2019

PREFACE

From the Virginia Mason Historical Society

Historically, medical institutions have striven to establish and maintain a reputation for clinical excellence, service and efficiency. Internationally and throughout the United States, there are certain medical systems that have been profoundly successful in developing and maintaining a reputation for cutting-edge clinical excellence and academic productivity. In the United States, medical systems belonging to this group include Mayo Clinic, Harvard/Massachusetts General Hospital, Cleveland Clinic and Stanford University. It is interesting to note that these elite medical centers have also had a persistent and dedicated commitment to documenting their history and including their previous historical accomplishments as a routine component of their modern-day delivery systems.

The leaders of The Mason Clinic, and now Virginia Mason Health System, have also shared the belief that the history of the medical center and its employees should be a routine component of its institutional infrastructure. The Virginia Mason Historical Society has existed in a variety of formats since the Second World War. It has been an active participant in preserving and promulgating the history of The Mason Clinic and Virginia Mason Hospital while highlighting and preserving the many institutional, clinical and academic achievements attained over the last 100 years.

Virginia Mason is currently celebrating its centenary and has produced two previously published histories documenting the evolution of the medical center at 50 years and again at 75 years. As we celebrate our 100th year anniversary, the Historical Society continues to provide the infrastructure for these celebrations in addition to its regular activities, which include contributing historical perspectives with presentations during Grand Rounds as well as vignettes on the back page of the Virginia Mason *Bulletin*, and producing informative historical displays throughout the Medical Center, including most recently, The Jones Historical Wall Display.

These regular contributions provide a unique perspective to new employees of Virginia Mason. When new immigrants to the United States applied for citizenship, they were, as a matter of course, presented with the uplifting history of the world's foremost democracy. New employees at Virginia Mason come to work experiencing an environment that fosters current clinical excellence while also celebrating a history of accomplishments. The most recent *Bulletin* historical article outlined the incorporation of Virginia Mason Hospital, where one of the goals of the founding group of physicians was to create the "Mayo Clinic of the West." The Virginia Mason caregivers highlighted in this sectional history are some of the individuals responsible for this prediction largely becoming a reality.

The sectional histories outlined in this book provide a perspective of the accomplishments of the individual sections at Virginia Mason and are filled with stories of physician leaders who not only helped shape Virginia Mason, but also their national professional societies and the evolution of their medical and surgical specialties. The Virginia Mason Historical Society has provided support not only for this outstanding publication but also the previous and current Virginia Mason historical narratives. This centennial celebration will dominate the scene in 2020. In 2021, Virginia Mason will move into its second century, and the history of Virginia Mason will continue to be chronicled and preserved by the Historical Society and the Archives.

The Virginia Mason Archives and its current archivist, Jeni Spamer, are a critically important component of not only the centenary celebration but also serve as a visible expression of Virginia Mason's commitment to the well-known statement: "You can't understand where you are going until you understand where you have been."

Virginia Mason continues to distinguish itself with its internationally recognized clinical and administrative infrastructure, its dedicated and accomplished physicians and staff, and its commitment to conserving and highlighting its illustrious past. As President of the Virginia Mason Historical Society, I would like to take this opportunity to thank and congratulate John Kirkpatrick, Katherine Galagan, Jeni Spamer and all of the contributing authors for producing this outstanding narrative of the sectional histories of Virginia Mason.

Donald E. Low, MD
President, Virginia Mason Historical Society
Seattle, WA
January 15, 2020

Virginia Mason Medical Center:
The First 100 Years

Volume 1

1

The Department of Medicine: An Overview

by John Kirkpatrick, MD

It is difficult to date the beginning of the Department of Medicine at Virginia Mason, since two of the 1920 founders of The Mason Clinic, John Blackford, MD, and George Dowling, MD, were general internists, and another, James Tate Mason, Sr., MD, listed general internal medicine and surgery as his specialties. One might therefore state that the department was present at the beginning. Diabetologist Lester Palmer, MD, who joined in 1920 as the youngest partner when Dr. Mason personally endorsed a loan to fund his partnership, was the only subspecialist in medicine at that time. The American Board of Internal Medicine wasn't established until 1936. However, many of the generalists developed specialty interests, and became experts in various disciplines.

In the first 40 years, there were so few partners that there was no designated Chief of Medicine, although historically, Lester Palmer, Bob King, MD, and Joseph Crampton, MD, were each referred to as the "Chief" at times. In a retirement tribute, Dr. Palmer is described as Chief of Medicine from 1944–1955 (from a tribute piece by Arthur R. Colewell, MD, titled "Medical Practice, Teaching, and Research," that appeared in the *Bulletin of the Mason Clinic* vol. 11(4), December 1957), while Dr. Robert King stated in an oral history interview that he took over the Chief position from Dr. Blackford, who died in 1945. Despite these uncertainties, it appears clear that the Department of Medicine was in existence at this point. By the 1960s, recruitment of physicians with added training was a priority and gradually filled out the specialty sections; ironically, at that point there were no designated general internists, although many of the partners in the various sections delivered generalist care. Eventually, leaders saw the importance of supporting generalist care directly, and the Section of General Internal Medicine was established in 1973.

The various sections that we know today came into existence as medical practice evolved and patient volumes grew. Some sections at The Mason Clinic were manned by a single physician early on (such as Cardiology, 1931; Neurology/Neurosurgery, 1934; Hematology/Oncology 1944; Gastroenterology, 1948; Dermatology, 1954; and Physical Medicine and Rehabilitation, 1974), while others were not declared "sections" until the second specialist arrived (such as Endocrinology, which had a partner with that expertise from the beginning, but didn't become a section until 1947 with the arrival of Joseph Crampton, MD). Some sections were part of other sections in their early days. For example, Nephrology was originally part of Endocrinology until the arrival of a second nephrologist, Robert Hegstrom, MD, in 1964, and Rheumatology and Immunology was part of Allergy and Immunology until 1964 with the arrival of Kenneth Wilske, MD. The Pulmonary Section, which formed in 1950 when Edward Morgan, MD, joined The Clinic, was the birthplace of several current sections, including Hyperbaric Medicine (1989), Infectious Disease (2000), Critical Care (2003, although the final separation in titles was not until 2012), and Sleep Medicine (2003). Radiation Oncology arose from the Radiology Department (present from the beginning) in 1948 when Thomas Carlile, MD, established the first nuclear medicine department in the Northwest.

Contained in the following chapters are the back stories of these 16 specialty sections of medicine that helped to make The Mason Clinic the main tertiary referral center of the Northwest. In the 1960s and 1970s, patients from around the Northwest, including Alaska, came to "go through the clinic", and other communities in Washington, such as Aberdeen,

4

developed strong referral relationships with our specialists. The diabetes school became the model for teaching diabetics how to live with their disease - patients and other doctors from around the country came to The Mason Clinic to learn from our endocrinology group. Gastroenterologists and cardiologists developed national reputations. The Virginia Mason Research Center provided a unique opportunity for bench-to-bedside research that enhanced patient care. The Graduate Medical Education programs flourished as The Mason Clinic recruited physicians with a strong interest in teaching in addition to providing excellent patient care, with the added bonus of protected research time.

In 1962, a formal process for the election of chiefs began and Clarence "Pete" Pearson, MD, was the first elected Chief of Medicine. He served two terms and was followed by John Allen, MD (1970–1990); David Dreis, MD (1991–1999); Robert Mecklenburg, MD (2000–2007); Joyce Lammert, MD, PhD, (2007–2013); Michael Gluck, MD (2013–2016); and Mariko Kita, MD (2017–present). It is remarkable that there have only been 7 to have held this position in 60 years, each providing exceptional leadership!

Working together, learning together, teaching together, they created an unmatched environment of respect, collaboration, and camaraderie that is difficult to emulate in today's medical world.

2

Asthma, Allergy and Immunology

by David M. Robinson, MD

Allergy and Immunology (AI) is a relatively young organized specialty in internal medicine. The American Board of Allergy and Immunology was organized in 1971 as a conjoint board of the American Board of Internal Medicine and the American Board of Pediatrics, recognizing the broad age ranges impacted by allergic disorders. The first institutional recognition of AI in Seattle was in the mid 1950s at the University of Washington (UW) when Robert Williams, MD, Chair of the Department of Medicine, told Paul Van Arsdel, MD (then trained as an endocrinologist) that the medical school needed an allergist.

The first allergist/immunologist at Virginia Mason (then The Mason Clinic) followed shortly thereafter with the arrival of **H. Rowland Pearsall, MD**, in early 1956. Rowland was universally admired by both patients and colleagues until his untimely death in 1974 at age 58. Ken Wilske, MD, wrote of Dr. Pearsall: he "was a gentleman, physician and scientist, in the best sense of each." He recruited **D. Robert (Bob) Webb, MD**, from SUNY Rochester (mentor John Condemi, MD) to join the Clinic in 1973 and grow the section of AI. Bob Webb also served in the Air Force and Reserves where he held the rank of Colonel. The section initiated the

AI fellowship at Virginia Mason soon after his arrival and fellows included **Britton Georges, MD**, and **Jack Hill, MD** (after Dr. Pearsall's death). Britt Georges had a long career as a solo practitioner in Bellevue until 2014 and Jack Hill practiced in Lexington, KY until 2018. Bob Webb left VM in 1998 for private practice in Bellevue/Kirkland.

Dr. Pearsall was an academic who provided the first descriptions of human T and B cells in the literature (*Bulletin of The Mason Clinic*). He also was the first to describe allergic alveolitis in bird owners and made one of the earliest associations between rheumatoid arthritis and interstitial lung disease as well as nitrofurantoin pulmonary toxicity. He served on national working groups within the specialty, defining best practices for testing penicillin and other drug allergies. His wife, Nancy, a mycologist and laboratory technician, established a medical training program in Africa that continues to this day.

Michael F. Mullarkey, MD, was recruited from Scripps Clinic to replace Dr. Pearsall in 1975. He had trained at Boston University in medicine and did a fellowship at the National Institutes of Health (NIH). He trained with Eng Tan, MD, at Scripps, an expert in defining antinuclear antibodies in rheumatologic disorders. Mike had diverse interests and was instrumental in the working relationship between the Sections of Rheumatology (Drs. Wilske, Healey and Stage) and AI. This relationship, along with the work of Stan Sumida, PhD, in the clinical immunology laboratory, helped provide improved diagnostics for rheumatologic disorders. The relationship between Rheumatology and AI also helped provide the drive to recruit **Gerald Nepom, MD, PhD**, to the Virginia Mason Research Center (VMRC) in 1985, which became the Benaroya Research Center (BRI) in 1999.

Mike will always be remembered for his wicked sense of humor and infectious laugh. He had research projects in aspirin-sensitive asthma and nasal polyps as well as then cutting-edge topics such as Interleukin-1 (IL-1), IL-3 and tumor necrosis factor (TNF). He and Bob Webb published the first description of eosinophilic non-allergic rhinitis and the first description of angiotensin-converting-enzyme (ACE) inhibitor-associated cough with Gene Pardee, MD, and Dick Paton, MD. He pioneered the use of methotrexate in steroid-dependent asthma (published in the *NEJM* and *Annals of Internal Medicine*). He left the clinic in 1991 for private practice, and then joined the Polyclinic until his retirement in 2001. Mike continues to serve as attending at the AI clinic at the UW where he continues to mold new generations of AI students and fellows.

David A. Stempel, MD, was recruited by Mike Mullarkey in 1980 to fill a need for competent pediatric allergy services. David had completed his AI training at Stanford and had a broad interest in pediatric pulmonary diseases, particularly cystic fibrosis. He was active in the pediatric pulmonary community at Children's Hospital. He formally joined our group in 1988, after first being a member of the Pediatric Section. David left VM in 2000 to work with United Care and Glaxo-Smith-Klein to help improve asthma care and appropriate medication utilization. He was first author on a recent large study in *NEJM* regarding the safety of inhaled corticosteroids and long-acting bronchodilators.

Dr. Mullarkey revived the AI fellowship program in Seattle single-handedly in 1986 for me (**David M. Robinson, MD**) and **Joyce K. Lammert, MD, PhD**. I was tasked with delving into the immunogenetics of aspirin-sensitive asthma and was provided a home by Jerry Nepom. We had collaborative relationships with William Henderson, Jr., MD, at UW along with Paul Gladstone, PhD, at Immunex. While at VMRC (VM Research Center), I also performed studies clarifying the HLA associations with type 1 diabetes in multiplex families. Funding was from the HRP Fellowship Fund and American Lung Association of Washington as well as VMRC. Joyce was focused on methotrexate and asthma studies resulting in the definitive publication in *Annals of Internal Medicine* in 1990. The AI fellowship program has continued to this day (now at UW) and has trained dozens of AI physicians. The fellowship training sites included all UW sites, Children's, Northwest Asthma and Allergy, Madigan and Virginia Mason.

My first VM experience was as a 4th year medical student on the wards with Phil Menasche, MD, as my resident in 1982. Dr. Lammert had a simi-

8

lar experience on the wards a year later with resident Chris Matthews, MD. I remember that we were all impressed by Joyce, and particularly that she rode a BMW 650 motorcycle. We both completed our internal medicine residency at VM before the AI fellowship. I joined the clinic in 1989 and Joyce in 1990. Joyce went on to become a physician administrator in many capacities including Section Head of AI, Section Head of General Internal Medicine, Chief of the Department of Medicine, Executive Medical Director of the Hospital, interim Director of Medical Education, head of the Physicians' Compact Committee, Chair of the Compensation Committee, and other positions within the Medical Center. She was the first woman to receive the **James Tate Mason Award**. I, on the other hand, continued to toil in the trenches as an RPU (revenue-producing unit).

Our practice was greatly enhanced with the addition of **Susan Holt, PAC,** in 2001. Susan had trained at Yale and brought a broad range of skills to our section, quickly becoming an expert in travel medicine as well as general allergy. This continued a long tradition of ARNPs and PAs in the Medical Center that included Irene Olason, ARNP in AI and Betty Backes, ARNP in Rheumatology, all valued colleagues. Susan developed the flow tools and protocols that are still used for travel medicine throughout the VM system.

Mary L. Farrington, MD, joined our section in 2002. She had been our fellow in the early 1990s and remained a good friend. She came from Pacific Medical Center to VM to expand our pediatric expertise. She completed her pediatrics training at Children's and did research with Hans Ochs, MD (father to Ulrike Ochs in Dermatology) into CD40/ligand-related immune deficiencies. She has proven herself to be an expert in food allergy research, diagnosis and treatment. Mary is retired from active clinical practice but continues an active role with our allergy research projects at BRI.

David K. Jeong, MD, joined our section in 2013 after 3 years with an excellent AI group in Washington, DC. David completed his AI fellowship training locally at UW and spent some of his clinical cross-training time with us at VM. He was the second AI fellow to spend a research year at BRI, exploring T cell epitopes of common food allergens (walnut in David's case). We have had 5 UW fellows spend a year with us at BRI and they have all been very productive (**Kelly Hetherington-Simpson, MD** – peanut; Dr. Jeong – walnut; **Sally Newborough, MD** – shrimp; **Fatima Kahn, MD** – milk; and **Lisa Winteroth, MD** – egg). David is currently Section Head of AI and has been named a Top Doc in the *Seattle Met Magazine* for 4 years in a row.

I would be remiss to not mention our outstanding allergy nurses. While we have had many work with us over 60+ years, our head nurses deserve special mention. **Louise Hutmacher, RN,** taught everybody everything. **Kelly Ross, RN,** is the glue that has held us together for over 30 years as well as **Lynn Collins, RN**.

Allergy research has been strong at VM/BRI since 2007. We (myself and Drs. Farrington and Jeong) have been working with **Bill Kwok, PhD,** and **Erik Wambre, PhD,** and their laboratories on a number of projects and built a patient registry and biorepository of over 500 participants across the allergic spectrum. The BRI group has become the "go to" lab for mechanistic studies of allergy therapeutics and has collaborations with groups around the world. Some notable publications have shown how allergen immunotherapy works (clonal deletion of allergen-specific T cells as opposed to induction of regulatory T cells) as well as specific cell markers that define the allergic phenotype at the T cell level. We have a number of projects in the pipeline including evaluation of novel therapeutics for food allergies as well as defining the mechanisms and immunologic signatures of eosinophilic esophagitis and other disorders.

I would like to give special thanks to Dr. Mullarkey for background information.

3

Cardiology

by John R. Holmes, MD

The Section of Cardiology has delivered superb care to cardiac patients at Virginia Mason for more than eight decades. The service has expanded from one physician in 1931 to the current team in 2019 of 11 physicians and 11 ARNP/PA providers.

I joined the practice in 1985, attracted by the section's remarkable teamwork, atmosphere of collaboration and clinical excellence. Today, bi-weekly conferences discussing challenging clinical cases with our cardio-thoracic surgical colleagues have resulted in improved outcomes and have fostered a team approach that is the envy of our competitors. It truly is the spirit of "Team Medicine" that distinguishes this practice from those at other institutions.

The following paragraphs are my attempt to tell the story of the evolution of cardiac care from 1931 to present with a parallel story outlining the growth and development of the Section of Cardiology at Virginia Mason Medical Center. At the end of the chapter are brief biographies of the cardiologists who have practiced at Virginia Mason over the decades.

The Early Days of Cardiology at Virginia Mason:
1931 - 1959

Robert King, MD, arrived in Seattle in 1931. He was recruited by John Blackford, MD, and Joel Baker, MD, to establish the Section of Cardiology at The Mason Clinic and the first cardiology specialty practice in the Pacific Northwest. Dr. King left a burgeoning academic practice at the University of Virginia to join the eight-member Mason Clinic for the "princely sum of $250 per month". In 1931, cardiology was a subspecialty of internal medicine without any formal board certification process. Treatment options included rotating tourniquets for acute pulmonary edema, phlebotomy, thoracentesis and pharmaceuticals like digitalis and ethacrynic acid (an early loop diuretic). This was well before beta-blockers and angiotensin converting enzyme (ACE) inhibitors for congestive heart failure (CHF). Cardiology practice in 1931 largely revolved around office visits and house calls. Inpatient care was only a small portion of Dr. King's duties. Common cardiac diagnoses included CHF, rheumatic fever and its complications including chronic mitral valve disease. Dr. King was the sole cardiologist at Virginia Mason for many years but was aided in his work by George D. Capaccio, MD, who came to Virginia Mason in 1936. Dr. Capaccio was trained in surgery and internal medicine but had a special interest in cardiology, and was a younger classmate of Dr. King. He eventually left Virginia Mason in 1948, and was involved with the cardiology services at Children's Orthopedic Hospital for many years, beginning in 1944.

The next trained cardiologist was Fred Cleveland, MD, who joined the 10 partners of The Mason Clinic in 1948. Drs. King and Cleveland established the Electrocardiography Laboratory at The Mason Clinic and established the Clinic as a referral center for cardiac patients throughout the Pacific Northwest. Both men were known regionally and nationally for their clinical and leadership skills. Robert Paine, MD, joined them in 1952 and brought skills in right and left heart catheterization from his training in Baltimore that were essential for the study of valvular and congenital heart lesions.

The Advent of Invasive Cardiology: 1960 - 1984

The 1960s saw the advent of the coronary care unit for the management of patients with acute myocardial infarction. This was a time when hypertension was first identified as a risk factor for cardiovascular mortality. Common anti-hypertensives in the 1960s included hydrochlorothiazide, propranolol, reserpine and hydralazine. The first ACE inhibitor (captopril) was released in the early 1970s. The first statin (lovastatin) received FDA approval in 1976. Open heart surgery (utilizing cardiopulmonary bypass) began with treatment of congenital and valvular heart disease followed in 1962 by the advent of coronary artery bypass surgery. Myocardial infarction (MI) management was revolutionized in the mid 1970s with the use of intravenous thrombolytic agents. Prolonged hospitalizations of four to six weeks for MI patients were transformed into four to seven day hospital stays. Standard protocols were developed for the use of intravenous streptokinase and later tissue plasminogen activator as "clot busters". Mortality rates for MI patients plummeted.

The first board-certified cardiologist at Virginia Mason was Leo Hughes, MD. Dr. Hughes was trained at the University of Alabama under Tinsley Harrison, MD, of *Harrison's Principles of Internal Medicine*. He joined The Mason Clinic in 1960 and eight years later was awarded his subspecialty boards in cardiovascular disease.

Drs. Robin Johnston, Robert CK Riggins, and John Graber followed. They performed the early coronary angiograms at The Mason Clinic, which served to diagnose coronary artery disease and were used as the "road maps" for the early coronary bypass operations performed by Hugh Lawrence, MD, and Richard Anderson, MD (see history of Cardiothoracic Surgery in volume 2).

Cardiology Subspecialization,
The Alliance and Satellite expansion: 1985 - 2005

The practice of cardiology was revolutionized in the 1980s by catheter-based interventions to dilate and stent coronary arteries, and procedures to ablate cardiac tissue responsible for the development of cardiac arrhythmias. Subspecialization within cardiology accelerated during these years with separate board certifications for electrophysiology, interventional cardiology, echocardiography and nuclear cardiology. Virginia Mason cardiologists were at the forefront of these new subspecialties and technologies. Robin Johnston, MD, performed the first coronary angioplasty in Seattle in 1984. Percutaneous transluminal coronary angioplasty (PTCA) outcomes improved markedly two years later with the release of the first intracoronary stent. Virginia Mason opened the first all-digital cardiac catheterization laboratory in Seattle in 1997 and catheterization volumes rose rapidly. Industry relationships were strengthened and new technologies such as drug-eluting stents (developed to prevent restenosis of coronary arteries after stent implantation) were soon offered to patients.

In 1986, Chris Fellows, MD, established what was to become the busiest electrophysiology (EP) laboratory in the Pacific Northwest. Pacemaker and automatic cardioverter defibrillator implantation moved from the operating room to the EP Lab. Cardiac surgical involvement in device implantation ended as cardiologists assumed responsibility for the entire procedure. Ablation of atrial fibrillation also started as a collaboration between cardiac surgery and cardiology (Dan Paull, MD, and Chris Fellows) utilizing an open chest approach. Percutaneous approaches performed by cardiologists have now virtually eliminated the need for surgical incisions. A similar transition from cardiac surgery to cardiology has been seen in the closure of atrial septal defects and in balloon valvuloplasty for the treatment of rheumatic mitral stenosis.

Cardiology and the Group Health-Virginia Mason Alliance
From 1995 to 2015, a close collaboration existed in the cardiology service line between Group Health Cooperative and Virginia Mason Medical Center. All Seattle-based coronary interventions and "device therapies" for both organizations were performed at Virginia Mason Hospital. A shared call rotation existed for interventional cardiology procedures and Group Health cardiologists referred patients to Virginia Mason cardiac surgeons for surgical therapy. Group Health cardiologists rounded on Group Health

patients at Virginia Mason Hospital and shared office space adjacent to VM physicians on Lindeman 3.

Cardiology Outreach and the Satellite Strategy

Cardiology has been active in outreach to suburban sites for many years. Fulltime cardiology satellite service started at Federal Way with Dennis Hansen, MD, in 2003. The program expanded rapidly to include services at Viginia Mason Kirkland and briefly at Virginia Mason Port Angeles. Further growth followed with clinic programs in Lynnwood, Issaquah, Bellevue and Bainbridge Island. Cardiology has also staffed freestanding outreach clinics in Aberdeen, Yakima, Wenatchee and Ellensburg. The most active non-Virginia Mason satellite clinic location is in Juneau, Alaska where bi-monthly clinic services are offered by VM cardiology providers. Due to these efforts the SE Alaskan region remains a high volume source of referrals for cardiology and cardiac surgery.

Cardiology at Virginia Mason: 2005 - 2015

Growth and change have characterized the last decade of cardiology care at Virginia Mason. Up until this time, all VM cardiologists had been males. As barriers preventing women from choosing the cardiovascular field slowly diminished, the demographics in cardiology training programs changed dramatically. The result has been that six of the last eleven cardiologists hired at Virginia Mason are women. This has been especially appreciated by our female patients who often prefer a female provider.

As is exemplified throughout the Medical Center, the Section of Cardiology strives for clinical excellence in all areas of practice including patient outcomes and patient service. Recognition of clinical excellence has been the norm. Focused quality improvement efforts have allowed us to improve upon already excellent results. For example, in 2014 and 2015, the section received numerous awards including: top 10 percent nationally for coronary intervention mortality; top 10 percent nationally for door-to-balloon time for acute myocardial infarction (47 minutes); top 10 percent nationally in appropriateness criteria for elective coronary intervention;

15

Washington State Award of Excellence in Healthcare Quality for care of heart attack victims; and Healthgrades 5-star recipient for treatment of heart attacks and congestive heart failure.

Clinical research has always been a part of the cardiology program at Virginia Mason. Research efforts have expanded rapidly within the past few years. Multiple active research protocols are administered within the section. These range from studies of anticoagulants post-coronary stenting, to device protocols in the EP Lab, to optimal management strategies for patients with congestive heart failure. Plans are also in motion to add bench research projects.

2016 and Beyond

The future of cardiology at Virginia Mason is bright. Cardiovascular disease remains the leading cause of mortality in the United States and given the emerging epidemic of obesity, hypertension and diabetes in the country, we anticipate further growth. Catheter-based therapies continue to develop at astonishing rates. Virginia Mason providers, in collaboration with partners at Evergreen Medical Center, have established a rapidly growing transcatheter aortic valve replacement (TAVR) program for treatment of aortic stenosis. This technology has exploded in the last few years. Done in collaboration with our cardiac surgical colleagues, we are now able to offer effective treatment to many patients previously felt to be too ill, too frail, or too old for standard aortic valve replacement surgery with sternotomy. Similarly, selected patients with mitral insufficiency can now also be treated by catheter-based techniques. Additional trans-catheter structural heart procedures available at Virginia Mason also include atrial and ventricular septal occlusion, and left atrial appendage intervention.

Physician Biographies (1931 - present)
Robert L. King, Sr., MD (1931 - 1969)

Robert King was born and raised in Virginia. He earned his medical degree at the University of Virginia and taught there before moving to Seattle to join The Mason Clinic in 1931. His starting salary was $250 per month. He was the first Chief of Cardiology at Virginia Mason and also served as Chief of Medicine prior to the institution of formal elections for this position in 1962. Known as an innovator, he established the Virginia Mason electrocardiogram (ECG) service and performed and interpreted the first 12-lead ECG on the West Coast. An active faculty member of the University of Washington, Dr. King became the first person honored with an endowed, namesake chair at the UW School of Medicine. He was the founder and first president (1947-1950) of the American Heart Association, Washington affiliate. Dr. King published original research on whale electrocardiograms with his friend and colleague, Paul Dudley White, MD, founder of the American Heart Association.

Fred E. Cleveland, MD (1948 - 1982)

A graduate of the University of Virginia, Fred interned at Virginia Mason Hospital in 1940. His medical training was interrupted by World War II, when he served in the United States Army from 1941 to 1945. He then returned to an internal medicine residency at Virginia Mason Hospital and later joined the 10 partners of The Mason Clinic in 1948. His starting salary was $450 per month. Along with Robert King, MD, he developed the Section of Cardiology and was active in establishing the electrocardiography laboratory at the clinic. During his 34 years with Virginia Mason, he was elected as President of the Medical Staff, Chief of Staff and served five terms on the Executive Committee, including one term as Chairman (1976 - 1980). He was active in the American Heart Association as President of the Washington affiliate and later served on the national Board of Directors. Dr. Cleveland retired from practice in 1982 and passed away in 1989. He was an avid outdoorsman, who enjoyed bird hunting and fly fishing. He was also a connoisseur of good food and fine wine. One of his strengths was his sense of fairness. Robert Riggins, MD, remembered Fred this way, "First and foremost, he was always forthright and honest. If you asked him a question, and he didn't know the answer, he'd say so. If he gave you an answer, it was what he believed to be true, and he'd always stand behind his statement or commitment. He was a gentleman and had a strong sense of integrity. He didn't partake in gossip, especially if the conversation was derogatory to a colleague or to the institution, of which he was very proud. His patients loved and respected him, feeling that he was always their advocate."

Robert M. Paine, MD (1952 - 1985)

A graduate of Bowdoin College in Maine, Robert Paine attended the College of Physicians and Surgeons, Columbia University, interned at Evanston Hospital, and trained as a resident at Johns Hopkins before starting his long and successful practice in internal medicine and cardiology at The Mason Clinic. He introduced invasive hemodynamics (right and left heart catheterization) at Virginia Mason. Bob was a life-long amateur radio operator (W7RX).

M. Leo Hughes, Jr., MD (1960 - 1985)

Leo Hughes trained at the University of Alabama under Dr. Tinsley Harrison of *Harrison's Principles of Internal Medicine*. He was awarded board-certification in cardiology in 1968. He was a Fellow of the American College of Cardiology, the American Heart Association and the American College of Chest Physicians. He retired from clinic practice in 1985 just prior to the dissolution of the partnership and the creation of the current Virginia Mason Health System corporate structure. Dr. Hughes is remembered as a soft spoken, Southern gentleman.

Robin R. Johnson, MD (1965 - 2000)

Robin Johnston completed medical school, residency and fellowship at the University of Washington School of Medicine. Robin was the director of the Cardiac Catheterization Laboratory at Virginia Mason for many years. He performed the first coronary angioplasty in Seattle. He served as Section Head for many years and also was President of the American Heart Association, Washington affiliate from 1982 - 1984. An avid alpine skier and member of the Ski Patrol, Robin has spent countless weekends skiing the back bowls at Crystal Mountain.

Robert C. K. Riggins, MD (1970 - 1996)

Bob Riggins was born and raised in Manhattan. He graduated from Columbia University, College of Physicians and Surgeons in 1961. He completed his fellowship in cardiology at The New York Hospital-Cornell Medical Center and then moved to Seattle to join The Mason Clinic. While at Virginia Mason, Dr. Riggins published manuscripts on stress testing, coronary bypass surgery outcomes and on the efficacy of intra-aortic balloon counterpulsation. He served as section head for many years and spearheaded the creation of the sabbatical program. In retirement, he moved to Lopez Island where he and his wife ran a successful sheep ranch. He later moved to Atlanta, GA.

John Graber, MD (1974 - 2009; outreach til 2014)

John Graber was born and raised in Iowa. He served as resident in internal medicine and fellow in cardiology at The Johns Hopkins School of Medicine. He was recruited by Dr. Riggins to come to The Mason Clinic in 1972. He was viewed as a master diagnostician and expert of the bedside cardiac exam. He maintained an extensive teaching file of electrocardiograms for the benefit of the residency program. Dr. Graber retired from clinical practice in 2009 but continued to support the institution by offering cardiology outreach clinics in SE Alaska for several years.

Edward F. Gibbons, MD (1985 - 2009)

A native of Massachusetts, Ted attended the University of Chicago School of Medicine. He completed his clinical fellowship in cardiology at Massachusetts General Hospital and stayed on for an additional year of research in echocardiography. He joined Virginia Mason in 1985. Ted served as the director of the Echocardiography Laboratory for many years and also developed and directed the Virginia Mason Anticoagulation Clinic. He was a multi-year recipient of the "Teacher of the Year" award from the internal medicine residency. Ted also served as Section Head of Cardiology and Deputy Chief of Medicine before leaving Virginia Mason to join the faculty at Harborview Medical Center. The consummate "foodie", Ted hosted many cardiology holiday parties at his home on Capitol Hill.

John R. Holmes, MD (1985 - 2017)

A native of Washington State, Dr. Holmes attended the University of Washington School of Medicine and completed his internal medicine residency at the same institution. He then moved to New York City and served as a fellow in cardiology at New York Hospital-Cornell Medical Center. He returned to Seattle in 1985 and joined the Section of Cardiology. Echocardiography has remained a major focus throughout his career. Dr. Holmes served as Section Head for 12 years. His non-medical pursuits include windsurfing in the Columbia Gorge, jazz piano, and fly fishing.

Christopher L. Fellows, MD (1986 - present)

Dr. Fellows attended medical school at Oregon Health Sciences University in Portland, OR. He considered a career in pathology but instead opted for a residency in internal medicine at Massachusetts General Hospital. He then moved to Seattle for cardiology training at the University of Washington. Chris joined Virginia Mason in 1986 and established the Electrophysiology Laboratory, which quickly became the highest volume program in the Pacific Northwest. Dr. Fellows performed the first catheter-based atrial fibrillation ablation and the first transvenous automatic cardioverter-defibrillator implant at Virginia Mason. Dr. Fellows was elected President of the Washington Chapter of the American College of Cardiology and has also served as Section Head of Cardiology for many years. In 2017, he received the **James Tate Mason Award**, Virginia Mason's highest honor. Chris can be seen in the gym and weight room at the Washington Athletic Club at 5:45 am each workday and can be found water-skiing with friends on weekends.

D. Dennis Hansen, MD (1987 – 2002)

Dennis Hansen established the cardiology satellite clinic at Virginia Mason Federal Way in 1987. He practiced clinical cardiology there (1987 – 2002) but maintained his interventional cardiology practice at the downtown campus. He graduated from the University of Washington School of Medicine in 1976 and then stayed on to complete his internal medicine residency and cardiology fellowship at the same institution.

Kevin W. Judge, MD (1990 – 1998)

Kevin Judge received his medical degree from the University of Chicago and completed his residency and fellowship at the University of Washington. He practiced at Virginia Mason Federal Way for eight years and then left clinical practice to enter the pharmaceutical industry. He is currently Vice-President of Medical Affairs at Becton-Dickinson Biosciences.

Gordon L. Kritzer, MD (1992 - present)

Gordon Kritzer is a native of Southern California. He completed medical school at UC San Diego, then moved to Boston where he served as a resident in internal medicine at Peter Bent Brigham Hospital followed by a cardiology fellowship at Massachusetts General Hospital. He briefly practiced interventional cardiology in New Haven, CT before being recruited to join Virginia Mason in 1992. He served as Director of the Cardiac Catheterization Laboratory for many years and performed many "firsts" at Virginia Mason (e.g., percutaneous balloon mitral valvuloplasty, catheter-based atrial septal defect closure, etc.). Gordon is a cycling enthusiast who has completed many marathon rides and races throughout the Pacific Northwest.

Kenneth Mahrer, MD (1995 - 2008)

Kenneth Mahrer attended medical school at the University of Southern California and graduated in 1988. This was followed by a fellowship in cardiology and interventional cardiology at Cedars Sinai Medical Center in Los Angeles. Ken practiced at Virginia Mason from 1995 to 2008 before moving to San Francisco to join the interventional cardiology team at Kaiser-Permanente. Ken was an accomplished/competitive tennis player and "ski bum" prior to his career in medicine.

James Fritz, MD (1997 - 2004)

Jim Fritz practiced as an interventional cardiologist at Virginia Mason from 1997 to 2004 followed by his return to practice at Group Health. He attended the University of Washington School of Medicine, graduating in 1976. He continued at UW for his residency and fellowship. In retirement, he completed training as a merchant marine and has taken multiple long-distance sailing trips with friends and colleagues (including Dan Paull, MD, CT surgery).

Michael Belz, MD (1998 - 2005)

Michael Belz practiced as a cardiologist/electrophysiologist at Virginia Mason from 1998 until 2005 when he joined Group Health. He attended the University of Kansas School of Medicine graduating in 1987, and completed his residency in internal medicine at the Medical College of Virginia. Dr. Belz was a fellow in cardiology and electrophysiology at the same institution.

Patrick J. Reagan, MD (1998 – 2008)

Jack Reagan practiced as an interventional cardiologist at Virginia Mason Federal Way for 10 years. He attended Creighton University School of Medicine and completed his internal medicine residency and cardiology fellowship at the same institution.

Michael J. Longo, MD (1999 - present)

Mike Longo is the only Virginia Mason cardiologist to have pitched a no-hitter in Little League. He was recruited to pitch for Cornell University but injured his arm and decided to focus his efforts on academics. He graduated with honors. He completed medical school at the State University of New York, Buffalo. Mike then served as resident, chief resident and fellow in cardiology at Yale University. He joined Virginia Mason in 1999 and has served as Director of the Echocardiography Lab for many years. Dr. Longo is another Virginia Mason cardiologist who is a multi-year recipient of the "Teacher of the Year" award from the internal medicine residents.

Joseph V. Condon, MD (1999 – 2002)

Dr. Condon graduated from the University of Miami School of Medicine in 1987. He then moved to Chicago where he completed his internal medicine residency and cardiology fellowship at Rush University Medical Center. Dr. Condon practiced in Bellevue before and after his tenure at Virginia Mason.

Wayne S. Hwang, MD (2003 - present)

Wayne Hwang attended medical school at the Indiana University School of Medicine and then completed his residency at the Baylor College of Medicine. He moved to New Haven, CT where he was a fellow in cardiology and interventional cardiology at Yale University. Wayne joined Virginia Mason in 2003. He is the current Director of the Cardiac Catheterization Laboratory. In addition to his interventional cardiology skills, Dr. Hwang also has subspecialty training in nuclear cardiology and management of peripheral vascular disease. Outside of work he can often be found playing competitive tennis.

Elizabeth Gold, MD (2007 - present)

Elizabeth Gold joined Virginia Mason in 2007 as a part-time cardiologist at the Issaquah satellite clinic and at the main campus in Seattle. She has a parallel career as a bench scientist doing research into the underlying causes of atherosclerosis. Dr. Gold attended Yale University Medical School followed by a residency in internal medicine and a fellowship in cardiology at the University of Washington. She has a special interest in cardiovascular risk factor reduction and women's cardiovascular health. Her free time is spent as an avid horse owner and equestrian.

James S. Lee, MD (2008 – 2011)

James Lee practiced interventional and nuclear cardiology during his three-year stay at Virginia Mason. He attended Loma Linda School of Medicine and graduated in 2002. He completed his internal medicine residency at the Cleveland Clinic followed by cardiology training at UCLA (San Fernando Valley Program) and Mount Sinai in New York.

Sara Weiss, MD (2009 - present)

Sara Weiss joined Virginia Mason in 2009 and established the Congestive Heart Failure Clinic. She attended medical school at Columbia University, College of Physicians and Surgeons, graduating in 2001. Her internal medicine residency, cardiology and heart failure fellowships were completed at the University of Colorado. She has special interests in echocardiography and women's cardiovascular disease. Dr. Weiss is an exercise enthusiast and local champion in Crossfit competitions.

J. Susie Woo, MD (2010 - present)

Susie Woo joined Virginia Mason in 2010 after completing her internal medicine residency and cardiology fellowship at the University of Washington. While at the University she did additional training in congestive heart failure and the management of patients with heart transplants. She attended Duke University School of Medicine and graduated in 2002. Dr. Woo is an accomplished classical musician (flute) who performs with various local orchestras. She has special expertise in echocardiography and nuclear medicine. She practices at the regional medical centers in Seattle and Bellevue.

Elizabeth Y. Chan, MD (2011 - 2017)

Elizabeth Chan graduated from the University of Medicine and Dentistry of New Jersey, Robert Wood Johnson Medical School in 2002. She completed her internal medicine residency at UCLA and then moved to Seattle where she was a fellow in cardiology at the University of Washington. She has expertise in invasive cardiology, nuclear cardiology and echocardiography and practiced at the Main Campus and at VM Federal Way before her departure in 2017.

Drew Baldwin, MD (2012 - present)

Drew Baldwin is an interventional cardiologist with additional interest and training in the management of peripheral vascular disease. He graduated from Tulane University School of Medicine and then completed his residency in internal medicine at New York University School of Medicine in 2004. He completed his cardiology fellowship at the University of Pittsburgh followed by an interventional fellowship at Brown University in 2008. He was on faculty at Tulane prior to joining Virginia Mason in 2012. Dr. Baldwin has become an expert and advocate for patient safety efforts, quality improvement and outcomes research.

Robert W. Rho, MD (2013 - 2018)

Robert Rho graduated from Loma Linda University School of Medicine in 1992 followed by a residency in internal medicine at the University of Massachusetts. He completed his cardiology and electrophysiology fellowships at the University of Pennsylvania in 2002. He was on faculty at the University of Washington for several years prior to joining Virginia Mason in 2013. Dr. Rho has a special interest in the management of complex ventricular arrhythmias and ventricular tachycardia ablation. He served as the Director of Cardiovascular Research while employed at Virginia Mason. Outside of work, Dr. Rho is an accomplished jazz pianist and recreational sailor.

Diana Revenco, MD (2017 – present)

Diana Revenco joined our cardiology team in 2017 when she moved with her family from Boston, Massachusetts. She graduated from State Medical and Pharmaceutical University, Moldova in 2003, followed by a residency in internal medicine and a cardiology fellowship at Tufts University, St. Elizabeth's Medical Center, Boston, MA. She practiced general cardiology and supervised the echocardiography laboratory at Wentworth Douglass Medical Center in Dover, NH for several years prior to joining Virginia Mason in 2017. Dr. Revenco has a special interest in echocardiography, nuclear cardiology, valvular heat disease and management of cardiovascular disease in women. Outside of work, Dr. Revenco enjoys hiking with her family, skiing and gardening.

Mariko W. Harper, MD, MS (2017 – present)

Mariko Harper received her medical degree from the University of British

Columbia in 2011. She then moved to Seattle where she completed her residency in internal medicine and her fellowship in cardiology at the University of Washington. She also has a master's degree in Human Nutrition from Columbia University. She joined Virginia Mason in 2017 and has established an active practice in general cardiology, echocardiography and nuclear cardiology. She has a special interest in managing hypertrophic cardiomyopathy and other genetic cardiac conditions. She sees patients at the downtown Seattle campus and at Virginia Mason Lynnwood. When not working, she enjoys spending time with her husband, two children, and dog as well as traveling to see extended family in her native Canada and Japan.

Adam Mohmand-Borkowski, MD (2018 – present)

Dr. Borkowski graduated from the Medical University of Lodz, Poland in 1997. He completed his cardiovascular fellowship at Lankenau Hospital, Philadelphia followed by subspecialty training in electrophysiology at Boston University Medical Center and the Cleveland Clinic. He also completed a fellowship in advanced heart failure management and cardiac transplantation while in Cleveland. Dr. Borkowski specializes in cardiac arrhythmia therapies with special interest in ablation of ventricular tachycardia and atrial fibrillation. When not busy at work or with family activities in Seattle, Dr. Borkowski makes frequent trips back to his native Poland to visit his extended family. He is an avid skier and enjoys long-distance running.

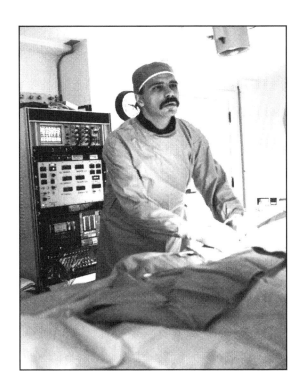

Chris Fellows, MD, in the Electrophysiology Laboratory (PH 6493, VMHA)

4

Dermatology

by Charles J. Hammer, Jr., MD, and David Wilma
with contributions from Ulrike Ochs, MD

Although the Virginia Mason Hospital and Clinic was established in 1920, the first dermatologist – **Robert A. Pommerening, MD** – was not hired until 1954. From 1945 to 1952, the number of partners at The Mason Clinic grew from ten to sixteen reflecting the growth in patient care. Dermatology patients were referred to consultants and a dedicated dermatology section had to wait until new clinic space was available, which finally occurred in 1954. Dr. Pommerening had received his degree from the University of Michigan School of Medicine and was practicing nearby with Joseph Shaw, MD, in offices on Boylston Street near Swedish Hospital. The new dermatology practice that he began at The Mason Clinic expanded to treat more than 6,000 patients in 1957 and the partners looked ahead to adding another physician.

Charles J. Hammer, Jr., MD, joined the section in 1960, which then consisted of the two physicians and one nurse, **Delores Froehling**. Interns rotated through the clinic as part of their education. Dr. Hammer graduated from the University of Maryland Medical School, interned at the University of Michigan and served in the United States Air Force for two years. While serving on Guam, he became interested in dermatology after seeing tropical diseases treated there.

The patient load grew steadily through 1968, at which point it was double the 1957 level. Besides their busy practices, Dr. Pommerening became a clinical professor of medicine at the University of Washington, a consultant with the Veterans Administration, and headed the dermatology clinic at Children's Orthopedic Hospital. Dr. Hammer served on the faculty of the Division of Dermatology of the University of Washington and also helped out at Children's and Harborview one afternoon a week. Dr. Pommerening's wife Betsy helped found the volunteer program. Sadly, late in 1968, Dr. Pommerening passed away suddenly at the age of 53, and Dr. Hammer was suddenly in solo practice.

Dr. Hammer, as the new Section Head, hired **Robert E. Kellum, MD**, the following year from the faculty at the University of Oregon. In 1970, the two physicians moved to a newly remodeled area of the 8th Floor of the clinic (Buck Pavilion). By 1974, some 14,000 patients were treated by Drs. Hammer and Kellum. In 1975, the section moved into new office space in former meeting rooms and the old clinic auditorium, 8 North.

In approximately 1972-73, **Frank Parker, MD**, joined the section from the University of Washington faculty but left two years later to head the Department of Dermatology at the University of Oregon. **Ivor Caro, MD,** from the faculty at the University of North Carolina, joined the section in 1978. Dr. Caro was a graduate of the University of Witwatersrand in South Africa. He left in 1988 and returned in 1993 for an additional 6 years, during which he served as Section Head from 1994 – 1999.

When Bob Kellum decided to work as a consultant at the King Fiasal Hospital in Ryad, Saudi Arabia, **Allan Kayne, MD,** was recruited to join the section in 1982. Dr. Kayne graduated from Cornell University and was a vital part of the section for twenty-one years.

Satellite clinics became an important part of the Virginia Mason Health Care System in the 1980s. As the medical center grew and multiple satellite clinics were added throughout the Puget Sound area in the 1990s, the section endeavored to supply dermatological coverage at the larger satellites, which required expanding the staff. **Lauri Tadlock, MD; Alice Ormsby, MD; Kelli Arntzen, MD; Christine Ng, MD; Brian Kumasaka, MD**, and **Rebecca Smith, MD,** were added to fill the need for dermatologists in these satellite locations. All of these individuals stayed for varying periods before leaving to go into private practice.

Early on, these dermatologists practiced primarily at the main clinic and would see patients in the satellites one or two days a week. However, this soon became insufficient, so in 1990, Dr. Arntzen opened the dermatology clinic at Virginia Mason South in Federal Way. Issaquah's Dermatology program followed in 1993. Although these satellite clinic dermatologists were based primarily in their satellite location, the section has developed the format of having these dermatologists also practice one day every week in the main clinic, which helps to build cohesion with colleagues and to develop a standard level of practice.

Frederick Leaf, MD, joined the section downtown in 1990. He graduated from Stanford University Medical School and became a mainstay in the teaching program until his departure in 2006. He also served as Section Head from 1999 – 2002 after Dr. Caro stepped down.

Early advances in therapy included sclerotherapy for treatment of small "spider" veins, which was begun by Dr. Caro in 1994. In addition, Drs. Tadlock, Ormsby, and Arntzen had a special interest in cosmetic treatments, which were popular among patients and profitable. In February 1996, the dermatologists began using an argon laser to treat broken blood vessels on the face. As interest in these cosmetic procedures increased, nurse-manager **Sharon Wells** encouraged the physicians and the medical center to start an aesthetician program. Not long before, the section had moved to 2 north in the Buck Pavilion, which provided more space for this idea. Thus, in 1998, two licensed aestheticians were hired to counsel patients on skin care routines and resources about alternative treatments for the skin. Other services included therapeutic facials, glycolic peels and other customized body treatments. Therapeutic massage was performed by registered nurses who also were licensed massage practitioners. This practice gradually expanded to become the Medi-Spa where patients could receive treatments and purchase high-quality skin care products. Services in the section now include Cosmetic Dermatology, Cosmetic Surgery, Phototherapy and the Medi Spa. In 2004 the team moved to Lindeman 9 and the section became The Skin Care Center at Virginia Mason.

In 1997, there were eight physicians on the team (Drs. Hammer, Caro, Kayne, Leaf, Arntzen, Kumasaka, Ormsby and Smith) and Dr. Leaf served as Section Head. Not only were the dermatologists busy with a clinical practice, but they also took call for the hospital and emergency room, which was unusual in the Seattle dermatology community. **Ulrike (Sires) Ochs, MD**, joined the section that year. At that time, all medical records were on paper and some charts were inches thick. Doctors dictated their notes onto small recorders, and the transcripts were printed out and pasted into the charts. Experiments with telephone dictation were less successful, but over time, more innovations were tested until the medical records became entirely computerized.

Dr. Hammer stepped away from fulltime practice in 1997, but worked as a locums for the section for the next 4 years. Dr. Caro left in 1999 and was replaced by **Kendell C. Wilske, MD,** who practiced in the section for the next 12 years. Dr. Leaf stepped down as section head in 2002 and Dr. Ochs became the new section head; new dermatologists in the 2000s included **John R. Streidl, MD** (2001 – 2004); **Diane S. Chiu, MD** (2004 – 2008); **Edwin Y. Rhim, MD** (2004 – present and now serving as Section Head after Dr. Ochs stepped down in 2016); **Nobuyoshi Kageyama, MD** (2006 – 2008); and **Alison Z. Young, MD, PhD** (2007 – 2014), who is board-certified as both a dermatologist and dermatopathologist, and was part of an experiment in conjunction with the Pathology Department in which she split her time between seeing clinic patients and evaluating dermatopathology specimens. After 5 years, she decided to limit her practice to dermatology, and left 2 years later to join Dermatology Associates of Seattle. A full-time Mohs surgeon was also hired – **Ravi S. Krishnan, MD**, joined the group in 2008, making this procedure available to VM patients.

The last 10 years have seen several dermatologists come and go–

Christina M. Wahlgren, MD (2010 – 2014); **Jane Yoo, MD** (2012 – 2016); **Viet Quoc Nguyen, MD** (2013 – 2014); and **Catherine Pham, MD** (2014 – 2017). Currently, the section has 7 dermatologists: Drs. Rhim, Ochs, Krishnan, and **Edward M. Esparza, MD, PhD** (2011); **Cathryn Z. Zhang, MD** (2014), **Tracie Chong, MD** (2016), and **Eric Brum-well, MD** (2017). Dermatologists have also served the various satellites as listed below.

Short Physician Biographies

(with medical school, primary place of practice and tenure)

Downtown

Robert A. Pommerening, MD: University of Michigan School of Medicine, 1954 – 1968; Section Head 1960 – 1968

Charles J. Hammer Jr., MD: University of Maryland Medical School, 1960 – 1997; back as locums 1997 – 2001); Section Head 1968 - 1994

Robert E. Kellum, MD: 1969 – 1981

Frank Parker, MD: approximately 1972 – 1977

Ivor Caro, MD: University of Witwatersrand in South Africa, 1978 - 1988, 1993 - 1999; Section Head 1994 - 1999

Allan L. Kayne, MD: Cornell University, 1982 - 2003

Lauri M. Tadlock, MD: University of Washington School of Medicine, 1988 - 1995.

Frederick A. Leaf, MD: Stanford University Medical School, 1990 – 2006; Section Head 1999 -2002

Kelli R. Arntzen, MD (and Federal Way): St. Louis University School of Medicine, 1990 - 2006

Christine S. Ng, MD: Loma Linda University School of Medicine, 1993 - 1995

Ulrike I. (Sires) Ochs, MD: Northwestern University Medical School, 1997 - present; Section Head 2002 - 2014

Kendell C. Wilske, MD: Medical College of Wisconsin, 1999 - 2011

John R. Streidl, MD: St. Louis University School of Medicine, 2001-04

Diane S. Chiu, MD: University of Washington School of Medicine, 2004 - 2008

Edwin Y. Rhim, MD (and Issaquah): University of Washington School of Medicine, 2004 –present; Section Head 2016 - present

Nobuyoshi Kageyama, MD: University of Hawaii John A. Burns School of Medicine, 2006 -2008

Alison Z. Young MD, PhD: Weill Cornell Medical College with PhD, at Memorial Sloan Kettering Cancer Center, 2007 – 2014

Ravi S. Krishnan, MD: Baylor College of Medicine, 2008 – present

Christina M. Wahlgren, MD: University of Washington School of Medicine, 2010 - 2014

Jane Yoo, MD: Washington University School of Medicine, 2012 – 2016

Viet Quoc Nguyen, MD: University of Washington School of Medicine, 2013 – 2014

Catherine Pham, MD: University of Texas Medical School, 2014 – 2017

Cathryn Z. Zhang, MD: Case Western Reserve University School of Medicine, 2014 – present

Tracie Chong, MD: University of Hawaii John A. Burns School of Medicine, 2016 - present

Bainbridge Island

Reuben Makala Anders, MD: Loma Linda University School of Medicine, 2006 - 2007

Simone Ince, MD: University of Arizona College of Medicine, 2009 - 2016

Eric Bramwell, MD: Case Western Reserve University School of Medicine, 2017 - present

Bellevue

Frank J. Baron, MD: University of Washington School of Medicine, 1998 - 2001

DeEtta M. Gray, MD (also Issaquah 1999 - 2001): University of Saskatchewan College of Medicine, 1999 - 2004

Peter J. Jenkin, MD (also at Issaquah): McGill University Faculty of

Medicine, 2002 - 2009

Janie M. Leonhardt, MD: Northeast Ohio Medical University, 2010 - 2014

Edward M. Esparza, MD, PhD, (also Federal Way): Washington University School of Medicine, 2011 – present

Federal Way

Brian H. Kumasaka, MD: University of Washington School of Medicine, 1993 - 2001

Suseela V. Narra, MD: Albert Einstein College of Medicine, 2001-11

Christine D. Ambro, MD: Jefferson Medical College, 2005 - 2006

Issaquah

Rebecca L. Smith, MD: Baylor College of Medicine, 1995 -1999

DeEtta M. Gray, MD: University of Saskatchewan College of Medicine, 1999 – 2001; moved to Bellevue 2001 – 2004

Allison L. Hughes, MD: Chicago Medical School, 2006 - 2007

Amy S. Cheng, MD: Washington University School of Medicine, 2009 - 2010

Arlo J. Miller, MD: Harvard Medical School, 2010 - 2012

Kirkland

Alice M. Ormsby, MD: Duke University School of Medicine, 1989 - 2002

Renata M. Jenkin, MD: McMaster University Michael G. DeGroote School of Medicine, 2002 - 2012

Sarah Dick, MD: Harvard Medical School, 2007 - 2015

Sequim

Claire L. Haycox, MD, PhD: University of Washington School of Medicine, 1999 - 2002

5

Endocrinology

by Paul Fredlund, MD, and Katherine Galagan, MD

The Early Days: 1920 - 1966

Lester Palmer, MD, was one of the original founding physicians of The Mason Clinic; he was recruited by James Tate Mason, MD, and became the youngest partner in the group. From the beginning under the direction of Dr. Palmer, VMMC was a regional leader in the care and treatment of patients with diabetes. Prior to the discovery of insulin by William Banting, MD, and Charles Best, MD, in Toronto, Canada in 1921, fully established Type 1 diabetes was uniformly fatal with a life expectancy of less than one year. Because Dr. Palmer was a nationally respected authority on the management of diabetes, he was able to obtain insulin directly from Dr. Banting and as a result he was the first physician to administer life-saving insulin to a patient in the Pacific Northwest. [1]

The Mason Clinic was founded by a group of physicians dedicated to the importance of life-long continuing medical education and academic excellence with a goal of rapidly adopting new medical breakthroughs developed in academic medical centers. Consequently, patients treated at the Mason Clinic from the beginning received comprehensive "state of the art" care. Dr. Palmer's early administration of insulin to Mason Clinic patients is a noteworthy example of the vital importance of academic excellence and over the past 100 years, delivery of "state of the art" care has proved to be a model governing the care of all Mason Clinic patients.

Dr. Palmer understood the essential role diabetes education plays in successful management of diabetes. In 1922, he instituted a free class for his patients, which he personally conducted, inspiring them with his enthusiasm and interest. Drawing upon his personal relationship with a growing numbers of patients and friends, he was able to establish The Diabetic Trust Fund, which helped finance activities for the welfare of diabetic patients, including summer camps for diabetic children - one on Vashon Island, and the other on Hood Canal. The diabetes camps and outpatient diabetes education program are described in a 1957 issue of *The Bulletin*:

"In addition to furnishing these young children an opportunity to camp out for two weeks while receiving instruction and guidance in proper diets and administration of insulin, the Hospital-Clinic Diabetic program is very active throughout the year. Approximately 300 diabetic outpatients from all over the Northwest and Alaska receive a concentrated two-week course of instruction in administration of insulin, proper diet and planned exercise. The Hospital-Clinic program is one of the oldest and most successful diabetic schools in the country. The diabetics attend lectures by specialized doctors, nurses and dieticians. Wives, mothers and other relatives of pupils often attend the classes and learn how to weigh food and give insulin injections." [2]

Dr. Palmer also established *The Diabetes Monthly*, a newsletter for patients and their families. In addition, he was a founder of the Washington State Diabetes Association. In addition to his devotion to patients with diabetes, Dr. Palmer played an essential leadership role at VM over the years as he served terms as Chief of the Department of Medicine, President of the Board of Trustees of the Virginia Mason Hospital, and Chief of Staff of the VM Hospital.

In 1947, Joseph Crampton, MD, joined the new "Section of Endocrinology and Metabolism" at The Mason Clinic. Dr. Crampton's vision, enthusiasm and organizational skills were highly valued at the Mason Clinic and he was largely responsible for the Clinic's interest in teaching and research, being instrumental in the founding of the Virginia Mason Foundation for Medical Research (later known at the Virginia Mason Research Center) along with the encouragement and support of pathologist Hugh Jones, MD. The first donation to the Foundation of $5,000 was from The Mason Clinic. [3] The Virginia Mason Research Center was incorporated on March 8, 1956 with the goal of improving "health and medical care to the people of the Northwest". [3] Dr. Crampton was also active in the national American Diabetes Association (ADA), serving that organization in many capacities (ADA Board of Directors [five years] and secretary of the ADA). [4] When Dr. Palmer retired in 1955, Dr. Crampton became Section Head of Endocrinology and Metabolism, a position he held until his death in 1966. Much of the long-term success of the VM Endocrine Section can be attributed to the wise leadership of Joe Crampton.

Robert Reeves, MD, joined the section in 1952, and William Steenrod, Jr, MD, was hired in 1953. Dr. Reeves was particularly interested in research. There are several notations in the Chairman's Reports and *Bulletins* of the era mentioning various grants that he was awarded, often along with Dr. Crampton and Angela J. Bowen, MD, as co-investigators. Dr. Bowen served as Coordinator of Metabolic Research of the VM Research Center [5] and was one of only 4 women graduating in the UW medical school class of 1963. She had a long and distinguished career as a researcher in endocrinology while later maintaining a practice in Olympia, authoring books and sponsoring workshops on nutritional health. In 1968, Dr. Bowen established the Western Institutional Review Board to protect patient safety during human clinical research trials. Currently the Western IRB is the largest, independent medical review board in the world. [6]

All of the members of the endocrine metabolic section were involved in research and teaching while maintaining active clinical practices. In 1956, the following notice appeared in the professional journal *Diabetes:*

"The following members of the American Diabetes Association will participate in The Clinical Meeting of the American Medical Association to be held in Seattle, Washington, November 27-30 ... On November 28 William J. Steenrod, Jr, MD, and Robert L. Reeves, MD, Seattle will discuss "Present Day Management of Diabetic Coma." ... Lester J. Palmer, MD, Seattle will serve as Moderator of a panel on diabetes November 30 with Joseph H. Crampton, MD, Seattle, Blair Holcomb, MD, Portland, Oregon, Henry B. Mulholland, MD, Charlottesville Virginia, Robert H. Williams, MD, Seattle and Edward H. Rynearson, MD, Seattle." [7]

Robert Nielsen, MD, joined the Section of Endocrinology and Metabolism in 1957. Dr. Nielsen graduated from Harvard Medical School in 1951; completed an internal medicine residency at King County Hospital in Seattle; and post-residency was trained in endocrinology and diabetes at the Massachusetts General Hospital under the direction of Fuller Albright the "Father of American Endocrinology".

Dr. Nielsen brought cutting edge new endocrine clinical skills to VM and immediately became an active investigator at the VM Research Center while maintaining a busy clinical practice. He continued the section's passion for diabetic patient education, and was instrumental in expanding the Diabetes Camping program, volunteering two weeks each summer at Camp Parsons and at the YMCA Camp Orkila. He was president of the Washington and Alaska Diabetes Association for many years, and founded the nonprofit Diabetic Health and Education Foundation, which created dozens of educational TV programs for people with diabetes and other diseases.

All early members of the Endocrine Section were committed to the pursuit of continuing medical education and academic excellence. During his entire Mason Clinic career (1952-1967), Dr. Reeves continued his passion for clinical research, serving as the President of the Northwest Society of Clinical Research, as noted in the 1959 VM Chairman's report [8]. In addition, he was chairman of several committees at VM including the Research Committee [9], the Procedures and Records Committee [10], and the Professional Relations and Post-Graduate Education Committee. [11] Dr. Reeves was elected to the Board of Trustees of the King County Medical Society [9] in 1966. That same year, he became Section Head when Dr. Crampton became ill, and was nominated and elected to serve the remainder of Dr. Crampton's term of office on the Executive Committee. [9] Sadly, Dr. Crampton died that same year.

Team Medicine at its Best: 1967 – 2000

Dr. Reeves left Virginia Mason in September 1967 to start an endocrine/diabetes practice in Olympia and Dr. Nielsen became Section Head, serving in that capacity until 1982. Dr. Reeves remained active as a principal investigator in the VMRC until 1971 as he and Dr. Angela Bowen were co-Principal investigators in the landmark multi-center University Group Diabetes Program study (UGDP: studying the long-term outcome of patients with diabetes treated with various oral agents). In 1971 Dr. Nielsen was appointed as a Principal Investigator for the UDGP (assuming the roles previously held by Drs. Reeves and Bowen) and continued in that role until the study was completed. [12]

Up until 1968, with the arrival of pediatric endocrinologist C. Patrick Mahoney, MD, the physicians in the Endocrinology Section had been responsible for both adult and pediatric endocrinology patients. Dr. Mahoney, with board certification in both pediatrics and endocrinology, brought additional expertise to VM, and was at the forefront of advances in management of childhood diabetes and growth problems. James R. Hansen, MD, another pediatric endocrinologist, joined him briefly in 1991, but left in 1993 when Dr. Mahoney retired from VM and took a position as Chief of Endocrinology at Childrens' Orthopedic Hospital (see Pediatrics chapter for more information in this volume).

Dr. Nielsen was a leader with a long-term vision to build a nationally recognized endocrine section respected for providing both expert tertiary care for complex endocrine issues and at the same time every day primary care for patients with both Type 1 and Type 2 diabetes. In ad-

40

dition, he promoted active clinical research with the aim of publishing landmark studies in the most prestigious medical journals (*New England Journal of Medicine, JAMA,* etc.). Dr. Nielsen was supremely confident and approached recruiting with a plan to hire highly qualified candidates and he was never frightened of adding partners who might compete with him for referrals of patients with complex fascinating endocrine problems. Because of Dr. Nielsen's vision, he helped build a remarkably cohesive section of academically-oriented endocrinologists/diabetologists. At its peak, VM had seven board-certified endocrinologists. Each physician attempted to develop specific areas of clinical expertise with the goal of providing "cutting edge" treatment to patients with any endocrine/metabolic problem (patients were often referred to a specific section member depending on their endocrine diagnosis).

From the first days of The Mason Clinic, the Endocrinology Section was widely applauded as a regional leader in the education and management of patients with diabetes. As noted above, besides focusing on diabetes, Dr. Nielsen's vision was to recruit an equally skilled group of general endocrinologists. In 1969, Dr. Nielsen recruited Robert Metz, MD, PhD. Dr. Metz earned his MD in South Africa and completed a PhD, in physiology in Toronto, Canada, where he worked under the direction of Charles Best, the co-discoverer of insulin. In 1969, Dr. Metz was a rising star in U.S. academic endocrinology. Immediately before joining The Mason Clinic he was Chief of the Department of Diabetes and Metabolism at Cook County Hospital, Chicago; Chief of the Medical Division at Northwestern University Medical School, and Assistant Chief of Medicine at Passavant Memorial Hospital. Dr. Metz brought further endocrine expertise to VM and almost immediately after arriving became President of the VM Research Center and earned a joint appointment as a Clinical Professor of Medicine at UW. In addition Dr. Metz was charismatic and proved to be an extraordinary VMMC recruiter. For years he played a vital role on the VM Recruiting Search Committee, interviewing nearly every prospective VM physician candidate. He was often called upon to be the "closer" to recruit academically-gifted Mason Clinic applicants.

John Leonard, MD, a talented University of Washington fellow, joined the section briefly in 1971, but left in 1973 to return to UW before becoming a partner. Even though Dr. Leonard's tenure at VM was brief, he left an important mark on the section because he was an astute clinician and an exemplary teacher of house staff.

In 1974, Bob Mecklenburg was completing a senior endocrinology fellowship at UW under the direction of Robert H. Williams, MD. Bob Nielsen and Bob Metz quickly recognized Dr. Mecklenburg's clinical skills and his impeccable resume in both clinical and research endocrinology (endocrine fellowship at the National Institutes of Health). Dr. Mecklenburg joined the section in 1974, immediately adding energy and further endocrine academic excellence to the Endocrine Metabolic sSction.

At that time Paul Fredlund, MD, was a fellow in endocrinology at the NIH, one year behind Dr. Mecklenburg. Dr. Fredlund was offered a permanent position at the NIH but his strong preference was an "academically oriented" clinical practice position with the possibility of active participation in the education of internal medicine residents. He joined the section in September 1975. Shortly after arriving at VM, Dr. Fredlund became the Director of Graduate Medical Education {responsible for providing the overall direction of the multiple VM residencies (internal medicine, general surgery, anesthesia and radiology)}.

Dr. Fredlund's roommate from 1968 to 1973 (during medical school, internal medicine residency and NIH) was Jim Benson, MD. In 1975 Dr. Benson was completing his endocrine fellowship at UW. After meeting Bob Nielsen and Bob Metz, Dr. Benson was convinced that The Mason Clinic was the best employment opportunity in the country for a practicing endocrinologist. Dr. Benson received his BA from Stanford University with Great Distinction (Biology) in 1966 and his MD from Harvard Medical School (magna cum laude, AOA) in 1970. Although VM administrators argued that the projected patient volumes did not support the addition of three endocrinologists in three successive years, Drs. Nielsen, Metz, Steenrod, Mecklenburg and Fredlund were 100% supportive of adding Dr. Benson and even proposed expanding their practice to include general internal medicine patients if the volume of patients with endocrine/diabetes issues was insufficient. After reviewing Dr. Benson's stellar credentials, the VM Executive Committee approved his position and Dr. Benson joined the section in 1976.

By 1976, the Endocrine Section had extraordinary manpower with six full-time well-trained endocrinologists/diabetologists. In addition, endocrinology was flourishing nationally in the late 1970s due to the advent of radioimmunoassay (facilitating the precise diagnosis of endocrine disease) and simultaneously the introduction of self-blood glucose monitoring, which was revolutionizing the management and treatment of patients with diabetes.

Under the leadership of Drs. Nielsen and Metz along with the three new recently trained endocrinologists, interest in the weekly diabetes class exploded (teaching on average each week 10 to 15 patients and their families diabetes management skills). In addition every section member was actively involved in VM resident education and simultaneously served as clinical professors at the University of Washington. Finally the section actively participated in annual Endocrine or Diabetes Post-Graduate Education Courses offered at Virginia Mason.

In 1982, Dr. Nielsen passed the leadership of the section to Dr. Metz. In addition Dr. Steenrod retired in 1982 and the section was fortunate to recruit Ed Benson. Dr. Benson (no relationship to Dr. Jim Benson) was an outstanding VM internal medicine resident from 1975-78 (chief resident in 1977/78). He won the Joseph Crampton Award as the outstanding intern in 1975 and received the Robert Pommerening Award for Outstanding Graduating Resident in 1978. Following residency, Ed was recruited by the section to serve as an endocrine fellow under the direction of Dr. Metz with the collaboration of all section members. After finishing his VM fellowship, Ed completed post-doctoral training in endocrinology at the University of Auckland in New Zealand (1980/81) and at the University of Hong Kong (1981). Ed joined the Endocrine Section in 1982, and immediately brought new energy and expertise to the endocrine section.

Team Medicine has long been a marketing tag line for VMMC. In many ways "Team Medicine" was the Endocrine Section's guiding principle from 1967 to 2006. Several noteworthy examples are outlined below:

1. *The Critical Role Played By Nurse Clinicians, Nutritionists and Pharmacists as Part of the Diabetes Treatment Team*

From the beginning Nurse Clinicians were the key to success of the weekly Diabetes Classes. In this regard the Endocrinology/Diabetes Section was far "ahead of the curve" in utilizing not only nurses but also clinical nutritionists and pharmacists to extend care and expertise. The success of the Diabetes Classes was directly linked to coordinated education by RNs, nutritionists, pharmacists and physicians working together. In 2020, every field of patient care has confirmed the value of coordinated management by allied health practitioners working together. The Endocrine Section fully realized this necessity and opportunity in 1967.

The three nurse clinicians of this era, Nancy Becker/Lencioni, ARNP; Pat Brazel/Vinje, ARNP; and Carolyn Sannar, ARNP, deserve much of the credit for making the Mason Clinic a nationally respected Diabetes Center. (Nancy describes some of this work in the chapter on Outpatient Nursing in this volume.)

2. *Every Challenging Endocrinology Referral Received Six Consultations*

Section members were confident that patients with complicated endocrine or diabetes issues could receive equal or better care at VMMC compared to famous academic research centers. The section had a formal meeting every week devoted to planning treatment strategy for challenging problems (similar to Institutional Tumor Boards in oncologic care). In addition, the diabetes class curriculum was continually updated and new programs were aggressively pursued. The section functioned cohesively partly because Drs. Mecklenburg, Fredlund, Jim Benson and Ed Benson were close friends before they joined The Mason Clinic, and also because of the visionary leadership of Drs. Metz and Nielsen.

3. *Implementation of Insulin Pump in Clinical Practice Resulting in Lead Articles in the New England Journal of Medicine (NEJM) and Journal of the American Medical Association (JAMA)*

In 1979 pediatric endocrinologists at Yale introduced the insulin infusion pump capable of delivering insulin subcutaneously with tiny doses administered by a steady basal rate and also with the capacity to administer larger insulin boluses before dinner. The original Yale publication reported the results of seven patients, each treated by a single individual endocrinologist assigned to each patient. Academic diabetes authorities applauded the breakthrough but were skeptical that the insulin pump could be safely managed in everyday clinical practice.

As mentioned above, the VM Endocrine Section firmly believed that The Mason Clinic was the ideal medical center to test and perfect the implementation of major medical breakthroughs in everyday clinical practice. The section believed that they had everything necessary to test the feasibility that the insulin pump could be utilized by not only academic diabetologist but also by practicing diabetologists. The reasons for this confidence were as follows:

a. VM had a large population of motivated, intelligent patients with Type 1 diabetes.

b. VM had a well-trained team of three nurse clinicians who could provide education, motivation and encouragement to maximize safety and compliance.

c. The Endocrine Section had six well-trained academically-oriented diabetologists.

After consulting with the team at Yale, the VM Section of Endocrinology designed a rigorous research protocol to test the feasibility of using the insulin pump in everyday clinical practice. Dr. Robert Mecklenburg was the driving force, leading the insulin pump research with steady undeterred perseverance. In short order, 100 patients were enrolled with truly astonishing success. The insulin pump dramatically improved diabetes glycemic control and the patients also benefited from a notably improved quality of life. In addition, insulin pump therapy was associated with a low incidence of complications. Three major publications in two of the most prestigious medical journals definitively proved that the insulin pump was effective when used by a team of: 1) motivated educated patients, 2) nurse clinicians, and 3) diabetologists. The publications in the *NEJM* and *JAMA* brought world-wide acclaim to the VM Endocrine Section and include:

1. Clinical Use of Insulin Infusion Pumps in 100 Patients with Type 1 Diabetes." *NEJM* 1982; 307:513-518.

2. "Acute Complications Associated with Insulin Infusion Pump Therapy: Report of Experience with 161 Patients." *JAMA* 1984; 252:3265-3269.

3. "Long Term Metabolic control with Insulin Infusion Pump Therapy: Report of Experience with 177 Patients." *NEJM* 1985; 313:465-468.

Dr. Metz continued to lead the Endocrine Section with unwavering wisdom, integrity and vision until 1986 when Dr. Mecklenburg became Section Head. After the insulin pump research was published, endocrine/diabetes referrals to the section increased and the section started a recruitment search. More than 50 candidates applied to fill the open position and the section was thrilled to hire Norm Rosenthal, MD. Dr. Rosenthal received his MD from Thomas Jefferson Medical College in Philadelphia and completed his residency in internal medicine at Alton Ochsner Medical Center in New Orleans. Following residency he completed fellowship training at Yale (1982-85). Dr. Rosenthal brought energy, keen clinical judgment and innovation. He immediately became a vital force in the section and provided important leadership in academic pursuits.

Under Dr. Mecklenburg's leadership, metabolic research thrived. In fact, Dr. Mecklenburg deserves much of the credit for the highly successful Virginia Mason Research Center's Diabetes Research program. Bob was the physician providing meticulous care for the grandson of the great Seattle philanthropist Jack Benaroya. Mr. Benaroya focused on Type 1 diabetes as a major philanthropic interest and his generosity enabled the Virginia Mason Research Center to recruit Gerald Nepom, MD, PhD, to head immunologic research at Virginia Mason. Dr. Nepom had a hugely successful career and in 1999, through the generosity of the Benaroya family and multiple other philanthropists, the 100,000 square foot Benaroya Research Institute (BRI) was opened on the Virginia Mason campus. Over the years, the focus of research at the BRI expanded from Type 1 diabetes to include other auto-immune diseases.

The late 1980s and the early 1990s were a time of transition in the Endocrine Section as first Dr. Nielsen retired in 1987 and then Dr. Metz in 1991. In addition, VM was becoming more focused on business efficiency and physician financial productivity. In the early days, VM physician salaries were determined by a formula based in equal weight to productivity, academic excellence and seniority. By 1990, the formula was tilting strongly toward a primarily productivity-driven formula. This decision (driven largely by outside market forces) palpably changed the tenor of life in the Endocrine Section. Inevitably the prior emphasis on academic pursuits (educating talented dedicated residents, clinical research and community service) was replaced with a push for increased productivity and efficiency. This change in philosophy had consequences as Dr. Rosenthal resigned in 1999 and accepted a position as Clinical Director of Research at Johnson and Johnson and, in 2000, Dr. Paul Fredlund started a new career as Clinical Director of Research at a local biotechnology company ICOS. The Endocrine Section, however, responded to these lossses and was fortunate to add Ken Gross, MD, in 1999, an astute gifted endocrinologist trained at the University of Washington, and Paul M. Mystkowski, MD, in 2001 from his endocrinology fellowship at the University of Washington, who added significant clinical expertise and began a thyroid cancer tumor board at VMMC.

Transition Years: 2000 - 2007

With the addition of Drs. Gross and Mystkowski, the section was thriving. Dr. Gross became Section Head in 2000. However, the amount of available clinical hours for patient care began to decrease as Dr. Mecklenburg accepted the position of Chief of Medicine and only practiced part-time. Jim Benson had already assumed the position of program director for the internal medicine residency and was also practicing half-time. Dr. Fredlund had left to pursue other research opportunities, and in 2003, Ed Benson left to become Chief of Endocrinology at Group Health. Attempts to work out call schedules with other endocrinologists in the community were not successful and by 2006, the prospect of a section manned by only 2 full-time and 2 part-time endocrinologists was untenable for both Drs. Mystkowski and Gross, who left in 2007 for positions at the PolyClinic.

Dr. Mecklenburg then took a full-time administrative position at VM in 2007, which temporarily left the section without a full-time board-certified endocrinologist. Lucy Sutphen MD, an internist with an interest in endocrinology, stepped into the gap until new endocrinologists could be hired and re-establish the practice.

Rebuilding: 2007-present

The next five years saw the arrival and departure of several endocrinologists, most of whom stayed at VM for only 3-4 years. Farideh Eskanari, MD, was hired in 2007 from her fellowship at Pennsylvania and Michael Williams, MD, joined her in 2008 from the University of Virginia. Dr. Eskanari left in 2010 and was replaced by Monica Rodriguez, MD, from the University of Arkansas. Anna Marina, MD, from the University of Washington was hired in 2011 but left the following year. Dr. Williams left the same year and Dr. Rodriguez left a year later in 2013. It wasn't until the hiring of Grace Lee, MD (UCSF), Elizabeth Reilly, MD (Virginia Commonwealth) and Jonathon Stoehr, MD, PhD, (OHSU) in 2012 that the section began to stabilize, and these three represent the core group today. Gal Omry-Orbach, MD, and Jessica Brzana, MD (OHSU) were both short-term additions. Janet Leung, MD (Brigham Womens) and Francisco Perez Mata. MD (Mount Sinai St. Luke's Roosevelt, New York) are the latest to join the section, which now provides endocrinologic expertise to the downtown clinic, Edmonds, Bainbridge and Federal Way. Kim Erickson PA-C and Diane Osborn, ARNP and Gregor Derupe, PharmD, also provide important care and expertise for diabetic patients.

Physician Biographies
Lester J. Palmer, MD (1920 – 1955)

Lester Palmer was born in Peabody, Kansas on October 15, 1890. "He grew up in the Yakima area and completed his undergraduate training at the University of Washington." [1] He received his MD at Northwestern University in Chicago, graduating in 1914. It was at this time that he became interested in diabetes, working with Elliott Joslyn, MD, a pioneer in the field. [1] Dr. Palmer interned at Cook County, and did his residency at St. Lukes in Chicago. During WW1, he served as Chief of Medicine at a military hospital in France. [1]

He was one of the original partners of the Mason Clinic, coming to Seattle in 1920. He was recruited by James Tate Mason, MD, who personally endorsed a loan to allow him to join, making him the youngest partner [1]. It was an exciting time in Endocrinology, as insulin had been discovered by Banting and Best in 1921. Dr. Palmer was the first physician to administer insulin to a patient in the Pacific Northwest. [1]

Dr. Palmer devoted his career to the treatment and study of diabetes. He showed an interest in education of the diabetic patient and instituted a free class for his patients, which he personally conducted, inspiring them with his enthusiasm and interest. With growing numbers of patients and friends, he was able to organize The Diabetic Trust Fund, which helped finance activities for the welfare of diabetic patients, including summer camps for diabetic children - one on Vashon Island, and the other on Hood Canal. He also established *The Diabetes Monthly* and was a founder of the Washington State Diabetes Association. Within VM he found time to be the Chief of the Department of Medicine, President of the Board of Trustees of the Virginia Mason Hospital and Chief of Staff of VM Hospital for many years. In his later years, he was also a Clinical Professor of Medicine at the University of Washington. He retired from the Mason Clinic in 1955. "At the time of his death, November 29, 1959, at the age of 69, Mr. John Dare, the administrator of the Mason Clinic, described Dr. Palmer as 'unquestionably the outstanding physician in his field'." [1]

Joseph H. Crampton, MD (1947 – 1966)

Joe Crampton was born in Spokane, Washington on April 26, 1917. [2] He graduated from the University of Idaho in 1938 and Vanderbilt Medical School in 1941. He did his internship at Vanderbilt under Hugh J.

Morgan, MD, his medical residency under the greatly respected Tinsley H. Harrison, MD, [2] at North Carolina Baptist, and later at the University of Texas Southwestern Medical College at Parkland Hospital in Dallas. In 1947, he joined Dr. Palmer in the two-man Section of Endocrinology and Metabolism at the Mason Clinic. Following Dr. Palmer's retirement in 1955, he became Section Head. His vision, enthusiasm and organizational skills were highly valued at the Mason Clinic and he was responsible for the Clinic's interest in teaching and research, being instrumental in the founding of the Virginia Mason Foundation for Medical Research. He was extremely active in the American Diabetes Association (ADA) serving as Chairman of the Committee on Detection and Education for 5 years, was on the Board of Directors for 5 years and also was Secretary of the ADA, being elected to a second term even though disabled. At The Mason Clinic, he presided over the Diabetes Trust Fund and the Diabetes Teaching and Research Foundation. A colleague described him as "truly a gentleman as well as a forthright, intelligent and conscientious physician who loved people and helped all who were in need". [2] He passed away in 1966 at the age of 49.

Robert L. Reeves, MD (1952 – 1967)

Robert Reeves, MD, joined the section in 1952, and was particularly interested in research. The Virginia Mason Research Center was incorporated on March 8, 1956. [3] There are several notations in the Chairman's Reports and Bulletins of the era mentioning various grants that he was awarded, often with Dr. Crampton and Angela J. Bowen, MD, as co-investigators. He also worked on the UGDP as a Principal Co-investigator with Dr. Bowen. [14] Dr. Reeves served as the President of the Northwest Society of Clinical Research, as noted in the 1959 VM Chairman's report [8], and was Chair of several committees at VM including the Research Committee [9], the Procedures and Records Committee [10], and the Professional Relations and Post-Graduate Education Committee. [11] He also served as the ex-officio Medical Advisor to the new Exeter House, and was asked by the Executive Committee to assess the issues related to the increasing number of senior citizen homes that were being developed. [10] In November 1965, he headed a diabetes detection drive, as the state coordinator of the Washington Diabetes Association, which sponsored the campaign. [15]

Dr. Reeves was elected to the Board of Trustees of the King County Medical Society in 1966. [9] That same year, he became Section Head when Dr. Crampton became ill, and was nominated and elected to serve the remainder of Dr. Crampton's term of office on the Executive Committee. [9] Sadly, Dr. Crampton died that same year.

The Seattle Times reported that Dr. Reeves and Lucius Hill, MD, thoracic surgeon at VM, attended a national conference on air pollution in 1966. Dr. Reeves had "led the (King) county society's legislative committee on medical aspects of air and water pollution." [16]

Dr. Reeves left Virginia Mason in September 1967 to start a practice in Olympia, WA. He remained active as an investigator in the VM Research Center until approximately 1971, when Dr. Nielsen was appointed as a Principal Investigator for the University Group Diabetes Program at VMRC, replacing co-Principal Investigators Drs. Robert Reeves and Angela Bowen. [12]

William J. Steenrod, Jr. MD (1953 – 1982)

William Steenrod was born Dec 25, 1920 in Michigan [17]. He attended the University of Michigan for medical school, graduating in 1946 [18], and then did his residency in internal medicine in Ann Arbor at the University of Michigan. He joined The Mason Clinic in 1953 and was active in the ADA and education, and continued the tradition of the summer camps at Camp Parsons. He and his wife Florine had 4 children, and he died 2/9/1998 in Nordland, Jefferson, Washington. [19] [20]

Robert L. Nielsen, MD (1957 – 1987)

Robert Nielsen was from Livingston, Montana. During the depression, his family lived in a tent in Yellowstone National Park. Stationed in England during WW II as a laboratory technician, he was accepted to Harvard

Medical School and graduated in 1951. He did his residency at King County Hospital in Seattle, and then a fellowship in endocrinology at the Massachusetts General Hospital. He joined The Mason Clinic in 1957 and was Head of the Endocrinology Department from 1967 to 1982. He continued the section's passion for diabetic patient education, and was a major part of the Virginia Mason team to pioneer the use of the insulin pump. He also volunteered two weeks each summer at Camp Parsons and later at the YMCA Camp Orkila, introducing diabetic children to camp life. He was President of the Washington and Alaska Diabetes Association for many years, and founded the nonprofit Diabetic Health and Education Foundation, which created dozens of educational TV programs for people with diabetes and other diseases. Around VM, he was known as a "devil's advocate" who was not willing to back down from any controversial issue, and was nicknamed "Bullet" for his legendary quick comments, literally shot from the hip and often "brutally honest"! Following retirement he donated his services to the University of Washington, teaching medical residents and seeing patients without remuneration at Harborview Medical Center. He passed away in 2010. [21]

Winston Tustison, MD (1964 - 1968)

Winston Tustison attended Washington University School of Medicine in St Louis and graduated in 1960. He left Virginia Mason in 1968 after being voted into partnership, and entered private practice in Riverside, CA.

Robert J. S. Metz, MD (1969 – 1991)

Robert Metz grew up in South Africa, where he went to medical school. He came to the U.S. from London where he and his wife had lived and worked for two years. He received an MS degree in 1959 from Northwestern University in Chicago and his PhD in physiology in 1962 from the University of Toronto, where he worked under Dr. Charles Best, the co-discoverer of insulin. Upon his return to Chicago, he quickly rose to become Chief of the Department of Diabetes and Metabolism at Cook County Hospital, Chief of the Medical Division at Northwestern University and Assistant Chief of Medicine at Passavant Memorial Hospital. He joined The Mason Clinic in 1969 where he served as the President of the VM Research Center for several years, mentored scores of physicians (including his section peers) and nurses, co-authored many articles and textbooks, and spoke eloquently at medical conferences, imparting great wisdom with keen intellect and humor. Bob became Endocrine Section Head in 1982 and lead the section with a steady hand until 1986. Dr. Metz died suddenly in November 2006 and his passing was a tragic loss for family and friends.

John Leonard, MD (1971 – 1973)

John Leonard came to The Mason Clinic in 1971 and although he was only briefly in the section (leaving in 1973 to join the endocrine faculty at UW), he was a role model because of his skills as an astute endocrinologist and exemplary teacher of housestaff and medical students.

Robert Mecklenburg, MD (1974 – 2007 in Endocrinology; 2007 – present in Administration)

Bob Mecklenburg grew up in Illinois and earned his BA in Biology at Northwestern with Highest Distinction. He continued at Northwestern for medical school and graduated in 1969 (AOA). Following his internal medicine residency at Presbyterian-St. Lukes' Hospital (Chicago) he completed his fellowship in endocrinology at the NIH. In addition, Bob spent an additional year of fellowship under the direction of Robert H. Williams at UW.

Bob joined the Mason Clinic in 1974 and from the onset took the lead in developing an effective clinical diabetes research program. Under Bob's leadership, the VM Endocrine section demonstrated to the world's diabetes community that the newly developed breakthrough insulin pump therapy could be safely implemented in everyday clinical practice. The insulin pump research resulting in three lead articles in the *NEJM* (2) and *JAMA* would never have been published without Dr. Mecklenburg's vision, energy and perseverance.

Bob served as Section Head from 1986-2000 and as Deputy Chief of Internal Medicine from 1989-99. In 2000 he was appointed Chief of Medicine and continued in that role until 2007. In recognition of his contributions to VMMC, Dr. Mecklenburg was awarded the **James Tate Mason Award.** In 2007, Bob assumed the administrative role of Medical Director, Center for Health Care and he continues to contribute to the success of VM.

Paul Fredlund, MD (1975 – 1999)

Paul Fredlund graduated from Harvard College (magna cum laude) in 1966 and Harvard Medical School (cum laude) in 1970. He completed his training with a residency in internal medicine at Harvard Medical School's Peter Bent Brigham Hospital and a clinical fellowship in endocrinology and metabolism at the National Institutes of Health. He is board-certified in internal medicine and endocrinology. [22] He joined Virginia Mason in 1975 and was a vital member of the section and made a contribution to the Clinic as a whole as he served as Graduate Medical Education Director (1976 - 1979), Continuing Medical Education Director (1995 - 1999). He received the Teacher of the Year award in 1976, 1977 and 1996. He was involved in research activities within the section, and was co-author of numerous peer-reviewed articles. He also had an appointment as Clinical Professor of Medicine at the University of Washington School of Medicine.

Dr. Fredlund retired from the Mason Clinic in 1999 and subsequently has worked in biotechnology pharmacologic research designing clinical research trials. In 2000 he joined ICOS Corporation and as a Director of Clinical Research, he was actively involved in the clinical development and the successful worldwide registration of Cialis (tadalafil) for erectile dysfunction. In 2003/2004 Dr. Fredlund was the Co-director of the Lilly/ICOS U.S. Affiliate Cialis™ Product Development Team responsible for the commercialization of Cialis and the design and implementation of Phase 4 Cialis clinical trials. Since 2004, he has continued to work in clinical drug development with a focus on protecting the safety of human subjects participating in clinical trials.

James W. Benson, Jr. MD (1976 – 2015)

James W. Benson received his BA with Great Distinction (Biology) from Stanford in 1966 and his MD from Harvard Medical School magna cum laude in 1970. He completed his internal medicine residency at the Peter Bent Brigham Hospital and completed his fellowship in endocrinology at the University of Washington in 1975.

Dr. Benson joined The Mason Clinic in 1976 and was quickly recognized as an exemplary educator winning the Teacher of the Year in 1979. In 1990 Jim was appointed Chairman of the VM Education Policy Committee and he led post-graduate education with steady intelligent leadership through 2003. Dr. Benson's academic excellence extended to the University of Washington School of Medicine serving as a Clinical Professor of Medicine.

Dr. Benson retired from Virginia Mason in 2015 and finished his professional career at Group Health Seattle.

Edward A. Benson, MD (1982 – 2003)

Ed Benson received his BS (physics) from the University of Kansas in 1967. He was an outstanding undergraduate student and was awarded a Bell Laboratories Fellowship at Stanford where he earned a BS in applied physics in 1968. Ed continued his education at Columbia University in applied mathematics (1969-71). After a brief career in aeronautical engineering, Dr. Benson was accepted to medical school and graduated from the University of Washington School of Medicine in 1975.

Dr. Benson completed his internal medicine residency at Virginia Mason winning both the Intern of the Year and the Outstanding Resident Awards. After completing a Fellowship in Endocrinology at the University of Auckland (New Zealand) (1980-81) and at the University of Hong Kong (1981-82) Ed joined the VM Section of Endocrinology in 1982.

Ed was uniformly respected as a compassionate physician with superior clinical judgment and a unique ability to make important clinical observations resulting in clinical publications. He continued to be a loyal member of the Endocrine Section until 2003 when he accepted a position as Chief of Endocrinology at Group Health Cooperative Seattle.

Norman R. Rosenthal, MD (1987 – 1999)

Norm Rosenthal earned his MD from Thomas Jefferson Medical College in Philadelphia, PA. He did his residency in internal medicine at Alton Ochsner Medical Foundation in New Orleans and completed his Endocrinology Fellowship at Yale (1982-85). Dr. Rosenthal was a superb clinician and an outstanding teacher. He was a vital force in the Endocrine Section until 1999 when he accepted a position in the pharmaceutical industry at Johnson and Johnson.

David K. McCulloch, MD (1992 – 1994)

David K. McCulloch obtained his medical education at Edinburgh University, Scotland with additional postgraduate training at the University of Nottingham, England, and University of Washington, Seattle. He has worked in the field of clinical diabetes for over thirty years and published over 80 articles on a wide variety of diabetes-related topics [24]. Dr. McCulloch joined VM in 1992 as a research associate and served for two years before joining Kaiser Permanente Seattle where he works as a diabetologist leading clinical improvement efforts. [24]

Kenneth M. Gross, MD (1999 – 2007)

Kenneth Gross earned his medical degree from State University of New York at Stony Brook School of Medicine. He completed his residency in internal medicine at Tucson Hospitals Medical Education Program in Arizona and an endocrinology and metabolism fellowship at the University of Washington School of Medicine in Seattle in 1985 [25]. Dr. Gross joined Virginia Mason in 1999 and was uniformly respected as a superior clinician and an excellent teacher. He was the Section Head of Endocrinology from 2000 until 2007 when he left to take a position at the Polyclinic in Seattle.

Paul M. Mystkowski, MD (2001 – 2007)

Paul Mystkowski graduated from the University of Cincinnati School of

Medicine in 1994 and did his internal medicine residency at Northwestern Memorial in Chicago. His endocrinology fellowship was at the University of Washington. He started a thyroid cancer tumor board at Virginia Maosn and provided excellent care to diabetic patients. He was an avid cyclist and fan of nationally prominent Tour de France participants. He left VM in 2007 to join a private practice at the PolyClinic.

Farideh Eskanari, MD (2007 - 2010)

A graduate of Shiraz University Medical School in Iran, Dr. Eskandari completed her internal medicine residency at St. Luke's and an endocrinology fellowship at the University of Pennsylvania. She also earned a Masters in Health Sciences in Clinical Research from Duke and was a co-investigator in the ACCORD trial. After 3 years at VM, she left for a private practice in Kirkland.

Michael D. Williams, MD (2008 – 2012)

Michael Williams earned his medical degree at the University of North Carolina – Chapel Hill. He completed both an internal medicine residency and endocrinology fellowship at the University of Virginia. He was a trusted endocrinology consultant at VM and left after 4 years for a position at the PolyClinic in Seattle.

Monica C. Rodriguez, MD (2010 - 2013)

Monica Rodriguez completed her internal medicine residency at the University of Illinois and her endocrinology fellowship at the University of Arkansas. After her 3 years at Virginia Mason, she left for private practice in Phoenix, Arizona.

Anna L. Marina, MD (2011 – 2012)

After her internal medicine residency at the University of Pittsburgh, Anna Marina completed an endocrinology fellowship at the University of Washington and joined Virginia Mason. She left after just one year to join a private practice in Astoria, Oregon.

Elizabeth R. Reilly, MD (2012 – 2017)

Elizabeth Reilly graduated from Drexel University Medical School, and completed her internal medicine residency at George Washington University. Her endocrinology fellowship was at Virginia Commonwealth. She left VM after 5 years to join Kaiser in Tacoma.

Grace A. Lee, MD (2012 – present)

Grace A. Lee MD, graduated from Cornell Medical School, did her internal medicine residency at New York Presbyterian, and her endocrinology fellowship at UCSF. She has been the Section Head of Endocrinology since joining in 2012 and practices both downtown and in Edmonds.

Gal Omry-Orbach, MD (2012 – 2018)

Jonathan P. Stoehr, MD, PhD, (2012 – present)

Jonathan Stoehr graduated from the University of Wisconsin with his MD in 2004 and PhD in 2006. He completed his internal medicine residency at Yale in 2008 and his endocrinology fellowship at Oregon Health Sciences University (OHSU) in 2012. He has a strong interest in nutrition and is the Director of the Nutrition Center of Excellence. He lives on Bainbridge Island, and practices both downtown and in Bainbridge.

Jessica A. Brzana, MD (2013 – 2017)

Jessica Brzana graduated from New York Medical College in 2006 and completed both her internal medicine residency (2009) and endocrinology fellowship (2013) at OHSU. After 4 years at VM, she left to join Swedish Hospital in Issaquah.

Janet H. Leung, MD (2018– present)

Janet Leung graduated from the University of Michigan School of Medicine in 2010. Her internal medicine residency was at Stanford, and her endocrinology fellowship at Brigham and Women's/Harvard. She has special interests in quality improvement, technology and medical education.

Francisco J. Perez Mata, MD (2019 – present) Federal Way, Seattle

Francisco Perez Mata graduated from medical school in El Salvador. He also had training at the Latin American School of Medicine in Havana, Cuba. His internal medicine residency and endocrinology fellowship were at Mount Sinai St. Lukes-Roosevelt in New York. He is board-certified in both internal medicine and endocrinology. At VM, he sees patients in both Federal Way and downtown Seattle.

Kim D. Erickson, PA-C

Kim D. Erickson, PA-C trained at the University of Wisconsin and is a certified PA in Diabetes Care. She practices at VM Edmonds and in Seattle.

Diane Osborn, ARNP

Diane Osborn ARNP is a certified nurse practitioner in diabetes care, and practices at both downtown Seattle and Federal Way.

Gregor F. Derupe, PharmD

Gregor F. Derupe, PharmD, is another important member of the diabetes care team practicing in downtown Seattle.

References:

1. Low DE. "From the Archives, Our Founding Fathers: Lester J. Palmer, MD." *VMMC Bulletin*, 60(2), Summer 2006.

2. *The Virginia Mason Bulletin;* 1957.

3. Low DE. "From the Archives – Virginia Mason Research Center: The Early Years." *VMMC Bulletin*, vol. 63(1), Spring 2009.

4. "Joseph H. Crampton, MD" at http://diabetes.diabetesjournals.org/content/16/1/64; accessed February 10, 2019.

5. "Dr. Angela Bowen, Coordinatory of Metabolic Research of the Research Center, has been elected to the Board of Trustees of 'Citizens for Clean Air'." *Bulletin* (Virginia Mason Staff Newsletter), June 13, 1967; Virginia Mason Archives.

6. Obituary, Angela J. Bowen at: https://www.legacy.com/obituaries/theolympian/obituary.aspx?n=angela-j-bowen&pid=186618086&fhid=2237; accessed 2/15/19

7. . "Personals" in *Diabetes* 1956 Nov; 5(6): 521-522. At: https://doi.org/10.2337/

diab.5.6.521; accessed 2/14/19

8. 1959 Chairman's Report, Virginia Mason Archives.

9. 1966 Chairman's Report, Virginia Mason Archives.

10. 1962 Chairman's Report, Virginia Mason Archives.

11. 1964 Chairman's Report, Virginia Mason Archives.

12. "Dr. Robert L. Nielsen Appointed to Head UGDP". *Pulse,* February 1971.

13. Transcript from interview with Drs. Paul Fredlund and Jim Benson, July 9, 2015; Virginia Mason Archives.

14. UGDP at: https://jhuccs1.us/clm/PDFs/UGDPTrib_10Jul2015.pdf

15. *The Seattle Times,* "Diabetes Detection Drive Due Here:, November 9 ,1965 a t:https://infoweb-newsbank-com.ezproxy.spl.org/apps/news/document-view?p=WORLDNEWS&t=favorite%3ASEATTLE%21Seattle%2BTimes%2BCollection%2Bwith%2BHistorical%2BArchives&sort=_rank_%3AD&page=2&maxresults=20&f=advanced&val-base-0=Reeves&fld-base-0=alltext&bln-base-1=and&val-base-1=Robert&fld-base-1=alltext&docref=image/v2%3A127D718D1E33F961%40EANX-NB-12CC96170D97A461%402439074-12CC90B068667E17%4016-12CC90B068667E17%40; accessed February 21, 2019.

16. *The Seattle Times,* "Awareness Needed to Fight Air Pollution, Says Doctors", December 9 ,1966,at:https://infoweb-newsbank-com.ezproxy.spl.org/apps/news/document-view?p=WORLDNEWS&t=favorite%3A-SEATTLE%21Seattle%2BTimes%2BCollection%2Bwith%2BHistorical%2BArchives&sort=_rank_%3AD&page=1&maxresults=20&f=advanced&val-base-0=Reeves&fld-base-0=alltext&bln-base-1=and&val-base-1=Robert&fld-base-1=alltext&docref=image/v2%3A127D718D1E33F961%40EANX-NB-12CEE311E630E983%402439469-12CEDEB4054ADDF6%406-12CEDEB4054ADDF6%40; accessed February 21, 2019.

17. "United States Census, 1930," database with images, FamilySearch (https://familysearch.org/ark:/61903/1:1:X7ZH-2LF : accessed 13 February 2019), William J Steenrod Jr. in household of William J Steenrod, Kenmore, Erie, New York, United States; citing enumeration district (ED) ED 460, sheet 27A, line 16, family 719, NARA microfilm publication T626 (Washington D.C.: National Archives and Records Administration, 2002), roll 1437; FHL microfilm 2,341,172. Accessed February 13, 2019.

18. "Obituary Listing" *Annals of Int Med.* 1 Mar 1980; vol. 92(3).

19. "Find A Grave Index," database, FamilySearch(https://familysearch.org/ark:/61903/1:1:QV2Y-ZNZS : 13 December 2015), William J Steenrod, 1998; Burial, Nordland, Jefferson, Washington, United States of America, Sound View

Cemetery; citing record ID 78272183, Find a Grave, http://www.findagrave. com. Accessed February 13, 2019.

20. Obituary, Florine M. Steenrod, https://www.legacy.com/obituaries/Seat-tleTimes/obituary.aspx?page=lifestory&pid=86747256; accessed February 13, 2019.

21. "Passages: Robert L. Nielsen, MD, Res. '51" in the *UW Medicine Magazine* vol 33(2): 1, Fall 2010. At: http://depts.washington.edu/meddev/uwmedmagazine/ also-in-this-issue/passages/robert-nielsen.php. Accessed March 3, 2019.

22. "Paul Fredlund, MD" at: http://www.biopharma-cs.com/people.html#fred-lund; accessed June 22, 2019.

23. Low D. "Evolution, Education and Excellence: Graduate Medical Education at Virginia Mason." *The Virginia Mason Bulletin*, Vol. 57(2), Fall 2003.

24. "Kenneth McCulloch, MD, FRCP, Introduction." At http://www.diabetesin-control.com/dave-mcculloch-md-frcp-introduction/; accessed June 22, 2019.

25. "Ken M. Gross, MD." At https://polyclinic.com/providers/ken-gross; ac-cessed June 22, 2019.

6

Gastroenterology and Hepatology

by Richard Kozarek, MD; Julie Katz, RN;
Liz Moehrke, CGRN; Pat Pethigal, RN, BSN, and Patti Wilbur, RN,
with contributions from Michael Gluck, MD

The Gastroenterology (GI) Section at The Mason Clinic started with a couple of well-trained general internists who had an interest in GI diseases and has developed into one of the premier GI sections in the world.

Building a First-Class Section of Gastroenterology: 1948 – 1983
The GI Section was founded by a general internist, Clarence "Pete" Pearson, MD, who graduated from the University of Texas Medical School and did post-graduate training at the Mayo Clinic where he developed his subspecialty interest in gastroenterology. Described as suave in manner and an intelligent clinician, he added other internists who had an interest in GI disorders and had obtained more training than he had. As a contrast to today's resource observant gastroenterologists, he was noted for admitting patients to the hospital to undergo barium enemas.

During Dr. Pearson's tenure as Section Head, he hired Richard Jones, MD; Randolph Clements, MD; Francis Milligan, MD; Richard Stemler, MD; Fritz Fenster, MD; and Marty Gelfand, MD. Dr. Jones introduced colonoscopy to VM after watching a local proctologist, Bill Friend, perform them. Dr. Jones assumed the role of section head in 1970 [1] and continued to attract highly skilled gastroenterologists and hepatologists with formal training to the section. These included Terry Ball, MD; Len Rosoff, MD; and Bob Gannan, MD. Dr. Jones served as Chief of Staff at VM from 1976–1981 and was President of the Board of Directors from 1986–1988.

Fritz Fenster, and later the team of Fritz and Len Rosoff, provided a new dimension to the section with their expertise in hepatology. Marty Gelfand's main interests were in esophageal diseases and inflammatory bowel disease. He did upper endoscopies and took over the gastric lab, which was previously the purview of the thoracic surgery section led by Luke Hill, MD. The lab performed gastric analyses, secretin stimulation tests, and initiated esophageal motility studies. Marty Gelfand also ran a GI teaching conference for residents. He became Section Head in 1977 and served in that role for 23 years. [1]

Terry Ball brought endoscopic retrograde cholangio-pancreatography (ERCP) and endoscopic papillotomy for common duct stones to Virginia Mason and was the first to perform them in Washington state. Terry also established a formal well-run endoscopy unit that demonstrated the importance of both admitting and recovering patients in a safe and consistent manner. Its creation is described in the 1983 Chairman's report: "An endoscopy/minor surgery suite was constructed on 3 North in 1983. The need for this project stemmed from increasing volume in endoscopy procedures in Gastroenterology, with concurrent quality demands for better monitoring during the procedure and in the recovery period. In addition, with increasing demand for ambulatory surgery being imposed by the government and third party payers, general surgery head and neck surgery, and plastic surgery have also found increasing use for this facility." [2]

Building a World-Class Section of Gastroenterology: 1983 – 2006
The direction of the section over the ensuing 35 years and to the present day was strongly impacted by the arrival of Dick Kozarek, MD, in 1983. Dr. Kozarek was a pioneer in pancreatic endoscopy, providing the cutting edge work previously considered inaccessible or impossible. His work and subsequent publications brought an entirely new dimension to endoscopic

therapy that has continued to evolve to the present day. His rare technical expertise and leadership skills led to the creation of an internationally recognized Gastroenterology Section. He subsequently developed advanced therapeutic GI fellowships at VMMC. He served as Section Head of the GI Section as well as founding the Digestive Disease Institute (DDI) at VMMC, a noted combination of surgical, medical, endoscopic, hepatic, and nutritional Centers of Excellence in both the US and worldwide.. His work, and that of others whom he has hired, has brought national and international attention and acclaim to the section and Virginia Mason. During his leadersip in the section and at DDI, an additional 9 gastroenterologists were hired, some bringing specialty expertise on various GI or liver diseases. Although most of these physicians have now retired or moved on to other positions around the country, they helped build the section and expand their offerings. During these years, there were many important advances, with the section leading the way regionally, nationally and internationally. Some of these include:

1982: First in the **region** to perform percutaneous endoscopic gastrostomy.

1983: First in the **world** to perform endoscopic drainage of pancreatic pseudocysts.

1988: First in the **United States** to use tunable dye laser lithotripsy to treat choledocholithiasis.

1988: Published the longest follow-up study in the **world** on any benign disease entity: 20-year follow-up results on the Hill procedure.

1989: First in the **world** to report using methotrexate to induce remission in patients with refractory inflammatory bowel disease.

1991: First in the **world** to report endoscopic transpapillary therapy for disrupted pancreatic duct and pancreatic fluid collection.

1992: First in the **world** to place metallic, self-expanding stents in the duodenum.

1992: First in the **region** to use endoscopy to treat pancreatic duct stones and obstructive pancreatitis.

1994: First in the **world** to treat pancreatic ascites endoscopically.

1996: First in the **world** to describe gastroesophageal flap valve as an anti-reflux mechanism.

1998: Initially utilized in the mid-1980s, first in the **world** to describe percutaneous computerized tomography-guided catheter drainage of infected acute necrotizing pancreatitis.

1998: First in the **United States** to report the use of extra-corporeal shock wave lithotripsy for treatment of pancreatic stones.

2002: First in the **world** to link paraesophageal hernia repair to routine improvement in pulmonary function.

2003: First in the **world** to develop a specialized protocol for the chemotherapeutic radiation treatment of patients with resected pancreatic cancer.

2003: First in the **world** to report that partially covered metallic stents could be removed from the esophagus.

2005: First in the **region** to adopt double-balloon enteroscopy to diagnose and treat very distal small bowel lesions.

The Digestive Disease Institute: 2007 – present

In 2007, Richard Kozarek was named Executive Director of the new Digestive Disease Institute (DDI) at Virginia Mason, which was formed with the goal of enhancing excellence through multidisciplinary collaboration between GI, surgery, oncology, radiology and pathology in the care of patients with digestive disorders. Building on years of national and international breakthroughs, DDI's focus on education, research, innovation and quality anchored work in four Centers of Excellence: Pancreas, Esophageal, Liver and Therapeutic Endoscopy. Shannon Diede was DDI's first administrative director, partnering with Dick to put the foundations of the Institute in place. The advanced endoscopy fellowship launched in 2007, with Shayan Irani, MD, as the first fellow. Dr. Irani was later hired as a therapeutic endoscopist and has served for many years as Associate Director of DDI's Pancreas Center of Excellence.

Since that time, DDI has grown to eight Centers of Excellence, adding Bariatric Surgery; Nutrition; Inflammatory Bowel Disease; and Liver, Pancreas and Biliary Surgical Centers of Excellence. Eight fellowships, both clinical and research, as well as a thriving Visiting Scholar program and three to five continuing medical education courses per year bring clinician scientists from around the world to study and collaborate with DDI physicians. Research includes 160+ Institutional Review Board (IRB)-approved studies ranging from clinical trials to retrospective chart reviews to bench and translational science. Dr. Kozarek has co-authored over 425 peer-reviewed publications, most with other leading DDI investigators. DDI's work is highlighted in *Gut Instinct*, a publication that showcases recent accomplishments and reaches 17,000 clinicians each year. The section currently (as of Fall 2019) has 19 gastroenterologists, 5 ARNPs, 6 PAs and one nutritionist supporting their practices.

Important advances during this time include:

2007: First in the **world** to combine an external catheter into walled-off pancreatic necrosis with transenteral stents to eliminate pancreatic-cutaneous fistulae.

2007: Utilizing standardized clinical pathways, first in the **world** to publish a large series of esophageal resections with a mortality rate under 1%, earning the *Journal of Gastrointestinal Surgery*'s Best Paper of the Year award.

2008: First in the **region** to endoscopically treat dominant and intrahepatic strictures in patients with primary sclerosing cholangitis (PSC), utilized since the 1990s.

2008: First in the **United States** to introduce T2*-weighted MRI for hepatic iron measurement.

2008: First in the **region** to study multiple new medication therapies for liver disease, including obeticholic acid, lambda IFN and NS5 polymerase inhibitors.

2009: First in the **region** to use simultaneous antegrade-retrograde endoscopy to reestablish patency of the completely obstructed esophagus and colon.

2009: First in the **world** to create the Salvage Procedure for internal drainage of disconnected pancreatic ducts.

2009: First in the **United States** to participate in the first study of a novel non-invasive method, susceptometry, to measure hepatic iron.

2010: Published largest study to date exploring the relationship between hepatic iron content and severity of fatty liver.

2010: Launched the first dedicated hepatology fellowship in the **Pacific Northwest.**

2012: First in the **region** to perform endoscopic submucosal dissection for the removal of GI cancers.

2013: First in the **region** to offer non-invasive FibroScan technology to evaluate disease stage in patients diagnosed with liver conditions.

2014: First in the **United States** to offer the use of SEDASYS (Computer-Assisted Personalized Sedation System) to patients needing minimum to moderate sedation prior to a colonoscopy or an examination of the esophagus.

2015: First in the **world** to report culture and quarantine of duodenoscopes to eliminate multi-drug resistant organism transmission by an endoscopic instrument.

2015: First in the **region** to use endoscope-delivered balloons for obese patients.

2015: First in the **region** to access the biliary tree by EUS and to drain bile duct and gallbladder, including stone removal.

2016 to current: numerous endoscopic procedures to treat bariatric surgical complications including leaks.

2016: First in **region** to fistulize stomach to jejunum for patients with malignant obstruction using Lumen-apposing metal stents.

2016 and 2017: First in **region** to remove submucosal lesions initially with combined surgical and endoscopic therapy, then with Endoscopy alone using over-the-scope clipping devices.

Current team members (as of August 2019):
The current physician and advanced practitioner team members are listed below along with their primary area of expertise:

Hepatology:	**Inflammatory Bowel Disease:**
Blaire Burman, MD	Michael Chiorean, MD
Asma Siddique, MD	Elisa Boden, MD

Christina Pham, ARNP

Therapeutic Endoscopy:
Richard Kozarek, MD
Andrew Ross, MD
Shayan Irani, MD
Michael Larsen, MD
Rajesh Krishnamoorthi, MD
Joanna Law, MD
Ella Sanman, MSN, ARNP

Hospitalist Team:
Omar Suwarno, PA-C
Rebekah Kooy, MMS, PA-C
Caroline Schildbach, ARNP

James Lord, MD, PhD
Tim Zisman, MD, MPH
Teresa Vasicek, PA

General Gastroenterology:
(several also see liver & IBD patients)
Geoffrey Jiranek, MD
Nanda Venu, MD, MS
Fred Drennan, MD
Qing Zhang, MD, PhD
Susan McCormick, MD
Otto Lin, MD
Sarah Sprouse, MD
Diana McFarlane, PA-C

Other Advanced Practitioners in GI:
Advanced practitioners have been a vital part of the gastroenterology section since the 2000s, contributing to the section's enormous growth and exquisite patient care over time. Some are listed above with their respective teams and others include:

Lacey Siekas, DNP, ARNP
Kathleen O'Conner, PA-C

Sophia Lichenstein-Hill, DNP, ARNP
Amy Ziegler, PA-C

Fellows in DDI have included:
Advanced Endoscopy Fellowship

2007 – 2008	Shayan Irani, MD
2008 – 2009	Kayode Olowe, MD
2009 – 2010	Rahul Pannala, MD
2010 – 2011	Mitch Schreiner, MD
2011 – 2012	Greg Lutzak, MD
2012 – 2013	Bryan Balmadrid, MD
2013 – 2014	Nanda Srinivasan, MD (EUS only)

2014 – 2015	Aaron Small, MD
2015 – 2016	Anthony Razzak, MD
2016 – 2017	Rajesh Krishnamoorthi, MD
2017 – 2018	Jennifer Higa, MD
2018 – 2019	Nadav Sahar, MD

Ryan Hill Research Foundation Fellowship

2005 – 2006	Chance D. Felisky, MD
2007 – 2008	Matthew Deeter, MD
2008 – 2010	Madhan Kuppusamy, MD
2010 – 2011	Philip W. Carrott, Jr., MD
2011 – 2012	Sheraz Markar, MD
2012 – 2013	Artur M. Bodnar, MD
2013 – 2014	Henner Schmidt, MD
2014 – 2015	Kamran Mohiuddin, MD
2015 – 2016	Mustapha El Lakis, MD
2016 – 2017	Andrea Wirsching, MD
2017 – 2018	Piers Boshier, MD, PhD
2018 – 2019	Fredrik Klevebro, MD, PhD

Hepatology Fellowship

2010 – 2012	Asma Siddique, MD,
2012 – 2014	Pushpjeet Kanwar, MD, and Nihar Shah, MD
2014 – 2015	Yasir Al-Azzawi, MD
2018 – 2019	Amulya Reddy, MD

Pancreas Cancer Research Fellowship

| 2014 – 2015 | Stephen Oh, MD |
| 2016 – 2017 | Zaheer Kanji, MD |

Pancreas Research Fellowship

| 2016 – 2018 | Nadav Sahar, MD |
| 2018 – 2019 | George Baison, MD |

HepatoPancreatoBiliary Surgical Fellowship

2012 – 2013	Sameer Damle, MD
2013 – 2014	Farzad Alemi, MD
2014 – 2015	Jesse Clanton, MD
2015 – 2016	Kimberly Bertens, MD
2016 – 2017	Jad Abou Khalil, MD
2017 – 2018	Zaheer Kanji, MD
2018 – 2019	Janelle Rekman, MD, MAEd
2018 – 2020	Morgan Bonds, MD

University of Washington-Virginia Mason Gastroenterology Fellowship Rotation

2012 – 2013	Mark Derleth, MD; Kevin Webb, MD; Adam Templeton, MD; Ashley Evans, MD
2013 – 2014	Lisa Kaiser Mathew, MD; Peter Liang, MD; Casey Owens, MD; Rebecca Fausel, MD
2014 – 2015	Alex Ende, MD; Jessica Fisher, MD; Anand Singla, MD; Rex Cheng, MD
2015 – 2016	Andrew Korson, MD; Jennifer Higa, MD; Margot Herman, MD; Justin Taylor, MD
2016 – 2017	Liz Rosenblatt, MD; Jennifer Higa, MD; Sarah Sprouse, MD; Steve Vindigni, MD; Joey Roberts, MD
2017 – 2018	Evan Tiderington, MD; Nina Saxena, MD; Sophia Swanson, MD; Brandon Dickinson, MD
2018 – 2019	Mitra Barahimi, MD; Daniel Bushyhead, MD; Jeff Jacobs, MD; Rebecca Kosowicz, MD

Visiting Scholars to DDI have included:

Visiting Scholar	Year of Appointment	Home Country	Sponsor
Rolf Jakobs, MD	1991	Germany	Kozarek
Francisco Vida, MD	1998	Spain	Kozarek
Hiroki Taoka, MD	1998	Japan	Traverso
Damon Bizos, MMed	1999	South Africa	Kozarek
Yuji Nukui, MD	1999	Japan	Traverso

Eduardo Gutierrez, MD	2000	Uruguay	Kozarek
Yuichi Kitagawa, MD	2000–2001	Japan	Traverso
Fouad Attia, MBBCH	2000–2002	Egypt	Kozarek
Julius Spicak, MD, PhD	2003	Czech Republic	Kozarek
Hiroyuki Shinchi, MD	2002–2003	Japan	Traverso
Ostein Hovde, MD	2003	Norway	Kozarek
Patrick Mosler, MD	2003	Germany	Kozarek
Rajkumar P. Wadhwa, MD	2003	India	Kozarek
Monica Almeida, MD	2007	Ecuador	Ayub
Jason Dominitz, MD	2008	United States	Kozarek
Nagammapudur S. Balaji, MD	2008	India	Low
Johannes J. Bonenkamp, MD	2008	Netherlands	Low
Ibrahim Aziz, MD	2009	Egypt	Kozarek
Deepak Bhasin, MD	2009	India	Kozarek
Russell Fleischer, PhD	2010	United States	Kowdley
Carmen Lim, MD	2010	Malaysia	Kowdley
Deepak Bhasin, MD	2010	India	Kozarek
Arthur Lau, MD	2011	Australia	Kozarek
Gulseren Seven, MD	2011–2012	Turkey	Kozarek
Dekey Lhewa, MD	2012–2013	United States	Kowdley
Jae-Myung Cha, MD	2013–2014	Korea	O. Lin
Hyun Phil Shin, MD, PhD	2015–2016	Korea	Kozarek
Varun Thiagarajan, MD	2016–2017	India	Ross
Kyong Ok Kim, MD	2017–2018	Korea	Chiorean
Jong Jin Hyun, MD, PhD	2017–2018	Korea	Kozarek

The History of Nursing in the Gastroenterology (GI) Section

When Virginia Mason opened its School of Nursing in 1922, no one could have envisioned the role and impact of nursing in the years ahead. As medical and technical tools and skills continued to advance, so did the need for the specialized nurse.

A multidisciplinary approach evolved to care for the GI patient, which included trained nurses with current advanced technologic understanding who could safely administer medications, use progressive patient education to help the patient and families understand the care that was given, and monitor the patient during complex procedures.

This approach evolved with the technologic advances over the last 50 years in the field of gastroenterology. As methods were developed to examine the internal surfaces of the GI tract, the gastroenterologist or internist began to perform simple diagnostic office procedures, such as proctoscopy and rigid sigmoidoscopy, with the help of a medical assistant.

Developments in fiberoptics, lens technology and other improvements led to the introduction of the flexible colonoscope and upper endoscope. As the care of the patient became more complex, a registered nurse (RN) began to exclusively fill the role of the assistant. The nurses required advanced knowledge and a good understanding of the patients' needs to keep them safe during these more complicated therapeutic GI procedures.

The role of the registered nurse also expanded as more sedation medications (Demerol and Valium) were used in conjunction with other adjunct medications such as atropine and glucagon. In the early days of endoscopy, sedation was usually given by the physician using straight intravenous injections. These patients were cared for in recovery by nurses who recorded patient blood pressure and pulse. The recovery period was brief and when the patient was stable, she/he would be discharged. The discharge criteria included stable orthostatic blood pressure (lying, sitting, standing) after which the patient was walked back to an area where the physician would discharge them to home. However, the need for titrated medications resulted in the use of small IV butterflies, which are placed by the GI nurse, and the need for more careful monitoring also became part of their duties.

In 1974 the Society of Gastroenterology Nurses and Assistants (SGNA) was established for the education and support of nurses and associates. The Pacific Northwest Society of Gastroenterology Nurses Association (PNWSGNA) became a chartered organization in the early 1980s. This organization helped to provide a format for education, patient safety, and sharing of ideas and information with the nursing practice. Throughout the Seattle area, education was held in the evening at different facilities.

Virginia Mason nurses provided leadership and education in this organization for many years.

At Virginia Mason, the GI department registered nurses developed a relationship with the Anesthesia Department in the late 1980s to develop safe practices for administering conscious sedation. These guidelines included using state-of-the-art monitoring devices such as oximeters, administration of oxygen, and the requirement that all patients have IV access during procedures.

When President Reagan was diagnosed with colon cancer in 1984, the demand for screening colonoscopy increased dramatically. At that time, some insurance companies started to cover screening colonoscopy, and patients were able to do bowel preps at home rather than on admission to the hospital, resulting in decreased cost of care. As the demand for procedures increased, the number of staff at Virginia Mason grew substantially to meet the needs of both a busy clinic and hospital. Virginia Mason saw the need to provide a small unit where GI procedures could be performed and constructed a dedicated Procedure Department for both outpatients and inpatients in the early 1980s. These procedure rooms included equipment for basic procedures such as upper endoscopy, dilation, and colonoscopy with biopsy. Liver biopsies were performed by trained hepatologists. Fluoroscopy with radiology assistance was performed on the 5th floor in radiology. Mobile carts were designed to carry equipment both to radiology and critical care for procedures. Often transport of equipment required 2 or 3 fully equipped carts!

By the late 1980s, the department had totally outgrown its footprint. A new facility was designed to meet the regulations of Medicare and JCAHO regarding space requirements and care guidelines for "Conscious Sedation" administration. The new facility was completed in the beginning of 1991 and became Medicare-certified in April 1991. The new design provided more efficient care and a very safe environment for the patient. With this new department, an array of new, cutting-edge procedures could be performed: endoscopic ultrasound, YAG laser treatments, photodynamic therapy, treatment of acute GI bleeding, and others. At the same time, a specific ERCP suite was designed on Level 5 Radiology. No more pushing mobile carts, a vast improvement from the days of rigid proctoscopy!

At this point, the majority of the GI nursing staff at VMMC were certified CGRN (the first GI Certification test was given in San Francisco in 1986). Active members held Regional PNWSGNA board positions and spoke at National SGNA conferences, sharing the advancements of the specialty to other GI nurses in the region and nation.

More structured patient education became necessary. Nurses were instrumental in providing education for procedures such as photodynamic therapy, ERCP, endoscopic ultrasound (EUS), and lithotripsy. For example, an acute pancreatitis pathway was created to help the patient understand how to manage their symptoms at home and when to call the clinic for help. The symptoms were listed as green, yellow or red. If the patient was experiencing yellow symptoms they would call the clinic for advice from the nurse. This resulted in the patient receiving care when needed and potentially avoiding a long and expensive hospitalization.

As demand continued for screening colonoscopies in the late 1990s, parameters were devised for low risk patients. In addition, the monitoring methods improved as technology advanced by including oxygen saturation measurements with pulse oximetry, oxygen support during procedures and EKG monitoring, all under the careful eye of the nurses and physicians to make sure the patient had a safe and successful outcome. In the past 10 years, sedation has evolved as well and now includes the administration of Propofol by VM RNs, one of the first places in the United States to adopt this pathway.

In 2010, a new space was created in the Jones Pavilion at Virginia Mason to better manage the medically sicker and less stable inpatients and outpatients. The goal was to bring the care to the patient rather than the patient being moved to a variety of medical units. Anesthesia, Radiology, and Endoscopy (multi-disciplinary) were located in one unit in the new Jones Pavilion.

Although there have been astounding advancements in technology and nursing care for GI patients over the last 50 years, one thing has been constant: the team of MDs, nurses, medical assistants, technicians, and management, all focused on giving the best possible care to their patients safely and effectively. As the specialty changed, the team constantly grew and developed. Because of this, the VMMC GI Department is now recognized as a premier center nationally and internationally, and is well positioned to provide cutting-edge GI care to their patients in the future.

NOTE: The authors of this GI nursing section are **Pat Pethigal, RN, BSN; Patti Wilbur, RN,** and **Liz Moehrke, CGRN,** all of whom are now retired. They would like to reognize the many team members, with decades of experience and commitment, who continue to work to provide exemplary care for their patients. One of the influential leaders in nursing care at VM was **Jill Ragsdale, RN,** who recently died in 2018. Her laser focus on patient care and safety was a guiding light both during and after her tenure. Her resolute mission and contributions have left an indelible impact on GI nursing care at Virginia Mason Medical Center.

Physician Biographies
Clarence "Pete" Pearson, MD (1948 – 1978)
Pete Pearson was born May 11, 1913, and grew up in Texas where he attended the University of Texas Medical School, followed by some post-graduate training at the Mayo Clinic. He joined The Mason Clinic in 1948, and despite no formal training in GI, founded the modern-day GI Section. Over the years, he added others, some of whom had more subspecialty training, to build the expertise of the section, including Richard Jones, Randolph Clements, Francis Milligan, Richard Stemler, Fritz Fenster, and Marty Gelfand. He achieved board certification in GI in 1956, probably qualifying on the basis of experience. [3] He stepped down as Section Head in 1970 and retired in 1978. [1] He died on February 13, 1992 in Seattle at the age of 78.

Richard Jones, MD (1954 – 1988)
Richard Jones was born in Seattle and graduated from Stadium High

School in Tacoma. He received his MD from the University of Oregon and served as a Navy flight surgeon for 2 years after WW II. He obtained advanced medical training at Mayo Clinic where he met his wife Marice. He joined Virginia Mason in 1954, and introduced colonoscopy to VM after watching local proctologist Bill Friend, MD, perform them. He served as Section Head from 1970 to 1977 [1], and as Chief of Staff at VM from 1976–1981. He was President of the Board of Directors from 1986–1988. He was a member of the North Pacific Society of Internal Medicine, and Fellow of the American College of Physicians (ACP) and the American Gastroenterological Association (AGA). He was a superb clinician and well-liked by all with a calm, thoughtful presence and demeanor. He never said an unkind word about anyone. He retired in 1988, and died of leukemia in 2001 at the age of 78.

Randolph Clements, MD (1956 – 1989)

Randolph (Randy) Clements was born October 1, 1924 in Lewiston, Idaho. He entered the University of Idaho in 1940, but was drafted into WWII and sent to Ft. Sill, Oklahoma into the field artillery division. After the war, he enrolled in the University of Utah for pre-med studies and then attended the University of Texas (UT) Medical School, graduating in 1949. He completed an internship at Virginia Mason Hospital and then returned to UT in the Department of Pharmacology where he co-authored numerous papers. He eventually returned to VM to begin an internal medicine residency, but was called to the Korean War and served as Captain in the Air Force in Selma, Alabama. At the end of his tour, he returned to VM to complete his internal medicine residency; he joined the staff in 1956 and practiced GI and internal medicine until his retirement in 1990. He was a fellow of the ACP. After retirement, he took up bridge and pursued his talent for painting. He died unexpectedly on February 29, 2004 at the age of 79. [4]

Francis Milligan, MD (1962)

Frank Milligan was born in Cumberland, B.C, a small village on Vancouver Island, in 1931. He spent most of his childhood in Victoria, B.C. He went to medical school at John Hopkins, graduating in 1957. He was then an intern at Toronto General Hospital, followed by an internal medicine residency at Hopkins. He did a two-year GI fellowship at Massachusetts General Hospital in Boston, finishing in 1962. Dr. Milligan was at The Mason Clinic for 4 months before returning to Canada due to an inability to obtain a proper work visa, despite the best efforts of both the medical center and himself. Dr. Milligan returned to Canada, and achieved his board certifications there. He then practiced in Victoria for 7 years, moved to Ontario, Canada for a short while, and then was at John Hopkins for the remainder of his career. He retired in 2011, and lives in Baltimore with his wife Ann. Despite his short tenure at Virginia Mason, he has fond memories of his time here, and speaks highly of Dr. Pearson (personal recollections, Dr. Frank Milligan).

Richard S. Stemler, MD (1964 – 1992)

Richard (Dick) Stemler was born on January 19, 1927. He received his MD from the University of Pennsylvania. He served his internship and residency at Geisinger Memorial Hospital in Pennsylvania and his GI fellowship at Indianapolis General Hospital and the University of Washington. He came to Virginia Mason in 1964 and practiced internal medicine and gastroenterology, doing minor endoscopic procedures. In the 1992 VM Chairman's report, he is described as "quiet and self-effacing … took good care of a loyal cadre of patients, handled a lion's share of the Sigmoidoscopy Clinic for years, and supported the Section and the Clinic throughout his tenure here. In spite of an unfortunate accident, which was judged to be a retiring disability, he returned to support a short-handed Gastroenterology section in time of need. He was a team player and he will be missed." [5] He lived on Bainbridge Island and retired in 1992. He died August 17, 2009.

L. Frederick Fenster, MD (1967 – 1997)

Fritz Fenster was born in San Francisco on October 31, 1931. He was the son of a well-known physician in San Francisco. He attended Stanford

University, receiving a BA in history in 1953. He graduated from Harvard Medical School in 1957. He did his internship and residency at Yale-Grace New Haven Hospital, and spent a third year there as a fellow in liver diseases under Gerald Klatskin, MD. He was chief medical resident at King County Hospital and the University of Washington, and then served 2 years as clinical associate at the NIH in Bethesda, Maryland. [6] He was recruited to the University of Washington by Robert Petersdorf, MD, but joined The Mason Clinic in 1967. He started the Sub-section of Hepatology at VM, which he headed for twenty years, and served as Section Head of Gastroenterology briefly as well. [1] He was an expert clinician and hepatologist with a comprehensive knowledge of liver histology. The pathologists always called Fritz to discuss his biopsies before finalizing their reports, and they learned many things from him. The histology laboratory cut an extra set of slides for Dr. Fenster, and he had an extensive file of these cases as well as hepatological literature, which were typewritten and which he continuously updated. He served as a resource for many colleagues and medical housestaff, and spent many hours teaching not only housestaff but also UW GI fellows and medical students, receiving several "best teacher" awards over his career.

Dr. Fenster initiated peer-review efforts in Washington state and devoted his later years to quality improvement efforts for VMMC, including serving as Medical Director of the Office of Value Assessment between 1991 and 1997, and as Associate Chairman of the QA Committee. He was a Clinical Professor of Medicine at the UW from 1975 – 1997. He was awarded the R.H. Williams Leadership in Medicine Award by the Seattle Academy of Internal Medicine, and in 1995, won the **James Tate Mason Award** at VM. In 1997, he received the annual "Distinguished Clinician" award given by the American Gastroenterological Association. He was married briefly to singer/actress Marni Nixon (her voice was dubbed in for Audrey Hepburn's in the movie *My Fair Lady*). Fritz enjoyed the Seattle Symphony and was a friend of conductor Milton Katims. He was also a very good tennis player. He retired in 1997, and died January 19, 2011. [6]

Martin Gelfand, MD (1969 – 2002)

Marty Gelfand was born in New York City. He attended Harvard College, and then Johns Hopkins University where he received his MD degree. He did an internal medicine residency at the second (Cornell) division of Bellevue Hospital and a GI fellowship at Yale under his beloved mentor, Howard Spiro, MD. He met Dr. Pearson, who was a consultant for the Armed Forces chapter of the ACP, at a GI section meeting in San Antonio. At that time, Dr. Gelfand was serving his Berry Plan military stint as the head of GI at Wilford Hall Hospital in San Antonio. Dr. Pearson offered him a position and he was welcomed as the first Jewish member of the Clinic. His main interests were in esophageal diseases and inflammatory bowel disease. He did upper endoscopies and took over the esophageal lab, which was previously the purview of thoracic surgery and Luke Hill, MD. He performed gastric analyses and secretin stimulation tests with the expert help of Lillian Neale. Dr. Gelfand initiated esophageal motility studies and ran a GI teaching conference for residents. He served as Section Head from 1977 to 1990 [1], as well as head of the Personnel Committee for many years at VM. He also served as Chair of the local Medical Advisory Committee of the Crohn's and Colitis Foundation and was awarded the national honor of Premier Physician of the Year. He sat on the boards of both the AGA and the American College of Gastroenterology, a rarity since both groups were continually at odds with one another. Dr. Gelfand retired in 2002.

Terrence Ball, MD (1975 – 2001)

Terry Ball grew up in Longview, Washington and graduated from WSU. He received his MD degree from Johns Hopkins Medical School, and did his·internship and residency at Hartford Hospital in Connecticut, followed by a GI fellowship at Yale. After joining VM in 1975, he quickly surpassed the array of complex procedures being done at the University of Washington, and was the first to do endoscopic retrograde cholangio-pancreatography (ERCP) and endoscopic papillotomy for common duct stones in Washington state. Thanks to his efforts, a formal well-run endoscopy unit was established at VMMC. He retired in 2001.

Leonard Rosoff, Jr., MD (1976 – 2006)

Len Rosoff grew up in Los Angeles and received his BS degree from Carleton College. He attended the University of Southern California for medical school, graduating in 1968. He then did two years of residency at Johns Hopkins Hospital and two years of a hepatology fellowship at USC and The Royal Free Hospital in London. Following his training, he spent two years as a physician in the Army from 1972 to 1974.

Dr. Rosoff came to The Mason Clinic in 1976, joining Fritz Fenster as a second hepatologist. During his tenure he performed over 1000 liver biopsies and reviewed all of them with pathology – the pathologists greatly valued his opinion and insights and made sure to call him before signing the cases out. He also maintained a large primary care practice.

Dr. Rosoff was Chairman of the Grand Rounds Committee for a number of years, and also served on the Quality Assurance Committee and The Graduate Education committee, which was responsible for choosing our medical residents. In addition, he was always involved in the medical resident teaching program. Dr. Rosoff retired in 2006.

Robert Gannan, MD, PhD (1978 – 1983)

Robert Gannan attended medical school at the University of Rochester, followed by a residency in internal medicine at UCSF. He was at VM for 4 – 5 years and left to pursue his interest in devices and the business aspects of GI medicine. He had a very successful career including serving as President and Partner of Northwest Gastroenterology Associates in Bellevue. He is now retired.

Richard Kozarek, MD (1983 – present)

Dick Kozarek grew up in Wisconsin, and attended college and medical school at the University of Wisconsin, graduating in 1973. He did his internship at Dalhousie University in Halifax, Nova Scotia, Canada, and an internal medicine residency at Good Samaritan Hospital in Phoenix, Arizona, which he completed in 1976. This was followed by a gastroenterology fellowship at Phoenix Veterans Administration Medical Center and the

University of Arizona. Dr. Kozarek has been a pioneer in pancreatic endoscopy, guiding the path of national and international therapeutic endoscopists, who hold him in highest regard. He possesses technical expertise and taught general surgeons rudimentary laparoscopy at Virginia Mason. He developed the GI fellowships at VMMC, and has served as esteemed Section Head of the GI Section as well as founder of the Digestive Disease Institute at VMMC, one of the most important GI endoscopy organizations in the US and worldwide. He is much in demand as a visiting professor and for invited lectureships around the world. Dr. Kozarek has co-authored over 425 peer-reviewed publications and is primarily responsible for the consistently high rating of the GI section in *US News and World Report* rankings. Dr. Kozarek has received numerous recognitions for his work, including the Eddy D. Palmer Award for Gastrointestinal Endoscopy from the William Beaumont Society, the **James Tate Mason Award** at VM in 1992, the Schindler Award for Lifetime Contributions to Gastrointestinal Endoscopy in 2005, and The Masters of the World Gastroenterology Organization Award in 2015. He has several areas of active research and sits on the editorial board of numerous Gastroenterology journals. He is Past President of the World Gastroenterology Organization, the Society for Gastrointestinal Intervention and the American Society for Gastrointestinal Endoscopy.

David J. Patterson, MD (1985 – 2011)

David Patterson received his medical degree from the University of Auckland, Faculty of Medicine and Health Science, New Zealand in 1975. This was followed by an internship and residency in internal medicine at the University of Auckland, and a fellowship at Baylor University in Houston, TX, which he completed in 1981. Dr. Patterson joined Virginia Mason in 1985; he had a special interest in inflammatory bowel disease. He left in 2011 to pursue other opportunities and currently works with the Swedish gastroenterology group in Seattle and Issaquah. [7]

Alin Botoman, MD (1986 – 1993)

Alin Botoman completed his GI fellowship at UW with mentor Charles

Pope, MD, in 1985. He worked at VM from 1986 until 1993. He published extensively in the *VM Bulletin* and served on the Therapeutic Nutrition Committee. When he left VM he took a position in Pittsburgh, and then moved to the Cleveland Clinic in Florida. He is currently working at Massachusetts General Hospital in Boston with expertise in motility disorders. He is an avid fly fisherman.

James E. Bredfeldt, MD (1988 – 2015)

Jim Bredfeldt received both his BA and MD, from Kansas University, making him a huge Jayhawks fan for life! His fellowship in GI was also at Kansas University with Norton Greenberger, MD, and he did a hepatology fellowship at Yale with Dr. Grossman. He practiced hepatology and gastroenterology at VM including endoscopies. He had multiple publications and served on the VMMC Institutional Review Board for many years, including as Chair until 2018. He also served as Chair of the VMMC Credentials Committee. Dr. Bredfeldt retired in 2015.

Geoffrey C. Jiranek, MD (1991 – present)

Geoffrey Jiranek joined Virginia Mason in 1991 as a staff gastroenterologist. He attended Dartmouth Medical School, where he received his MD degree in 1981. This was followed by an internal medicine internship and residency, as well as a year as chief resident at Dartmouth. In 1989, he completed a 3-year fellowship in gastroenterology at the University of Washington. Dr. Jiranek then took a position at Pacific Medical Center before joining Virginia Mason shortly thereafter.

Dr. Jiranek's special interests include endoscopic ultrasound, peptic ulcer disease, inflammatory bowel disease, gastroesophageal reflux, and malabsorption. He has 28 articles in peer-reviewed journals and multiple abstracts to date.

John Brandabur, MD (1991 – 2010)

Jack Brandabur received his medical degree from the University of Cincinnati in 1984. He did his internship and residency in internal medicine at Virginia Mason, followed by a GI fellowship at the University of Texas, Southwestern, which he completed in 1991; he subsequently took a staff position at VM. He left in 2010 and now practices with the Swedish gastroenterology group in Seattle and Issaquah. [8]

Herb Wolfsen, MD (1993 – 1995)

Herb Wolfsen graduated from Loma Linda University and did his internal medicine residency at Virginia Mason Medical Center from 1986–1989 and GI fellowship at Mayo Clinic from 1989–1992. He and his wife, Christine Eng, MD (dermatologist), joined Virginia Mason in 1993 before taking positions at Mayo Clinic Jacksonville in the mid-1990s.

Michael Gluck, MD (1997 – 2019)

Michael Gluck is the former Chief, Department of Medicine and former Section Head of Gastroenterology at Virginia Mason Medical Center. He is a graduate of UCLA School of Medicine (1981), and completed his internal medicine residency and fellowship training at the University of Washington in 1986. His research interests include pancreaticobiliary disorders, with special interests in severe acute pancreatitis and pancreatic necrosis. Currently he has been involved in both clinical and research work on eosinophilic esophagitis, fecal transplantation for recurrent *Clostridium difficile*, duodenoscope infections, and treatment of obesity. He is a fellow of the American Gastroenterology Society and American Society of Gastrointestinal Endoscopy. He joined Virginia Mason in 1997. During his tenure, he has authored or co-authored in excess of 100 scientific publications and spoken extensively on his research work. Dr. Gluck retired in 2019.

Drew B. Schembre, MD (1998 – 2010)

Drew Schembre received his medical degree from New Jersey Medical School in 1988. He did his internship and residency in internal medicine at the University of Utah, which he completed in 1991, followed by a GI fellowship there. He took a staff position at VM in 1998, was an expert in endoscopic ultrasound, and was appointed as GI Section Head from 2006 to 2009 before leaving for the Swedish gastroenterology group where he practiced until 2018, when he and his family relocated to Northern California to lead a gastroenterology section there. [9]

Susan E. McCormick, MD (1998 – present)

Susan McCormick joined Virginia Mason in 1998 as a gastroenterologist with special interests in general gastroenterology including gastroesophageal reflux disease, esophageal motility disorders, inflammatory bowel disease and colon cancer screening. She attended George Washington University for her medical degree, which she received in 1988. She did an internal medicine residency at Letterman Army Medical Center in San Francisco, followed by a GI fellowship at Walter Reed Army Medical Center in Washington, D.C., which she completed in 1995. She then served as a staff gastroenterologist at Andrews Air Force Base in Maryland for 2 years, followed by one year in private practice in Tacoma before joining Virginia Mason in 1998. She is a published author who has written both young adult literature and mystery stories.

Otto S. Lin, MD (2001 – present)

Otto Lin is the Medical Director of Quality Improvement at the Digestive Disease Institute of Virginia Mason Medical Center, and Clinical Assistant Professor of Medicine at the University of Washington School of Medicine, Seattle. He is originally from Taiwan and Hong Kong, and attended college at Stanford University in California, where he earned degrees in electrical engineering and biological sciences. After graduating from Harvard Medical School in 1994, he underwent residency training and subspecialty training in gastroenterology at Stanford University Hospital. He served as a visiting research fellow at Changhua Christian Medical Center in Taiwan from 1997 to 1998. He also holds a Master of Science degree in health services research from Stanford University. He has been the recipient of numerous awards, including two American College of Gastroenterology Clinical Research Grants, the Cabot Prize at Harvard Medical School, the Franklin Ebaugh Award for Outstanding Research at Stanford

Hospital, and three Clinical Research Chair Awards at Virginia Mason Medical Center from 2005 to 2011. Currently, he is a special consultant for the Medical Devices Advisory Committee of the United States Food and Drug Administration. In addition to his patient care responsibilities, he is active in clinical and outcomes research, having published over 50 peer-reviewed papers and 30 abstracts, many of which involve colon cancer screening and surveillance.

Klaus Mergener, MD, PhD, MBA (2001 – 2003)

Klaus Mergener attended medical school in Frankfurt and Hamburg, Germany, graduating in 1989, and completed his MD-PhD, thesis at the German Cancer Research Institute in Heidelberg, Germany. He then went to Duke University for his residency and a fellowship in gastroenterology, which he completed in 1998. [10] He joined Virginia Mason in 2001 and left in 2003. He currently is a partner at Digestive Health Specialists, Medical Director of Gastroenterology at MultiCare Health Systems in Tacoma, WA, and president-elect of the American Society for Gastrointestinal Endoscopy. [11]

Kamran Ayub, MD (2004 – 2008)

Kamran Ayub is a therapeutic endoscopist. He received his medical degree from the Kyber Medical College in Pakistan, and then came to the US for an internal medicine residency at Baltimore Medical Center. He underwent advanced endoscopic training at Baylor College of Medicine after his GI fellowship there. He joined the UW faculty as Chief of Endoscopy at Harborview, and moved to VMMC in 2004 before leaving for private practice in the Chicago area in 2008.

Fred Drennan, MD, MHA (2004 – present)

Fred Drennan joined Virginia Mason in 2004 as a staff gastroenterologist. Prior to that time, he worked at Group Health Cooperative as staff gastroenterologist and internist from 1988 to 1999 with several administrative responsibilities, followed by administrative positions at Providence Medical Center, Swedish Medical Center and PRO-West/Qualis Health, all in Seattle.

Dr. Drennan graduated from Yale University School of Medicine in 1982, followed by an internship and residency at Yale and fellowship training in gastroenterology at the University of Washington, which he completed in 1987. He received a Master's in Health Care Administration for Medical Executives from the University of Washington in 1999. His current interests are in general gastroenterology and hepatology, inflammatory bowel disease and functional GI disorders.

Kris V. Kowdley, MD (2007 – 2014)

Kris V. Kowdley, MD, joined Virginia Mason in 2007 as a hepatologist and Director of the Liver Center of Excellence and Director of Research at the Digestive Disease Institute at Virginia Mason Medical Center. He received his medical degree from Mount Sinai School of Medicine, and completed his internship and residency at Oregon Health Sciences University. He did a GI and hepatology fellowship at Tufts University School of Medicine in Boston. His consultative hepatology practice focused on chronic liver diseases including non-alcoholic fatty liver, hepatitis B and C, hepatocellular carcinoma, primary biliary cirrhosis and sclerosing cholangitis. Dr. Kowdley was also a research member at Benaroya Research Institute at Virginia Mason Medical Center where he managed several clinical trials, including NIH-funded studies, and conducted bench research on liver diseases. He has presented his findings at more than 100 national and international medical centers and scientific symposia and is the author of over 300 articles, book chapters, reviews and commentaries in liver disease. He left Virginia Mason in 2014 to take a position as Director of the Liver Care Network and Organ Care Research at Swedish Medical Center, from which he retired in 2019. [12]

Andrew Ross, MD (2007 – present)

Andrew Ross is the current Section Head of Gastroenterology and Hepatology, and Director of the Therapeutic Endoscopy Center of Excellence at the Digestive Disease Institute at Virginia Mason Medical Center. He is focused on treating patients with pancreatitis, pancreatic cancer, bile duct diseases, GI bleed, and esophageal disorders, including Barrett's esophagus. Dr. Ross received his medical degree at the Mount Sinai School of Medicine of New York University in 2000. He then did his internship and residency in internal medicine at Massachusetts General Hospital, followed by fellowships in GI and Advanced Therapeutic Endoscopy at the University of Chicago Medical Center, which he completed in 2007. He is the author of multiple peer-reviewed articles and book chapters and serves on the editorial board for the *Journal of Clinical Gastroenterology*. Driven by his passion for innovation and technology, he was also deeply involved in designing and developing a state-of-the-art therapeutic endoscopy unit for Virginia Mason that debuted in the spring of 2012. Dr. Ross is also the Director of the VMMC Growth Council, a major administrative position.

Shayan Irani, MD (2008 – present)

Shayan Irani, MD, is the co-director of the Pancreatic Center of Excellence at the Digestive Disease Institute at Virginia Mason Medical Center. He has special interests in pancreaticobiliary diseases, gastrointestinal oncology, Barrett's esophagus, gastrointestinal stenting, endoscopic mucosal resection, and other advanced therapeutic and emerging techniques. Dr. Irani received his medical degree from the Seth G.S. Medical College & K.E.M. Hospital in Mumbai, India in 2000. He completed a fellowship in gastroenterology at Temple University Hospital in Philadelphia in 2007 and a fellowship in advanced therapeutic endoscopy at Virginia Mason in 2008, joining the staff at VM the same year. He is a fellow of the American Society of Gastrointestinal Endoscopy, American Gastroenterological Association and American College of Gastroenterology. Dr. Irani has written many scholarly articles related to digestive diseases and is on the editorial boards of two journals, *Gastrointestinal Endoscopy* and *Gastrointestinal Intervention*.

Ian Gan, MD (2008 – 2017)

Ian Gan served as gastroenterologist and the Director of Education at the

Digestive Disease Institute at Virginia Mason Medical Center. He is a specialist in therapeutic endoscopy, including endoscopic ultrasound (EUS) and endoscopic retrograde cholangiopancreatography (ERCP). Certified by the American Board of Internal Medicine in gastroenterology and by the Royal College of Physicians and Surgeons of Canada, Dr. Gan completed fellowships at the University of Calgary in gastroenterology and at Massachusetts General Hospital and Brigham Women's Hospital in advanced endoscopy before joining the staff at Tufts University in 2003. He joined Virginia Mason in 2008. He has authored numerous articles and currently serves as an ad-hoc reviewer for *Gastrointestinal Endoscopy* and on the Endoscopy Committee of the World Gastroenterology Organization. He left in 2017 to take a position as Chief of Endoscopy at Vancouver General Hospital in British Columbia.

Johannes Koch, MD (2010 – 2019)

Johannes Koch received his medical degree from Tulane University in New Orleans in 1987. This was followed by an internal medicine residency and GI fellowship at the University of California, San Francisco, which he completed in 1992. He then did a year in the Clinical Scholars Program there before joining the faculty as Associate Professor of Medicine and Radiology, Director of the Endoscopy and Gastroenterology Clinics, and Director of the HIV/AIDS GI Nutrition Service. He left San Francisco in 2000 to become a staff gastroenterologist at Seattle Gastroenterology Associates, and General Partner at Integra Ventures in Seattle. In 2008, he received an MBA degree from Columbia University in New York. In 2010, he joined Virginia Mason; he left in 2019, to join the University of Washington Section of Gastroenterology based at Northwest Hospital.

Dr. Koch has special interests in gastrointestinal malignancies, esophageal disorders and clinical research. He has published 43 articles in peer-reviewed journals and 7 book chapters and reviews.

James Lord, MD, PhD (2010 – present)

James Lord joined the Section of Gastroenterology at Virginia Mason in

2010. Raised in New England, he moved to Seattle in 1992 to attend the University of Washington School of Medicine, where he received his PhD, in immunology in 1999 and his MD in 2001. After completing residency and a GI fellowship at the UW, Dr. Lord earned board certification in gastroenterology and now oversees the Inflammatory Bowel Disease Biorepository at the Benaroya Research Institute. His areas of medical expertise include general gastroenterology, inflammatory bowel disease, and general gastrointestinal endoscopy. His current research focuses on studying the immune system in the blood and intestinal mucosa of patients with inflammatory bowel disease, both to determine the fundamental pathogenesis of disease, and to define immune cell predictors and consequences of current therapy.

Elisa K. Boden, MD (2011 – present)

Elisa Boden joined Virginia Mason in 2011 as a gastroenterologist in the Digestive Disease Institute. She received her medical degree from the University of Chicago's Pritzker School of Medicine in 2003, and completed her residency at Brigham and Women's Hospital in Boston, followed by a fellowship in gastroenterology at Massachusetts General Hospital and an advanced fellowship in inflammatory bowel disease at Mount Sinai Hospital in New York, which she completed in 2011. She is certified by the American Board of Internal Medicine, with subspecialty boards in gastroenterology.

She currently sees patients with inflammatory bowel disease and celiac disease and performs translational research looking at biomarker development for these diseases. She sits on the local and national medical advisory board to the Crohn's and Colitis Foundation of America.

Carol Murakami, MD (2011 – 2013)

Carol Murakami was a gastroenterologist at Virginia Mason Medical Center for two years and practiced at the Kirkland clinic as well as our main campus in Seattle. She is fellowship-trained in both gastroenterology and hepatology. Certified by the American Board of Internal Medicine, Dr.

Murakami specializes in gastrointestinal motility and gastric motility disorders and also has expertise in the care of patients with liver disease. After returning to Dallas for additional research exposure, Carol is currently in practice in Everett.

Maximillian F. Lee, MD, MPH (2011 – 2012)

Maximillian Lee received his medical degree from the New York University School of Medicine in 2004. He did his residency in internal medicine and a GI fellowship at the Stanford University, which he completed in 2011. He also studied at the Harvard University School of Public Health, receiving an MPH degree in 2008. He took a staff position at VM in 2011 and left one year later. He currently practices with the Swedish gastroenterology group in Seattle and Issaquah. [13]

Michael Chiorean, MD (2012 – present)

Michael Chiorean grew up in Romania, where he attended the University of Medicine and Pharmacy "Iuliu Hatieganu" in Cluj-Napoca, Romania, graduating in 1992. He did an internal medicine residency and gastroenterology fellowship in Europe, followed by additional training at William Beaumont in Michigan and the Mayo Clinic, which he completed in 2003. He then took a position at Indiana University Health in Indianapolis, working there for 8 years before joining Virginia Mason in 2012.

Dr. Chiorean is the Director of the Inflammatory Bowel Disease Program in the Digestive Disease Institute at Virginia Mason Medical Center. He is a fellow of the American Gastroenterology Association and a board member of the Crohn's and Colitis Foundation of America, where he serves on the Patient Education Committee. Dr. Chiorean's medical interests include inflammatory bowel disease, Crohn's disease, ulcerative colitis, *C. difficile,* gastrointestinal bleeding and small bowel endoscopy.

Michael Larsen, MD (2012 – present)

Michael Larsen is a gastroenterologist within the Digestive Disease Institute at Virginia Mason Medical Center. He has special interests in bariatric endoscopy and pancreaticobiliary diseases, especially advanced therapeutic and emerging techniques. After graduating from Columbia University College of Physicians and Surgeons in 2005, he completed an internal medicine residency training at Stanford University, a gastroenterology fellowship at the University of California San Francisco, and an advanced therapeutic endoscopy fellowship at the Massachusetts General Hospital and Brigham and Women's Hospital combined program, which he completed in 2012. He joined Virginia Mason the same year. In addition to serving as the director of Virginia Mason's Advanced Endoscopy Fellowship Program, he is a member of the American Society of Gastrointestinal Endoscopy, American Gastroenterological Association and American College of Gastroenterology, and has written numerous scholarly articles on digestive disease.

Asma Siddique, MD (2012 – present)

Asma Siddique is a hepatologist and Director of Innovation at Virginia Mason's Digestive Disease Institute. Dr. Siddique received her medical degree from the Ramaiah School of Medicine in India in 1992. After completing a residency in internal medicine and a two-year fellowship in hepatology at Virginia Mason Medical Center, Dr. Siddique has engaged in a rigorous program of patient care, clinical research and publication in addition to serving as past director of the hepatology fellowship program. Her specialties include non-alcoholic fatty liver disease, cirrhosis, and primary biliary cholangitis. She is board-certified by the American Board of Internal Medicine and is author of numerous publications in hepatology.

Blaire E. Burman, MD (2014 – present)

Blaire Burman joined the Section of Gastroenterology and Hepatology at Virginia Mason in 2014. She is board-certified by the American Board of Internal Medicine with subspecialty certification in gastroenterology and is the Digestive Disease Director of Training and Education. Her areas of expertise include general hepatology, viral hepatitis, liver cancer, and general gastrointestinal endoscopy.

Blaire was born and raised in Seattle, and attended the University of Washington School of Medicine, graduating in 2008. She completed her residency in internal medicine at Columbia Presbyterian in NYC, followed by fellowship training in gastroenterology and hepatology at the University of California San Francisco, which she completed in 2014. Dr. Burman sees patients at both the downtown and Edmonds campus.

Nanda Venu, MD, MS (2015 – present)

Nanda Venu joined Virginia Mason in 2015 as a gastroenterologist in the Digestive Disease Institute, specializing in inflammatory bowel disease, esophageal diseases, colon cancer, therapeutic endoscopy and food allergies. Certified in gastroenterology by the American Board of Internal Medicine, Dr. Venu received his medical degree from Kasturba Medical College Mangalore, Manipal University, India. He then conducted gastrointestinal cellular research at Harvard, earned a Master's degree in clinical and translational science from the Medical College of Wisconsin, and completed a fellowship in gastroenterology, hepatology and nutrition at the University of Chicago before moving to Seattle via Milwaukee.

Qing Zhang, MD, PhD (2015 – present)

Qing Zhang was born in China, where she earned her MD at Hunan Medical University and then her Ph.D. in gastrointestinal oncology at Tongji Medical University following a fellowship in gastroenterology. She served 2 years as a resident in a GI motility laboratory at the Royal Adelaide Hospital of Adelaide University, Australia from 1998–2000. In 2006, she began a residency in internal medicine at Texas Tech University, followed by a GI fellowship at the University of Florida School of Medicine. She joined Virginia Mason in 2015 and practices at the Lynnwood and downtown campus. Her areas of interest include general gastroenterology, gastroesophageal reflux disease, dysphagia, and GI motility disorders.

Rajesh Krishnamoorthi, MD (2017 – present)

Rajesh Krishnamoorthi is a gastroenterologist at Virginia Mason Medical

Center, who specializes in advanced endoscopic treatments. He is originally from Chennai, India and graduated from Madras Medical College in 2006. He completed residency training at Wayne State University and served as the chief resident of Quality and Patient Safety (CRQPS) before pursuing a gastroenterology fellowship at the Mayo Clinic, Rochester. He did an additional fellowship in therapeutic endoscopy at Virginia Mason before joining as staff in 2017. Dr. Krishnamoorthi is a recipient of numerous awards, including a Mayo Clinic GIH research grant (2014) for developing decision aids for patients with Barrett's esophagus. He is an associate editor of the journal *BMC Gastroenterology* and an editorial board member of *Annals of Hepatology*. He is a member of several professional committees including the American College of Gastroenterology's (ACG) publication committee. In addition to his training responsibilities, Dr. Krishnamoorthi is active in clinical and "patient-centered" outcomes research, having published over 16 peer-reviewed papers, a textbook chapter, and 48 abstracts in journals such as *Gastroenterology, Radiology, Gastrointestinal Endoscopy* and *Alimentary Pharmacology & Therapeutics*. He has over ten oral presentations to his credit including a "Presidential Plenary" presentation at ACG 2015. While his research has focused on Barrett's esophagus, his clinical interests include management of hepatobiliary and pancreatic diseases.

Alexander Kuo, MD (2017 – 2018)

Alexander Kuo is a gastroenterologist/hepatologist who joined Virginia Mason in 2017 as Director of the Liver Center of Excellence. His special interests are in liver transplantation, cirrhosis management, liver cancer, hepatitis B, hepatitis C, primary sclerosing cholangitis, autoimmune hepatitis and fatty liver. He received his medical degree from the University of California, San Francisco in 2001, which was followed by a 3-year internship and fellowship at Massachusetts General Hospital. He returned to UCSF for a GI and hepatology fellowship, which he completed in 2007. He then joined the faculty of University of California, San Diego, where he held a variety of leadership positions in the Gastroenterology Department, particularly centered on hepatology. Besides his clinical duties there, he was involved in research and teaching, with 32 articles in peer-reviewed journals to date. Alex has recently left to become head of the Liver Transplant Team at Cedars Sinai in Los Angeles.

Joanna K. Law, MD (2017 – present)

Joanna Law is a gastroenterologist at Virginia Mason Medical Center with interests in advanced endoscopic treatments and premalignant and malignant lesions. She graduated from medical school at the University of British Columbia where she also did her internal medicine and gastroenterology training. There she served as chief resident and chief fellow during her training. She went on to do a therapeutic and clinical research fellowship at Johns Hopkins Hospital in Baltimore, before coming to Seattle.

Dr. Law has clinical and research interests in pancreatic cysts, pancreatic cancer and familial GI cancer syndromes. She currently is an active member of the Standards of Practice Committee for the American Society for Gastrointestinal Endoscopy (ASGE) and also the Economics of Practice Committee for AGA. For the past 3 years, she has served as Director for the First Year Fellows' course in Chicago.

Sarah A. Sprouse, MD (2017 – present)

Sarah Sprouse attended Dartmouth Medical College in New Hampshire, graduating in 2011. She then did an internal medicine residency followed by a fellowship in gastroenterology at the University of Washington, which she completed in 2017. At Virginia Mason, she practices general gastroenterology, seeing patients at the Issaquah satellite as well as downtown.

Timothy L. Zisman, MD, MPH (2019 – present)

Timothy Zisman joined the Virginia Mason GI section in 2019, further growing the inflammatory bowel disease team. He graduated from Virginia Commonwealth Medical School, obtained his MPH at Harvard, and then did his residency and GI fellowship at the University of Chicago. He was an attending at the University of Washington Medical Center until joining Virginia Mason Medical Center in 2009, and now continues to serve there as a Clinical Associate Professor of Medicine. He has lectured extensively on IBD, been highly involved in the Crohn's and Colitis Foundation, performed multiple clinical research trials, and published many manuscripts, book chapters, and abstracts.

Acknowledgements:

This chapter was a group effort and would not have been possible without the help of Drs. Ball, Gelfand, Gluck and Ross, as well as Julie Katz and Terri Davis Smith. Many thanks also to Patti Wilbur, Pat Pethigal and Liz Moerhke for writing the nursing section.

References:

1. The *VM Bulletin*, multiple years.

2. 1983 VM Chairman's report, VM Archives.

3. Clarence C. Pearson, MD, Professional Activities report, 1976, VMMC Archives.

4. Obituary of Randolph Clements, at: http://www.legacy.com/obituaries/seattletimes/obituary.aspx?page=lifestory&pid=1988081; Accessed 16 September 2018.

5. "Retirement of Richard Stemler", 1992 VM Chairman's Report.

6. Obituary of L.F. Fritz Fenster, at: https://www.legacy.com/obituaries/name/L.-Fenster-obituary?pid=148137134; Accessed 16 September 2018.

7. Dr. David J. Patterson, MD, Swedish Gastroenterology Group website, at: https://www.swedish.org/swedish-physicians/profile.aspx?name=david+j+patterson&id=158748; Accessed 20 September 2018.

8. John Brandabur, MD, healthgrades website, at: https://www.healthgrades.com/physician/dr-john-brandabur-2kfpx?referrerSource=autosuggest; Accessed 20 September 2018.

9. Drew Schembre, MD, healthgrades website, at: https://www.healthgrades.com/physician/dr-drew-schembre-xfxn8; Accessed 20 September 2018.

10. Klaus Mergener, MD, PhD, MBA, healthgrades website, at: https://www.healthgrades.com/physician/dr-klaus-mergener-2vrwg; Accessed 20 September 2018.

11. Klaus Mergener, MD, PhD, MBA, Becker's GI and Endoscopy website; at: https://www.beckersasc.com/gastroenterology-and-endoscopy/gi-physician-leader-to-know-dr-klaus-mergener-of-digestive-health-specialists.html; Accessed

20 September 2018.

12.Kris V. Kowdley, MD, Swedish Medical Center website, at: http://neuroscience-cme.com/cmea_popup_faculty.asp?ID=491; Accessed 20 September 2018.

13. Maximilian F. Lee, MD, MPH, Swedish Medical Center website, at: https://www.swedish.org/swedish-physicians/profile.aspx?name=maximilian+f+lee&id=247766; Accessed 20 September 2018.

7

Hematology / Oncology

by Robert Rudolph, MD; Patrick Ragen, MD, MS, &
Katherine Galagan, MD, with contributions from
Paul Weiden, MD, & Albert Einstein, MD

The Early History of the Hematology / Oncology Section
at Virginia Mason: 1949 - 1970

Hematology and oncology as specialties, and as a joint section at Virginia Mason, developed later than other specialties such as cardiology and gastroenterology. The lack of therapeutic options for blood dyscrasias and inoperable solid tumors was the reason for this.

In the 1940s, nitrogen mustard was available as a therapy and was soon followed by ACTH (adrenocorticotropic hormone) and cortisone. In the 1950s, methotrexate, purine antagonists and other antimetabolites became available. The first diseases to respond to treatment with these drugs were often hematological dyscrasias. One of the most common side effects of these drugs was bone marrow suppression. Thus hematology and medical oncology were destined to be closely associated.

The first member of the Hematology Section at Virginia Mason was Randolph Preston Pillow, MD; he originally came to Virginia Mason in October 1944 as one of four interns. He followed a path well traveled from the University of Virginia to Virginia Mason. Two of the original founders, who also served as the first two Clinic Chairmen, James Tate Mason,

MD, and John Minor Blackford, MD, were from the University of Virginia class of 1903. In addition, the first four interns from the University of Virginia arrived at VM in 1928: Joel Baker, MD; Louis Edmonds, MD; Robert King, MD; and John Wilkinson, MD.

Randy returned to Virginia for a year's residency followed by two years of active duty as a medical officer at Madigan Hospital. He then returned to Virginia again as assistant to the Chief of Medicine at the University of Virginia. During the Korean War he spent several months on active duty, serving in California. He was subsequently recruited to Virginia Mason in 1949 and became a partner in 1954.

It is unclear whether or not he had specific training in hematology. He practiced internal medicine with a special interest in hematology until his retirement in 1986 at age 65. In 1964 Randy saw an 18-year-old male with acute aplastic anemia. The patient had an identical twin. Dr. Pillow arranged for a bone marrow transplant, which was successful. This was one of the first successful marrow transplants.

Dr. Pillow was in charge of the house staff training program from 1952 until 1963. He traveled extensively in the Far East and was involved in many extracurricular activities. He not only supervised the medical care at the popular annual hydroplane races on Lake Washington, but also served as General Chairman of the races from 1967-1969. He drove smaller hydroplanes himself. He was active at the Washington Athletic Club and served as its president for one year.

Patrick A. Ragen, MD, joined the Department of Medicine at Virginia Mason in May 1959. He and Dr. Pillow formed a two-man Hematology Section. Dr. Ragen also preferred to practice internal medicine with a special interest in hematology. The clinic continued to grow rapidly in the late 1950s and 1960s leading to the third addition to the Hematology Section—John Huff, MD. Robert Petersdorf, MD, had recruited John to be chief resident at King County Hospital (Harborview) in 1959-60. Dr. Huff then majored in biochemistry at the University of Washington from 1960-62 and served as senior fellow at the University of Washington from 1962-63. For two years he was Hematologist-in-Chief at Harborview Hospital and attending physician at the Seattle Veterans' Hospital.

John Huff, MD, joined Virginia Mason in July 1965. He was the first Board-certified physician in hematology in the section. He chaired the section from 1968 until 1988. He was an excellent consultant. He was both Chief of Staff of Virginia Mason Hospital and on the Executive Committee of the Virginia Mason Clinic for many years. He also served as President of the Puget Sound Blood Bank and President of the King County Medical Society.

Medical Oncology Becomes a Recognized Specialty: 1971 – 2000

As medicine advanced in its abilities to treat cancer, it became apparent that a large percentage of the patients seen in the section had solid tumor malignancies rather than hematological disease. What was needed was someone with the desire, the training and the skill to be the first oncologist at Virginia Mason. The physician that filled that role in 1971 was Robert Rudolph, MD, who was the first of many oncologists.

Dr. Rudolph was recruited from his position on the faculty of the University of Washington School of Medicine. He had previously done a fellowship in hematology and oncology at the University of Washington. Following completion of the fellowship he continued in the lab and clinical programs of E. Donnall Thomas, MD, as an assistant professor. During this time Dr. Thomas and a small group of investigators established the feasibility of bone marrow transplantation, initially in animal models and subsequently in humans. Dr. Thomas was awarded the Nobel Prize in Medicine in 1990 in recognition of this pioneering work in establishing bone marrow transplantation as a successful therapeutic modality in the treatment of human malignancy.

Medical oncology was a new specialty when Bob joined Virginia Mason. The ability of combination chemotherapy to cure Hodgkin's disease had just been established; new chemotherapeutic agents were being developed and for the first time patients with advanced and/or metastatic cancer could be helped. In 1973, Bob took the Boards in medical oncology, the first time they were offered. The section expanded with the arrival of two other oncologists, Al Einstein, MD, in 1976 and Paul Weiden, MD, in 1981. In addition several oncology nurses were added to the section to assist with patient treatment and to accommodate the expanding number of cancer patients. The first of this group was Janet Appelbaum, followed by Bev Solberg and Patti Kwok.

Dr. Rudolph's focus during his 29 years at Virginia Mason was on patient treatment, teaching, and outreach to the community of physicians throughout Washington and Alaska. He was promoted to Clinical Professor of Medicine at the University of Washington in 1993 and established telephone tumor boards with medical communities in Washington and Alaska as well as travelling to many of these communities to give talks and serve as consultant at local tumor boards. Through this outreach program Bob developed a large referral practice and expanded the number of cancer patients seen and treated at VM.

Bob served in many administrative roles in local and state professional societies, as well as at VM. He served as Section Head of Hematology/Oncology from 1993 until 1997. During this time two oncology clinical nurse practitioners, Barbara Fristoe, ARNP, and Denise Bundow, ARNP, became members of the section.

Albert B. Einstein, MD, joined Virginia Mason in 1976. During the Vietnam War, he was a US Public Health Officer and served two years as clinical associate at the National Cancer Institute, National Institutes of Health in Bethesda, MD. Because of the NCI experience, he decided to pursue a career in medical oncology.

After a residency and fellowship at the UW, Al was working at the UW School of Medicine as an assistant professor in medical oncology, engaged in the research of tumor immunology with Alex Fefer, MD, who was an attending physician on the bone marrow transplantation service and had a small practice of general oncology patients. However, Al decided he wanted a career more centered on clinical practice, so he joined The Mason Clinic where he practiced medical oncology for 17 years. During this time, he continued to pursue his interests in clinical research and became interested in administrative medicine, serving in many leadership positions both within the medical center and within many professional societies, including serving as national President of the Association of Community Cancer Centers from 1992 -1993.

In 1993, Al resigned from The VM Clinic to accept the position of Associate Director for Clinical Affairs at the H. Lee Moffitt Cancer Center and Research Institute, and tenured Professor of Internal Medicine at the University of South Florida in Tampa, Florida. This career change was motivated by his desire to pursue a leadership role in the development of a new national cancer center program.

Meanwhile, in 1981, encouraged by Dr. Albert Einstein, who was a colleague at both the National Cancer Institute and the University of Washington, Paul Weiden, MD, joined Virginia Mason. He practiced both medical oncology and hematology and partnered with Tom Yarington, MD, and Lucius Hill, MD, respectively, to add chemotherapy to the initial therapy of patients with resectable head and neck cancer, lung cancer and esophageal cancer, new concepts in the 1980s. Paul also introduced, with the support of his colleagues, both autologous and allogeneic stem cell transplantation to Virginia Mason.

In the late 1980s, VM had the opportunity to open a Phase 1 clinical trial unit with a local biotechnology company, NeoRx Corporation. Paul was the Principal Investigator on these studies that utilized radiolabeled monoclonal antibodies to direct radiation therapy to sites of persistent tumor. Initially, the focus was on patients with lung or colon cancer and later on patients with lymphoma. Although progress was made and the technology improved thanks to the contributions of the many patients who came to VM from both near and far, the treatment was not sufficiently effective for commercial development and this collaboration ended in the late 1990s.

In 1993, with the departure of Dr. Einstein, Paul became the Principal Investigator of the VM Community Cancer Oncology Program, part of a national network of community cancer centers to facilitate the participation of patients in cancer clinical trials investigating new treatments, new prevention approaches and new ways to reduce the side effects of cancer therapy. This program and the NeoRx collaboration were the major components of the Cancer Clinical Research Unit, which also supported studies from the drug industry and from VM investigators. Paul led this unit until his retirement from VM in 2001.

During the 1970s and 1980s, the section consisted of Drs. Pillow, Ragen, Huff, Rudolph, Einstein and Weiden. These physicians formed a stable core group that accomplished many advancements in their field, both inside and outside of the medical center. The late 1980s brought change to the section with the retirement of Dr. Pillow in 1986, and his replacement by Vince Picozzi, MD, the same year; the addition of David Aboulafia, MD, in 1990; the retirement of Dr. Huff in 1992, the departure of Dr. Einstein in 1993 and the retirement of Dr. Ragen in 1994; and the arrivals of Andrew Jacobs, MD, in 1994 and Henry Otero, MD, in 1998. All of these new physicians, boarded in hematology and/or medical oncology, continued the excellent and innovative work of the section, and each set his own mark on the section as it entered the new millennium.

The Modern Era: 2000 – Present

Dr. Rudolph retired in May 2000, and the section added Thomas Malpass, MD, the same year; Jaqueline Vuky, MD, joined VM a year later, replacing Dr. Weiden who retired in 2001. The section now consisted of a new guard and the group didn't miss a step in continuing the excellent care for which the section was known. It was about this time that the Section of Hematology/Oncology became the Department of Cancer Care Services, partnered with the Cancer Registry, Oncology Infusion Center and Radiation Oncology, with Andrew Jacobs as Chief. In 2004, the Floyd and Delores Jones Cancer Institute provided them with new offices on the second floor of Buck Pavilion, although Radiation Oncology had a separate location in the basement. This department was short-lived; by the fall of 2007, the department became two sections in the Department of Medicine, which was a return to the status quo for Hematology & Oncology, but a new location for Radiation Oncology, which had previously been part of the Department of Radiology.

During these years, there were several physicians who joined the group for a few years, including Vikramsinh (Vik) M. Dabhi, MD (2004 – 2007); Hershel Wallen, MD (2006 – 2010); and Mary Pender-Schenck, MD (2007 – 2009). Astrid Pujari, MD, originally joined the General Internal Medicine Section in 2001, but started working in the Hematology/Oncology Section in 2006, where she practiced for several years before eventually leaving VM, but returning recently to head the new "Integrative Medicine" section, which is where her training and special interests lie.

Nanette Robinson, MD, joined the section in 2009 bringing the total number of physicians to 8. In 2011, Dr. Vuky left VM to return to Oregon Health Sciences University, where she had attended medical school, and 4 physicians joined the section: Craig R. Nichols, MD (2011 - 2015); Prakash Vishnu, MBBS (2011 – 2016); Bruce Lin, MD (2011 – present); and Joseph Rosales, MD (2011 – present). Gurkamal S. Chatta, MD, joined the section the following year, but left in 2016. Dr. Jacobs retired in 2015.

The section is currently comprised (as of August 2019) of 8 hematologist/oncologists: David Aboulafia, MD; John Paul Flores, MD; Bruce Lin, MD; Meaghan O'Malley, MD; Vince Picozzi, Jr, MD; Nanette Robinson, MD; Joseph Rosales, MD, and Marc S. Rosenshein, MD (who practices in Edmonds), all with special areas of interest in the broad specialties of hematology and oncology (see individual biographies below). Hagen Kennecke, MD, MHA (who currently serves as Section Head) joined the group in 2017 and practices medical oncology; Joshua Wilfong, DO, practices Medical Oncology, and Hospice and Palliative Medicine at the Federal Way satellite and downtown. Gayle L. Funk, PA-C, works as a physician assistant in the section as well.

Physician Biographies
Randolph Preston Pillow, MD (1954 – 1986)
Dr. Pillow was the first member of the Hematology Section at Virginia Mason and arrived in October 1944, initially as an intern. He was born January 18, 1921, in Roanoke, Virginia. Dr. Pillow received a Bachelor of Arts degree from the University of Virginia in 1942, although he had

started medical school there in the fall of 1941. Because of World War II, medical schools accelerated their programs and students were enlisted into the Army as privates, receiving commissions as officers upon graduation. Randy graduated September 14, 1944 and arrived to intern at Virginia Mason in October 1944 as one of four interns. His time at Virginia Mason is summarized in the first section above and will not be repeated here. Of note is his contributions to the development of the specialty of hematology at The Mason Clinic, his involvement in one of the first successful bone marrow transplants, his contributions to graduate medical education and international medical collaborations, and his involvement in hydroplane racing in Seattle. During his lengthy retirement, Dr. Pillow never missed a Friday's Grand Rounds until his death in January 2015.

Patrick A. Ragen, MD, MS (1959 – 1994)

Pat Ragen joined the Department of Medicine at Virginia Mason in May 1959. He and Dr. Pillow formed a two-man Hematology Section. Pat was born July 2, 1928, in Townsend, Montana. He graduated from Carroll College in Helena, Montana in 1948 and the University of Chicago School of Medicine in 1952. He interned at Harborview Hospital from May 1952 to May 1953. Pat was a 1st Lt. Medical Officer from August 1953 until August 1955. The majority of his time in the service was at the 5th General Hospital in Stuttgart, Germany and in several field units in Germany. He was a fellow at the Mayo Clinic from October 1955 until March 1959 and received an MS in medicine from the University of Minnesota. He studied anemia of chronic renal disease using isotopes and spent extra time in the Section of Hematology at Mayo. He preferred to practice internal medicine with a special interest in hematology. Dr. Ragen retired in 1994. He and his wife Mary Murphy Ragen remain in the beautiful city of Seattle where they raised their four children.

John Huff, MD (1965 – 1992)

John Huff was born January 10, 1930 in Texas and raised in Texas and Kentucky. He graduated from Center College in 1950 at the age of 20 and from the University of Louisville School of Medicine in 1954. He interned at Philadelphia General Hospital. After one year at Francis Delafield Hospital in New York he became a Captain and Flight Surgeon in the United States Air Force. From 1956-58 he was stationed in Newfoundland. John was a resident in internal medicine at Strong Memorial Hospital in Rochester, New York from 1958-59.

Dr. Robert Petersdorf recruited John to be chief resident at King County Hospital (Harborview) in 1959-60. Dr. Huff was a biochemistry major at the University of Washington from 1960-62 and then a senior fellow at the University of Washington from1962-63. For two years he was Hematologist-in-Chief at Harborview Hospital and attending physician at the Seattle Veterans' Hospital.

Dr. Huff joined The Mason Clinic in July 1965. He was the first Board-certified physician in hematology in the section. He chaired the section from 1968 until 1988. He was an excellent consultant. He was both Chief of Staff of Virginia Mason Hospital and on the Executive Committee of The Virginia Mason Clinic for many years. He served at President of the Puget Sound Blood Bank and President of the King County Medical Society.

John retired in 1992 and sadly, died at age 65 in 1995. John and his wife, Sheryn, who died in 2005, had three children.

Robert Rudolph, MD (1971 - 2000)

Robert Rudolph was the first of many oncologists and was recruited from his position on the faculty of the University of Washington School of Medicine in 1971. He grew up in Pittsburgh, Pennsylvania. Bob received his AB in chemistry at Dartmouth College where he was elected to Phi Beta Kappa in his junior year. In 1962 he graduated from the University of Pennsylvania Medical School where he was elected to AOA. After a rotating internship at the Hospital of the University of Pennsylvania, he took his residency in internal medicine at the University of Michigan Hospital. In 1966, he began a fellowship in hematology and oncology at the University of Washington. Following completion of the fellowship he continued in the lab and clinical programs of Dr. E. Donnall Thomas as an Assistant Professor. Dr. Thomas won the Nobel Prize in Medicine in 1990 for his pioneering work in bone marrow transplantation.

Medical oncology was a new specialty when Bob joined Virginia Mason in 1971. The ability of combination chemotherapy to cure Hodgkin's disease had just been established; new chemotherapeutic agents were being developed and for the first time patients with advanced and/or metastatic cancer could be helped. In 1973, Bob passed the Boards in medical oncology, the first time they were offered.

Dr. Rudolph's focus during his 29 years at Virginia Mason was on patient treatment, teaching, and outreach to the community of physicians throughout Washington and Alaska. The Virginia Mason house staff consistently recognized his teaching skills. Many medical residents elected specialty rotations with him in their second and third years. He received the Teacher of the Year award from the Virginia Mason house staff in 1992. Dr. Rudolph also established a 3-month clinical rotation program in the Hematology/Oncology Section for University of Washington fellows in medical oncology. This proved to be the most popular and sought after rotation in the University of Washington program. He was promoted to Clinical Professor of Medicine at the University of Washington in 1993.

Dr. Rudolph established telephone tumor boards with medical communities in Washington and Alaska at which physicians could receive consultations with Virginia Mason cancer specialists. He traveled to many of these communities to give talks and serve as consultant at local tumor boards. Through this outreach program Bob developed a large referral practice and expanded the number of cancer patients seen and treated at VM.

Administratively he served as President of the King County Unit of the American Cancer Society and then as President of the Washington State Division of the American Cancer Society from 1991-1993. He was President of the Seattle Society of Hematology for many years. Bob was Director of the N. Peter Canlis Cancer Care unit from its inception in 1979 until 1994 and chaired the Virginia Mason Tumor Board for many years. He served as Section Head of Hematology/Oncology from 1993 until 1997. During this time two oncology clinical nurse practitioners, Barbara Fristoe and Denise Bundow, became members of the section.

Dr. Rudolph retired in May of 2000. He and his wife, Beth, have one daughter.

Albert B. Einstein, M.D. (1976 – 1993)

Al Einstein was born in Baltimore, Maryland, on November 17, 1941. He received a public school education, an AB degree from Princeton University and an MD degree from Cornell University Medical College. From 1967 to 1969, he was an internal medicine intern and first-year resident physician on the Osler Medical Service at Johns Hopkins Hospital. During the Vietnam War, he was a US Public Health Officer and served two years as clinical associate at the National Cancer Institute, National Institutes of Health in Bethesda, Md. Because of the NCI experience, he decided to pursue a career in medical oncology.

Al and his family moved to Seattle, Washington, in 1971 to pursue his training in medical oncology. He first completed a second year of internal medicine residency at the University of Washington, followed by a two-year fellowship in hematology/oncology with Dr. E. Donnall Thomas, Chief of the Division of Medical Oncology at the UW. As noted above, Dr. Thomas later went on to receive a Nobel Prize in Medicine for his work in bone marrow transplantation for hematologic malignancies. After completion of his fellowship, Al and his family decided to make Seattle their home and he joined the UW School of Medicine as an assistant professor in medical oncology. He was engaged in research of tumor immunology with Dr. Alex Fefer, was an attending physician on the bone marrow transplantation service, and had a small practice of general oncology patients.

In 1976, however, Al decided he wanted a career more centered on clinical practice, so he joined The Mason Clinic where he practiced medical oncology for 17 years. During this time, he continued to pursue his interests in clinical research as the founding principal investigator for the NCI-funded VM Community Clinical Oncology Program that supported cooperative clinical trial research. He also served as the medical oncology chairman for the National Bladder Cancer Collaborative Group A. He was active in the medical oncology activities of the Southwest Oncology Group and the Cancer and Acute Leukemia Group B. Al also became interested in administrative medicine and served as medical director of the VM Cancer Center, President of the VM Research Center, member-at-large of the VM Executive Committee, medical director of the Business and Occupational Health Program, member of the VM Hospital Board of Directors, member of the VM Medical Center Board of Directors, member of the VM Foundation Board of Advisors, and chairman of the VM Marketing Committee. Among the many professional societies in which he participated, he was most active in the Association of Community Cancer Centers where he served as national president from 1992-1993.

In 1993, Al resigned from The VM Clinic to accept the position of Associate Director for Clinical Affairs at the H. Lee Moffitt Cancer Center and Research Institute and tenured Professor of Internal Medicine at the University of South Florida in Tampa, Florida. This career change was motivated by his desire to pursue a leadership role in the development of a new national cancer center program.

Dr. Einstein and his wife, Margery, have four children. He retired in 2012 and has been enjoying cruising on their sailboat, spending time with grandchildren, and traveling.

Paul Weiden, MD (1981 – 2001)

Paul Weiden was born in Portland, OR and raised primarily on the San Francisco peninsula were he went to public high school. He attended Harvard College and Harvard Medical School, was a house officer at University Hospitals in Cleveland and spent 2 years at the National Cancer Institute in Bethesda. In 1971, he came to the University of Washington as a fellow in medical oncology and over the next 9.5 years worked in pre-clinical and clinical stem cell transplantation, described "graft vs. leukemia" activity as an important component of allogeneic stem cell transplantation and became an Associate Professor, based at the Fred Hutchison Cancer Research Center.

In 1981, encouraged by Dr. Albert Einstein, who was a colleague at both the National Cancer Institute and the University of Washington, Paul joined Virginia Mason. He practiced both medical oncology and hematology and partnered with Drs. Tom Yarington and Lucius Hill, respectively, to add chemotherapy to the initial therapy of patients with resectable head and neck cancer, lung cancer and esophageal cancer, new concepts in the 1980s. Paul also introduced, with the support of his colleagues, both autologous and allogeneic stem cell transplantation to Virginia Mason.

In the late 1980s, VM had the opportunity to open a Phase 1 clinical trial unit with a local biotechnology company, NeoRx Corporation. Paul was the Principal Investigator of these studies that utilized radiolabeled monoclonal antibodies to direct radiation therapy to sites of persistent tumor. Initially, the focus was on patients with lung or colon cancer and later on patients with lymphoma. Although progress was made and the technology improved thanks to the contributions of the many patients who came to VM from both near and far, the treatment was not sufficiently effective for commercial development and this collaboration ended in the late 1990s.

In 1993 Paul became the Principal Investigator of the VM Community Cancer Oncology Program, part of a national network of community cancer centers to facilitate the participation of patients in cancer clinical trials investigating new treatments, new prevention approaches and new ways to reduce the side effects of cancer therapy. This program and the NeoRx collaboration were the major components of the Cancer Clinical Research Unit, which also supported studies from the drug industry and from VM investigators. Paul led this Unit until his retirement from VM in 2001.

Paul and his wife, Marty, had two children. After Marty's death Paul married Bev Solberg, a widow who worked at Virginia Mason as a physician's assistant.

Vincent J. Picozzi, Jr, MD, MMM (1986 – present)

Vince Picozzi attended Yale University, where he received his BS in chemistry in 1974. He then attended Stanford University Medical School, graduating in 1978. This was followed by an internship and residency in internal medicine at Harvard University, Brigham and Women's Hospital, and fellowships in hematology and oncology at Stanford, which he completed in 1984. Dr. Picozzi served as an Instructor at Stanford in the Divisions of Hematology and Oncology for 2 years before joining Virginia Mason in 1986.

During his time at Virginia Mason, Dr. Picozzi has developed special interests in pancreatic and GI malignancies, as well as genitourinary cancers, hematologic oncology (especially lymphomas) and myelodysplasia. He served as Section Head from 1988 to 1993, and has been Director of the Pancreas Center of Excellence in the Digestive Disease Institute since 2010, serving as Associate Director from 2006 to 2010. He has been a six-time member of the organizing committee of the World Pancreas Cancer Symposium, and was an honoree of the PANCAN Seattle Gala in 2007. Dr. Picozzi has one of the largest practices in pancreaticobiliary cancer in the nation. As he explains: "I have a particular mission with respect to pancreaticobiliary cancer. Serving patients with this disease to date has been the central ministry of my professional career. My colleagues and I at Virginia Mason have achieved some of the finest clinical outcomes in the world in this disorder. An immediate goal over the next five years is to assist in the transformation of perceptions and outcomes for this disorder, which has the poorest prognosis of any common cancer." His practice also involves direction of GI oncology coordination (concierge/navigation methodology), primary supervision of VM pancreaticobiliary/GI oncology clinical pathways, Co–chair of VM GI oncology interdisciplinary tumor boards, and supervision of the VM pancreas cancer database.

Dr. Picozzi is actively involved in clinical research, particularly in the area of pancreaticobiliary cancer, and has 51 peer-reviewed journal articles, and 8 book chapters to date (as of November 2018). He is an excellent teacher, receiving the Teacher of the Year Award at VMMC in 1995-1996, and serving as a clinical preceptor of the Oncology Fellowship Program at the UW/Fred Hutchinson Cancer Research Center. He served as Research Chair of the Benaroya Institute from 2004-2006 and 2007-2009.

Dr. Picozzi is a member of numerous medical societies, serving on various committees and boards over the years. He has been on the board of directors of the Providence Hospice of King County Foundation since 2005. He has also served on governmental committees at the state and national level, and has made several TV and radio appearances involving high visibility medical situations.

David M. Aboulafia, MD (1990 – present)

David Aboulafia graduated from the University of Michigan Medical School in 1983. He then undertook his internship and residency in internal medicine and fellowship in hematology and oncology at UCLA, finishing in 1989.

Dr. Aboulafia joined Virginia Mason in 1990, where he practices general hematology and oncology with a focus on AIDS/HIV and HIV-related malignancies, viral syndromes, disorders of coagulation and hemostasis, and hematologic malignancies. He is the medical director of Bailey-Boushay House, and Clinical Professor at the UW. He serves as Principal Investigator of the AIDS Malignancy Consortium, and has many peer-reviewed articles to date (as of November 2018). Dr. Aboulafia was the recipient of the **James Tate Mason Award** in 2009.

Andrew Jacobs, MD (1994 – 2015)

Andrew Jacobs attended medical school at University College at the University of London, graduating in 1977. He then served his internship in internal medicine at St. Thomas West Middlesex Hospital, followed by residency years at Charing Cross Hospital, Northwick Park Hospital and Royal Marsden Hospital, which he completed in 1980. Dr. Jacobs then "crossed the pond" to do a fellowship in hematology/oncology at UCLA School of Medicine, which he completed in 1983.

After his fellowship, Dr. Jacobs joined the UCLA faculty as an Assistant Professor conducting research in the treatment of acute leukemia and hairy cell leukemia. This was followed by several years in clinical practice and teaching at Cedars Sinai Medical Center in Los Angeles. He then joined Virginia Mason in 1994 where he practiced oncology and hematology with an initial focus on cancer of the pancreas and subsequently breast cancer. He served as Section Head from 1997-2001 when he was appointed Chief of Cancer Care Services, and served as Medical Director of Clinical Research at Benaroya Research Institute from 2002-2007. He was appointed Assistant Professor of Medicine at the University of Washington in 1994. He also served as Principal Investigator of the VM Community Cancer Oncology Program from 2001-2007.

In 2007, Dr. Jacobs became the first Chief Medical Officer at VM, serving in this position until 2013, when he took the position of Medical Director of Physician Engagement and Development. He retired from VMMC in 2015 and relocated to Philadelphia to be closer to children and grandchildren.

Henry Otero, MD (1998 – 2012); Virginia Mason Institute (2012 - present)

Henry Otero received his MD from Michigan State University College of Human Medicine in 1989 and then did an internship and residency in internal medicine at the University of Virginia. This was followed by a fellowship in hematology/oncology at the UW, which he completed in 1997.

Dr. Otero joined VM in 1998 and practiced primarily medical oncology in the section for the next 14 years. During this time, he became involved in the Virginia Mason Production System and became a Kaizen Fellow with certification. He left the section in 2012 to join the Virginia Mason Institute, and works as an Executive and Transformation Sensei in that group.

Thomas W. Malpass, MD (2000 – present)

Dr. Malpass graduated from the University of North Carolina Chapel Hill in 1971 with a BA in chemistry and received his MD from the University of Virginia in 1975. He did his internal medicine residency at the Medical University of South Carolina and then a fellowship in hematology and oncology at the University of Washington. After fellowship, he took a position as assistant professor of medicine at the University of Washington where he was involved with clinical and laboratory research in platelet function. In 1985 he moved to Wenatchee and practiced general hematology and oncology at Wenatchee Valley Clinic. In 2000 he took a position as a locums at VM with the intention of returning to Wenatchee when his wife finished law school at the UW. This was at a time when both Drs. Rudolph and Weiden were leaving the section; he was offered a permanent position a few months later, which he accepted. He practices general hematology/ oncology with a focus on palliative care. He served as Chair of the Medical Ethics Committee for a few years as well as one of the medical directors for Hospice of Seattle. He was also involved in initial attempts to set up a palliative care service at VM. He holds board certification in hematology, oncology and palliative care.

Dr. Malpass in partial retirement continues to commute to Juneau monthly for three days to participate in a hematology/oncology outreach clinic under Virginia Mason sponsorship.

Jacqueline Vuky, MD (2001 – 2011)

Jacqueline Vuky graduated from Oregon Health and Science University School of Medicine (OHSU) in Portland, OR in 1995. She then did an internship and residency in internal medicine at New York Presbyterian Hospital, followed by a fellowship in Oncology at the Memorial Sloan-Kettering Cancer Center in New York, which she completed in 2001.

Dr. Vuky joined VM the same year, and is board-certified in Oncology. At VM, she practiced general oncology, with a special focus on genitourinary malignancies and breast cancer. She left VM in 2011 to return to OHSU and Portland.

Vikramsinh M. Dabhi, MD, PhD (2004 – 2007)

Vikramsinh (Vik) Dabhi attended the University of Texas Southwestern Medical School, graduating in 1998. He then did his residency in internal medicine at Emory University, and a fellowship in hematology/oncology at the University of Washington. Dr. Dabhi joined VM in 2004. He practiced general hematology/oncology with a special interest in GI, hema-

113

tologic and breast malignancies. In 2007 he left VM to join the group at Pacific Medical Center.

Hershel D. Wallen, MD (2006 – 2010)

Hershel Wallen graduated from the University of Michigan Medical School in 1999, and then did his residency in internal medicine followed by a fellowship in hematology/oncology at the University of Washington. Dr. Wallen joined VM in 2006 and practiced there for 4 years, before moving to Oregon and now practices at the Providence Cancer Institute Franz Clinic in Portland.

Mary C. Pinder-Schenck, MD (2007 – 2009)

Mary C. Pinder "completed a medical degree at Stanford University School of Medicine in California," [1] graduating in 2002. "During medical school, she trained village health aides in the East Sepik Region of Papua, New Guinea and developed a women's health curriculum to be included in this training. Her postdoctoral training included residency in internal medicine at the University of North Carolina at Chapel Hill and a fellowship in medical oncology at the University of Texas M. D. Anderson Cancer Center in Houston, where she conducted breast cancer outcomes research." [1]

In 2007, Dr. Pinder-Schenck joined the section, with special interests in lung and breast malignancies. She left in 2009, taking a position "on the faculty of the H. Lee Moffitt Cancer and Research Center and the University of South Florida." [1] She also led "the clinical development of an epigenetic agent in early phase clinical trials for cancer" and then "transitioned to a global health role with GSK's Africa NCD Open Lab, where she works with researchers in Africa to develop translational research projects focusing on cancer and other NCDs in Africa." [1]

Nanette G. Robinson, MD (2009 – present)

Nanette Robinson received her medical degree from McGill University School of Medicine in Montreal, Canada. She then did a residency in internal medicine at Indiana University Medical Center in Indianapolis, followed by a fellowship in hematology/oncology at the University of Washington, which she completed in 1996.

Dr. Robinson joined Virginia Mason in 2009. She practices general hematology and oncology with a special interest in breast cancer and palliative care. She is a member of the American Society of Clinical Oncology, the American Society of Hematology, and the Southwest Oncology Group.

Joseph Rosales, MD (2011 – present)

Joe Rosales received his medical degree from UCLA Geffen School of Medicine in 1999. He then did a residency in internal medicine at St. Mary Medical Center in Long Beach, CA, followed by a fellowship in hematology/oncology at the City of Hope National Medical Center in Duarte, CA, which he completed in 2006.

Dr. Rosales joined VM in 2011. He specializes in thoracic and urologic oncology, with particular interests in lung, esophageal and prostate cancer. He is a member of the American Society of Clinical Oncology and the American Society of Hematology.

Craig R. Nichols, MD (2011 – 2015)

Craig Nichols attended Oregon Health Sciences University School of Medicine, receiving his MD in 1978. "After training in Medicine (Louisiana) and Hematology (Miami), he completed his specialty training at Indiana University where he focused on clinical trials in germ cell tumors and lymphoma, his clinical areas of expertise. He subsequently returned to Oregon where he joined the Oregon Health & Science University Cancer Institute and served as the division chief for hematology/oncology and vice chair for cancer clinical research." [2]

Dr. Nichols joined Virginia Mason Medical Center in 2011 "where he led the multi-disciplinary testicular cancer program and was the principal investigator for the Northwest National Cancer Institute Community Oncology Research Program." [2] He left VM in 2015, becoming Director of the "Precision Genomics Cancer Research Clinic at Intermountain Healthcare" in Utah, and remains clinically active.

"Over the last decade, Dr. Nichols has served on the board of LIVESTRONG and the Oregon chapter of the Leukemia/Lymphoma Society. He also runs a nonprofit dedicated to information and knowledge exchange in testicular cancer.

"Dr. Nichols continues to serve as the executive officer for one of the nation's largest cancer research groups — SWOG — for community based cancer research, adolescent and young adult oncology, survivorship, patient advocacy and digital engagement. He was recently elected to the board of the American Society of Clinical Oncology and serves on its executive committee." [2]

Prakash Vishnu, MBBS (2011 – 2016)

Prakash Vishnu attended Bangalore Medical College, India, where he received his MBBS in 2000. He then did a fellowship in Health Sciences, molecular medicine at the Faculty of Medicine and Health Sciences, University of Auckland, New Zealand, which he completed in 2005. This was following by an internship and residency in internal medicine at Wayne State/Detroit Medical Center, and a hematology/oncology fellowship at the Mayo Clinic, which he completed in 2011.

Dr. Vishnu then joined Virginia Mason and practiced there for 5 years, before taking a position at the Mayo Clinic, Jacksonville, FL. [3]

Bruce Lin, MD (2011– present)

Bruce Lin attended Vanderbilt University School of Medicine, receiving his MD in 2004. He then did a residency in internal medicine at University of Southern California, and a fellowship in hematology/oncology at the University of California at Irvine, which he completed in 2011.

Dr. Lin joined VM in 2011 where he specializes in hematology and medical oncology with a focus on liver, colorectal and other GI malignancies. He is a member of the American Society of Clinical Oncology, the American Society of Hematology, the American Association for Cancer

Research and the Southwest Oncology Group.

Gurkamal S. Chatta, MD (2012 – 2016)

Gurkamal Chatta received his MBBS in 1981 from the University College of Medical Sciences, Delhi University, India. This was followed by an internship in medicine, surgery and intensive care at Safdarjang Hospital, Delhi University and internal medicine at Mount Sinai Medical Center and the University of Wisconsin Medical School, which he completed in 1988. Dr. Chatta then did a fellowship in gerontology and another in hematology/oncology at the University of Washington, which he completed in 1996.

Dr. Chatta joined VM in 2012 and practiced general hematology/oncology, leaving in 2016 to take a position at Roswell Park Comprehensive Cancer Center in Buffalo, NY. [4]

Deborah M. Abrams, MD, MS (2016 - 2019)

A native Southwesterner, Deborah Abrams grew up in Albuquerque, New Mexico, but has enjoyed traveling throughout the country for school and medical training. She attended college in Georgia; she then attended the Hahnemann School of Medicine in Philadelphia, receiving an MS in Biological Sciences in 2002, and the University of Vermont College of Medicine, where she received her MD in 2006. This was followed by a residency in internal medicine at Maine Medicine Center in Portland, ME and a fellowship in hematology and oncology at the University of Vermont, which she completed in 2009.

Dr. Abrams was only at Virginia Mason for a few years, practicing general hematology/oncology, with a special interest in melanoma, sarcoma and breast cancer. She now practices at Harrison HealthPartners in Poulsbo, WA.

John Paul E. Flores, MD (2016 - current)

John Paul Flores attended Dartmouth College, receiving a BA degree in genetics, cell and developmental biology in 2005. He then attended med-

117

ical school at the University of Florida at Gainesville, moving on to Tufts Medical Center in Boston for his residency in internal medicine and fellowship in hematology and oncology, which he completed in 2016.

Dr. Flores practices general hematology and oncology.

Hagen F. Kennecke, MD, MHA (2017 – present)

Hagen Kennecke attended the University of British Columbia in Vancouver, BC (UBC) where he received a B.Sc. in genetics in 1990. He then served as a research assistant there for 2 years, and received a Master in Health Administration from UBC in 1994. He received his MD from Dalhousie University in Halifax, Nova Scotia in 1997. He did his internship in internal medicine at the University of Massachusetts at Amherst, and then a residency at Legacy Health Care System in Portland, OR, which he completed in 2000. He did a fellowship in medical oncology at UBC, which he completed in 2003.

Dr. Kennecke took a position as medical oncologist at the Vancouver Cancer Clinic that year and joined the Faculty of Medicine at UBC in 2009, rising to the rank of Associate Professor, Partner track. He has authored/co-authored 89 articles in peer-reviewed journals, and also 100 conference proceedings. In the past five years, he participated in 35 clinical studies, being national principal investigator on seven and site principal investigator on 11 trials.

In 2017, he joined Virginia Mason as Medical Director of the Cancer Institute where he serves as a medical oncologist as well.

Meaghan W. O'Malley, MD (2016 - current)

Meaghan O'Malley was born in California and attended Wake Forest University School of Medicine in Winston-Salem, NC, graduating in 2007. She then did an internship and residency at University of Michigan in internal medicine, followed by a fellowship there in hematology/oncology, which she completed in 2013.

Dr. O'Malley practices general oncology and hematology, with a focus on breast, lung, and head and neck malignancies. She is a member of the

American Society of Clinical Oncology and the American Society of Hematology. She and her family enjoy living in the Pacific Northwest.

Marc S. Rosenshein, MD (2018 - present)

Marc Rosenshein attended Jefferson Medical College in Philadelphia, PA, graduating in 1973. He then did an internship and residency in internal medicine at Temple University in Philadelphia, followed by a fellowship in hematology/oncology at the University of Washington, which he completed in 1979. Dr. Rosenshein joined VM in 2018 and practices general internal medicine, hematology and oncology in Edmonds.

Joshua M. Wilfong, DO (2017 - current)

Joshua Wilfong graduated from Lake Erie College of Osteopathic Medicine in Bradenton, FL in 2009. He then did an internship in internal medicine at the Cleveland Clinic followed by fellowships in hematology/oncology at the University of Michigan, and hospice and palliative medicine at Stanford University, which he completed in 2016.

Dr. Wilfong specializes in medical and hematologic oncology, and palliative care.

References:

1. "Mary Pinder-Schenck, MD, , Director, Clinical Development GlaxoSmith-Kline" at: https://www.fredhutch.org/content/dam/public/labs-projects/global-oncology/symposium/Mary%20Pinder-Schenck,%20MD.pdf; accessed April 13, 2019.

2. "Craig R. Nichols, MD, FACP." at https://intermountainphysician.org/UrologySeminar/Pages/Craig%20R.%20Nichols.aspx; accessed 5/1/19.

3. "Prakash Vishnu, MBBS" at https://www.mayoclinic.org/biographies/vishnu-prakash-m-b-b-s/bio-20213663; accessed April 13, 2019.

4. "Gurkamal Chatta, MD" at https://www.roswellpark.org/gurkamal-chatta; accessed April 13, 2019.

8

Hyperbaric Medicine

by Neil B. Hampson, MD; James Holm, MD
& John Kirkpatrick, MD

The term "hyperbaric medicine" refers to "the treatment of patients with high pressure air, which may be enriched or diluted, as the need arises, with oxygen or other gases." [1] While many may consider the therapy new, the medical use of pressurized air as treatment dates back to 1662 when "an English pastor and physician, the Rev. Henshaw, reportedly treated patients in a compressed air chamber ... although his theory for such therapy is not recorded.

"The French surgeon Fontaine built a pressurized operating room in 1879, and Dr. J. L. Corning introduced hyperbaric (high-pressure) treatment to the United States in 1891. After experimenting with hyperbaric oxygen to treat 'Spanish Flu' victims at the end of World War I, Dr. Orville J. Cunningham constructed an 88-foot long chamber in Kansas City ...

... "These ambitious pioneers were hampered by a poor understanding of the actual physiological effects and benefits of hyperbaric oxygen." [2] However, important advances in understanding occurred during WWII when the US Navy began studying human tolerance for pure oxygen in compression chambers. "Research was spurred in part by the spread of professional and recreational scuba diving after World War II, and a corresponding rise in cases of 'decompression disease'" or "the bends". [2] This condition is the result of gas bubble formation in blood and tissues and is treated by repressurization in a chamber.

Exploration "of oil reserves in the North Sea off Scotland and Norway in the late 1960s required extremely deep dives ... Oil companies made funds available for new research into the physiology of such dives and potential health hazards and treatments for divers." [2] Following acquisition of a standard deck recompression chamber in 1966, "the Virginia Mason Research Center entered this field with a study ... by its director, **Merrill P. Spencer, MD**, on the application of cardiovascular adjustments of diving mammals to human survival under severe environmental conditions." [1]

"Spurred by Dr. Spencer, Virginia Mason Medical Center sought and received funding for hyperbaric research with diving mammals." [2] Deep diving research was funded by "government, military, and corporate funding. These grants were augmented by substantial gifts from donors such as Jon M. Lindbergh, son of the famed aviator and a noted deep-sea diver in his own right." [2]

In the background, "the benefits of hyperbaric oxygen treatments in promoting healing after radiation therapy were noted in the 1950s ... The first scientific congress on hyperbaric medicine was held in 1963 and the Undersea (Medical) Society developed the first board-certification standards and exams for hyperbaric medicine specialists in 1976. Blue Cross/Blue Shield approved insurance reimbursement for the treatments the following year." [2]

In April 1969, Virginia Mason formally organized and dedicated its hyperbaric unit to Lindbergh in recognition of his support. The available chamber had the capability "of attaining pressures equivalent to 1,500 feet of sea water." It was "fifteen- and one-half feet long" with "an inside diameter of four- and one-half feet" and could uncomfortably accommodate a maximum of three persons. "In May 1970 the chamber was relocated in enlarged quarters in the south end of Blackford Hall," [3] formerly the bed-making laboratory of the Virginia Mason School of Nursing.

As noted in articles at the time: "Within a short period" after opening in 1969, "four cases were treated in the Lindbergh chamber, two patients with bends and two suffering from gas gangrene. In addition to the
patient therapy, work proceeded on three research projects that currently
make use of the chamber." [1] However, a single chamber resulted in lack
of flexibility and a second vertical cylindrical chamber, seven feet deep
and eight feet in diameter, was installed. As further described, **"Dr. Kent
Smith**, Director of Hyperbaric Research and Diving Physiology, has a
staff of ten professional and technical personnel ... Dr. Smith's research
projects include studies of aseptic bone necrosis, hyperbaric decompression by means of bubble detection, and inert gas elimination. **Dr. Brian
G. D'Aoust** will be junior investigator on the inert gas elimination study.
He comes to the Research Center from Oakland, California, where he was
assistant research physiologist at the Naval Biological Laboratory at the
Naval Supply Center. **Mrs. Phyllis Stegall,** biologist and nuclear medicine technologist, is working with Dr. Smith on the aseptic bone necrosis
project. Before joining the staff of the Research Center, Mrs. Stegall was
in the biodynamics branch of the USAF School of Aerospace Medicine
at Brooks Air Force Base, Texas. **Michael Newman** is manager of the
hyperbaric laboratory." [3]

During the first six months, "16 patients ... received 328 hours of
treatment for a variety of conditions, including osteomyelitis, gangrene,
senescence and diver's bends. The helistop, opened in February 1970 atop
Virginia Mason Hospital makes it possible to transport emergency patients
by helicopter to the Medical Center ... (and) increases the speed with
which hyperbaric treatment can be given." [3]

As noted, Merrill Spencer, MD, was the first director of the Hyperbaric Unit. He was originally the director of the Virginia Mason Research
Center, which has now become the Benaroya Research Institute at Virginia Mason. His interests and contributions to medicine were enormous in
the fields of basic science, especially in the application of Doppler principles to measure cardiac, neural and peripheral circulation. He left VM to
establish a lab at Providence Hospital in Seattle, and ultimately Swedish

122

Hospital. There is an endowed lectureship in his name at Swedish.

The mainstay of the staff was **Diane Norkool, RN.** She ran the clinical aspects of the Unit under Dr. Spencer, and subsequently during a time when there was no medical director. Diane's background was in critical care, and her love of research led her to recognize enormous possibilities for professional growth in the specialty of hyperbaric nursing. She developed and refined the nursing care aspects from the occasional scuba diver to the patient with problem wounds. She completed her Master's thesis on the "Effects of Intermittent Hyperbaric Oxygen on Full Thickness Burns in the Rat". From the 1970s to the mid-1980s, hyperbaric oxygen therapy was moving from a primary focus on diving medicine into the clinical arena. The Undersea Medical Society became the Undersea and Hyperbaric Medical Society (UHMS) and in 1985, thirty-five registered nurses established the Baromedical Nurses Association (BNA). The mission of the BNA was to work on an international basis to define and implement the standards of practice, promote education and support clinical research for the hyperbaric nurse. Diane Norkool became the first elected President of the BNA; in its first year, the BNA had 176 members and represented the first step in defining the specialty of hyperbaric nursing. Today the BNA has members in Europe, Asia, South and Central America, and the South Pacific. In 1995, Norkool was one of the co-authors of a chapter on hyperbaric nursing in the first edition of Eric Kindwall's textbook, *Hyperbaric Medicine Practice*. The Diane Norkool Award was created by the UHMS in honor of the advancements made in the profession of nursing through her leadership, research contributions, and educational efforts. She was instrumental in developing hyperbaric nursing standards of care and certification. Norkool co-authored many papers on a variety of hyperbaric subjects, cheerfully treated patients at all hours of the day, night and weekends, and worked tirelessly touting the benefits of this very specialized treatment. She was the first recipient of the Diane Norkool Award in 1996, given posthumously after her untimely death of cardiac arrest at the age of 53 in 1995.

Richard Dunford, MS worked with Diane Norkool, serving as technical manager while she was alive, and assuming her role of manager after her passing. He had earned his Masters of Science at USC and did his thesis in "Airway Dynamics in the Hyperbaric State" in 1974. He was also a research analyst at the Divers Alert Network.

In the late 1970s and early 1980s, the Unit was jointly co-directed by the Hyperbaric Committee, a group of interested physicians who had essentially "disease-specific" hyperbaric privileges – **Thomas Green, MD**, from Orthopaedics treated gangrenous wounds and chronic osteomyelitis, **Thomas Yarington, MD**, from Otolaryngology treated osteoradione-crosis of the jaw, and **John Kirkpatrick, MD**, from General Internal Medicine helped to treat carbon monoxide (CO) exposure. These providers were directed by the consistent expertise of Ms. Norkool. Dr. Kirkpatrick pointed out some of the dangers of gas furnaces and appliances in a series of newspaper articles and a subsequent review of cases in the *Western Journal of Medicine*. [4] From his suggestion, an inaccurate statement in *Harrison's Principles and Practice of Medicine* was corrected. He gave several Grand Rounds presentations at local hospitals in the Puget Sound area on CO poisoning.

Gerald Zel, MD, was the interim director of the Hyperbaric Unit from 1986 to 1989 under the auspices of the Department of Surgery. He graduated from Tufts Medical School, had further training in the US Naval Hospital, residency at St. Elizabeth's Hospital, and completed a urology fellowship. He did not practice urology at Virginia Mason.

Neil B. Hampson, MD, was assigned leadership of the Hyperbaric Unit in 1989. He had come to Virginia Mason from Duke University in 1988 as a pulmonary and critical care physician, joining the then Section of Chest and Infectious Disease. Under his guidance, the Hyperbaric Unit became the Hyperbaric Section and moved operationally to the Department of Medicine. Dr. Hampson assumed Medical Directorship in 1990. During twenty years as Medical Director, he authored over 100 papers related to hyperbaric medicine, more than 70 on carbon monoxide poisoning, a topic in which he came to be considered a world expert. He testified numerous times before state and government committees and made significant contributions to public health awareness of carbon monoxide sources. He was known for publicizing the risk of carbon monoxide poisoning for children riding in the back of covered pickup trucks and for convincing the Federal government to include a nonverbal warning label against indoor use on bags of charcoal briquettes. He published extensively on treatment of chronic radiation tissue injury with hyperbaric oxygen and was considered an expert in that area, as well.

During the 1990s, Dr. Hampson worked to raise the visibility of hyperbaric medicine and promote the use of hyperbaric oxygen therapy for appropriate, proven indications. This emphasis on credibility resulted in a dramatic increase in regional referrals and growth in patient treatment hours. By the year 2000, treatment of four routine patients was scheduled every two hours from 07:00 AM to 9:30 PM six days a week. Despite this, there was a waiting list for treatment. The program was renamed the Center for Hyperbaric Medicine in recognition of its regional prominence and status as the major referral center in the Northwest. Dr. Hampson was assisted at that time by **Robert Barnes, MD**, of Infectious Disease; **Allen Johnson, MD**, of Emergency Medicine; and **Steven Kirtland, MD,** of Pulmonary and Critical Care Medicine. **Claude Wreford-Brown, RN,** served as nurse manager. It was clear that demand was greater than capacity and the decision was made to build a new facility.

Dr. Hampson worked with **Connie Winberry** and later **Michael Vanderhof** of the VM Foundation, as well as **John Ryan, MD**, of the Department of Surgery to raise philanthropic funds. The campaign was quite successful and $4.2 million of the $7.1 million cost was raised through philanthropy. A new Center for Hyperbaric Medicine was built in "8,000 square feet of remodeled conference rooms and a former auditorium on the ground floor of Virginia Mason's main hospital wing on Seattle's First Hill," [2] space that was originally part of Terry Avenue running under the hospital and a hospital parking garage.

The new facility opened in 2005 and was widely considered to be the best state-of-the art clinical hyperbaric facility in the world. As described at the time, "the spacious main room features comfortable waiting areas for patients and family members, examination (and treatment) rooms, an impressive saltwater aquarium, and a large control console resembling something one might find at Cape Kennedy. The main room is dominated by the large" [2] triple lock cylindrical chamber, measuring 46 feet in overall length with an interior diameter of 10 feet, similar in size to a Boeing 737. The two main chamber locks were designed to "accommodate up to sixteen seated patients … plus two attendants. Patients typically sit in comfortable recliner chairs" reminiscent of first-class seats on an airline "and breathe oxygen through clear plastic helmets, or 'hoods', during two-hour sessions called 'dives'. The chambers can achieve maximum pressures equivalent to submerging 165 feet below sea level, or roughly six times the normal surface atmospheric pressure, although 'dives' of 45 … feet are most common. These pressures are generated by a complex system of compressors, air storage tanks, and piping in rooms adjacent to and below the chambers. It also features a fire suppression system that can flood the locks in seconds …

"At the time of the Center's opening in 2005, hyperbaric treatments were supervised by a large team led by Dr. Neil Hampson and including physicians **David Dabell, Tony Gerbino**, **Steven Kirtland**, and **Anne Mahoney**." [2] All were personally trained by Dr. Hampson and became board-certified in undersea and hyperbaric medicine. "They were assisted by specially trained technicians and registered nurses, many of whom were divers. **Douglas Ross, RN,** provided advanced wound care to complement the treatments." [2]

Within two years after opening, Dr. Hampson's self-defined "Holy Grail" for Virginia Mason's hyperbaric program of 10,000 patient treatment hours in a year was achieved. "The Center is staffed 24 hours a day, 7 days a week to handle emergencies, and it routinely carries out 100 patient treatments a week. Its capacity was put to the test by severe local storms in December 2006, when it handled some 70 victims of carbon monoxide poisoning over a four-day period" without canceling a single routine patient treatment. Those poisoned were "chiefly newly arrived immigrants who had sought to stay warm during power outages and were unfamiliar with the dangers of using charcoal cookers and heaters in enclosed spaces. The incidents led to aggressive community education efforts." [2]

Dr. Hampson served as President of the UHMS from 2002 - 2004 and served on or chaired many committees within that organization. When undersea and hyperbaric medicine became a board-certifiable specialty under the American Board of Medical Specialties in 1999, Dr. Hampson was asked to join the board certification committee and served in that role for nineteen years. He received numerous career achievement awards from regional and national organizations. In 2007 he was the recipient of the prestigious **James Tate Mason Award,** given to Virginia Mason's outstanding physician of the year. A library at Virginia Mason was named in his honor at the time of his retirement in 2010.

Dr. Hampson recruited **James Holm, MD**, a nationally known hyperbaric and wound care physician, to VM in 2009 anticipating that Dr. Holm would become Medical Director of the program after his retirement. Dr. Holm brought invaluable expertise in diving medicine, wound healing, and monoplace chamber operations. Dr. Holm grew up in Los Angeles and attended the University of California at Santa Barbara, majoring in Physiology and Cell Biology. His interest shifted to medicine and he attended Georgetown University Medical School, followed by a combined residency in emergency medicine and internal medicine at Northwestern University. He maintains board certification in those specialties as well as receiving boards in undersea and hyperbaric medicine in 2000. He has worked at monoplace and multiplace chambers, all with the capability of attending to emergency cases. He was previously at a well-respected program at Intermountain Medical Center in Salt Lake City, when Dr. Hampson recruited him to Virginia Mason Medical Center.

Dr. Holm has a keen interest in SCUBA diving and became a certified diver in 1969 at the age of 13. He worked in dive shops while in high school, became a diving instructor in 1978 and taught diving at UCSB while in college. He spent a year teaching diving on Grand Cayman Island before going on to medical school. Dr. Holm has been diving for 50 years and has over 3000 dives; he continues to dive and retains his passion for undersea medicine. He was the previous director of the yearly Physician Training and Diving Medicine course sponsored by the National Oceanic and Atmospheric Administration (NOAA) and UHMS. He was President of the UHMS from 2014 to 2016. He is also the co-director of the Diving Medicine courses sponsored by Divers Alert Network (DAN) and UHMS, holding courses twice a year. His enjoys sharing his passion for undersea and hyperbaric medicine with residents and colleagues. In 2010, Dr. Holm took over as the Medical Director for the Center of Hyperbaric Medicine. He continues to work with Dr. Hampson on research interests.

The Center for Hyperbaric Medicine has recruited and retained many staff that have worked there for over a decade including nurses **Diana Bodwin, Sue Dunn** and **Sandi Hamilton**, along with a mix of part-time nurses and technicians who help staff the program. **Chris Kramer** and **Todd Courtney** are the technical supervisors who operate the chamber as well as maintaining flawless performance – the chamber has remained operational without any "down time" since its opening. The facility is "accredited with distinction" as a level 1 hyperbaric chamber by UHMS since 2006, and was one of the first in the country to achieve this recognition.

References:

1. "In Quest of a Dream." *VM Review* Fall 1969, pages 4-5.
2. Crowley W. "Virginia Mason Medical Center opens expanded Center for Hyperbaric Medicine in Seattle on July 16, 2005. " at: https://historylink.org/File/8171; accessed 28 Sept 2019.
3. "Hyperbaric Chamber Serves the Pacific Northwest." *Research Quarterly*, summer 1970, page 2.
4. Kirkpatrick J. "Occult Carbon Monoxide Poisoning." *West J Med.* 1987; 146(1):52-56.

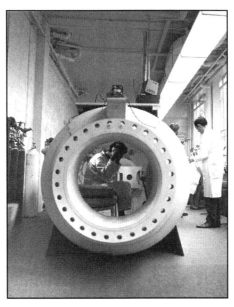

Hyperbaric Chamber, circa 1969 (PH 1244b, VMHA)

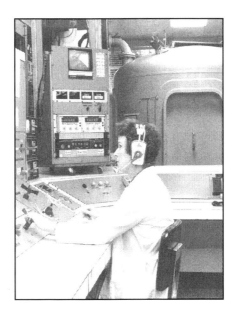

Diane Norkool operating hyperbaric equipment, circa 1981
(PH 1002, VMHA).

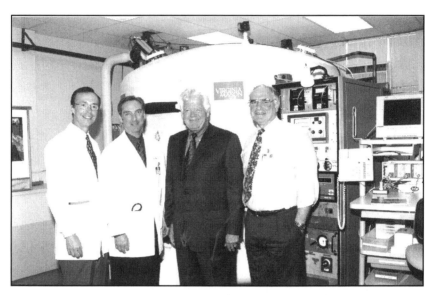

The Hyperbaric chamber with congressional visit, 2004
L to R: Neil Hampson, MD; Gary Kaplan, MD; Representative Jim
McDermott, MD; Richard G. Dunford, MS, manager (PH 6775, VMHA)

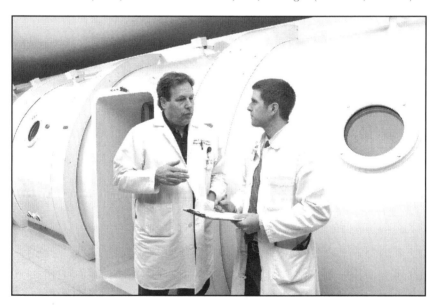

Modern Hyperbaric Chamber, 2013
James Holm, MD, (L) and resident Shawn Call, MD (PH 8997, VMHA)

9

Infectious Disease

by Margot Schwartz, MD

The Virginia Mason Section of Infectious Diseases (ID) was constituted at the turn of the millennium in 2000. However, its roots go back much further than that. Dick Winterbauer, MD, well known to many at Virginia Mason (VM) for his distinguished career in the Pulmonary Section, had also received infectious disease training in conjunction with his pulmonary fellowship, and did infectious disease consultations at VM along with his busy pulmonary practice. For many years thereafter, Dick was the de facto ID expert at VM. As he wasn't able to be on call 100% of the time, he roped in his pulmonary colleagues to also cover ID when they were on call, a duty they grudgingly accepted, and for which they did an admirable job considering their lack of subspecialty training. These pulmonologists included Gene Pardee, MD; David Dreis, MD; Steve Springmeyer, MD; Ken Casey, MD; Neil Hampson, MD, and Steve Kirtland, MD.

When Dick Winterbauer retired in early 1999, VM hired three physicians over a two-year period to replace him. One of these was Bob Rakita, MD, who became the first board-certified ID doc at VM in 1999. As one couldn't very well have a section of one, Bob joined the Pulmonary Section, and was forever grateful to those same pulmonologists for continuing to help with on-call coverage and for welcoming him into their fold. Not surprisingly, Bob was very soon overwhelmed with both clinical and administrative activities related to being the only ID specialist. Despite that, he managed to write a pro forma and convince the administration that another ID person was desperately needed. Margot Schwartz, MD, joined the group in 2000. With a critical mass of two ID docs, it was agreed that a separate section should exist, and the Section of ID was formally created that year. Because many at VM did not know that there was indeed a new ID section, our white lab jackets were (and some still are!) embroidered with "Pulmonary Section" in the collar! The Pulmonary and ID Sections continued to share space and staff in the Buck 7 clinic. It took a few years to teach our VM colleagues that ID was its own section, and not a part of the Pulmonary Section. Slowly the section grew and distinguished itself on its own merits.

Work continued to grow at an exponential pace, and Rob Barnes, MD, joined the section in 2001 after working for many years in Bellingham. He brought great experience to the section. For several years, this trio managed the growing clinical, administrative, and teaching duties of the section. However, Rob moved on to greener pastures at PeaceHealth in Eugene, OR in 2007. Chia Wang, MD, then joined the section and we continued to grow. Uma Malhotra, MD, next joined in 2008. In 2009, Dr. Rakita left after 10 years of being the first ID Section Head at VM, and took a position at the University of Washington to specialize in solid organ-transplant infectious diseases. Before Dr. Rakita left VM, he stepped down as Section Head and Tony Gerbino, MD, added the ID Section Head role to his resume in addition to his pulmonary responsibilities (ID couldn't quite escape the pulmonary connection!). Dr. Gerbino continued in that role until Michael Myint, MD, was hired in late 2009, serving as both section member and Section Head until 2013, when Dr. Schwartz took on the section head role. Hal Martin, MD, joined the group from Minnesota in 2011, but left in 2013 to work with Gilead, a pharmaceutical maker of HIV medications. Chris Baliga, MD, joined us in 2013, having previously worked with the ID Section in 2010 as a locums ID physician; he has been Section Head since late 2015. Shingo Chihara, MD, joined the section in 2014, and Sophie Woolston, MD, joined the ID Section in September of 2016. In January of 2018, the ID Section welcomed Lisa Roberts, PA-C, who specializes in travel medicine consultation. In 2019, Dr. Woolston moved to Portland, Maine to take a job closer to family. The ID Section has recently welcomed her replacement, Bob Geise, MD, to our ranks. Dr. Geise brings with him many years of experience as an ID physician at Evergreen Hospital. Thus, as of this writing, the section has 6 ID physicians and one PA – rapid growth for a section that didn't even exist 18 years ago!

Other people were critical to the success of the section over the years. As the clinical FTEs were never quite enough to cover all of the weekends, some of the weekends were covered by junior ID docs, typically senior fellows at the UW who were board-eligible in ID and helped as locums physicians. By and large, they were a great addition to the ID team, and many have gone on to prestigious careers in academia and private practice. In the early years, ID Pulmonary Section managers helped manage the ID Section, which worked well while we shared space and medical assistants (MAs). These included Sandy Tanski, Carol Vangelos and Claude Wreford-Brown. When the ID Section started hiring its own staff and prepared to move to its new space, Sara Martinez was hired as the first ID Section manager. After Sara left in 2014, Maria Rearick was briefly our manager before Fred De Leon became section manager in 2015 in addition to managing the Asthma and Allergy Section. The ID Section managed without a clinic nurse for many years, until they successfully lobbied to hire one; Rebecca Maxim, RN joined the group in 2015.

The Infectious Disease Section has several roles besides inpatient and outpatient ID consultation. We serve as primary care providers as well as consultants for patients with HIV. We see patients for pre-travel immunizations and prophylactic medications, and do post-travel ID consultations. We have played a significant role in selecting patients who may benefit from fecal transplantation for *Clostridium difficile* infection and screened donors for stool transplant before a commercial universal donor stool product was available. Our section members have administrative and committee roles in several areas including infection prevention and control, antimicrobial stewardship, employee health and travel medicine. We have been involved with high resolution anoscopy (HRA) screening for anal cancer in high-risk individuals. More recently, ID section members are working in the new Wound Care Clinic at the VM Seattle campus.

While clinical activities have occupied a tremendous amount of the ID Section's time, a variety of other efforts led by ID section members have contributed to the overall mission at VM. Soon after Dr. Rakita joined VM, he found himself on 13 committees. In fact, Karen, the pulmonary MA who handled scheduling for David Dreis, MD, the Chief of Medicine, told Bob that he had more meetings than David did. One of these areas related to utilization of antibiotics (what is now called antimicrobial stewardship), an area for oversight, which at that time was not widely recognized nationally. In conjunction with Roger Woolf from Pharmacy, and a number of his colleagues including Liza Vaezi, Bob founded the Antimicrobial Utilization Review Group (AURG – yes, say it out loud) as a subgroup of the P&T committee. This group instituted a variety of changes in how antibiotics were used at VM, including routine utilization reviews and antibiotic restriction policies. This led to more focused use of antibiotics, and saved the institution several hundred thousand dollars per year on an ongoing basis. On a more general level, Bob shared the outcomes of this effort with his colleagues at the UW, which subsequently led to the establishment of what have become flourishing antimicrobial stewardship efforts at all of the local institutions (UWMC, Harborview, Northwest, Children's, and Swedish, to name just a few). Antimicrobial stewardship activity is now a requirement for hospitals throughout the US; the VM ID Section was ahead of its time! Since 2013, Chia Wang has served as the Medical Director of Antimicrobial Stewardship at VM.

Infection control and employee health were two other areas that occupied a great deal of the section's efforts. For many years, Bob was the Medical Director for Infection Control and chair of the Infection Control Committee in conjunction with Gary Preston and his expert group of infection control practitioners - there was always a fire to put out! After Dr.

Rakita left, Mike Myint served in that capacity, followed by Chris Baliga, who is the current head of Infection Prevention and Control. The ID physicians have also served as Medical Directors of Employee Health, including Drs. Rakita, Barnes, Myint, Schwartz, Malhotra, and Baliga, and have had many great times with Bev Hagar and others in that group.

Some of the highlights of the ID Section's efforts with infection prevention and employee health include:

Ventilator-associated pneumonia (VAP): When Bob joined VM in 1999, the VAP rate in the ICU at VM was an astounding 21 (per 1000 ventilator days). By the following year, it was down to 12, and by 2004 it was at a respectable level of <2. Several of the pulmonary/critical care docs commented that this improvement was a tribute to the addition of a cadre of dedicated ID docs and infection control efforts. On top of the patient morbidity and mortality benefit, this also saved the institution several hundred thousand dollars per year.

Measles control: When an employee came down with this incredibly contagious infection in the early 2000s, and employee health records didn't document who was actually immune, a huge effort was undertaken to immunize employees in record time. The hospital almost closed due to this. But the team soldiered through, with Bob in meetings >14 hrs/day and Margot handling all of the clinical work. Sporadically, when patients at VM have been diagnosed with measles in recent outbreaks (some due to trends in underimmunization), the impact on the ID Section has been equally great with time-intensive meetings pulling our clinicians from their usual duties and other section members surging to cover the service.

Other infectious disease outbreaks: Similarly, cases of Legionella on campus have caused a flurry of activity in our section. When an immunocompromised patient came down with this serious infection, and it was found in the water supply of Cassel Crag where they had been staying, there was much consternation about what to do. Eventually, all was sorted out, and certain at-risk patients were no longer allowed to reside there.

Over the years, cases of pertussis, norovirus and tuberculosis exposure in the work environment, as well as needle-stick exposures to bloodborne pathogens, have involved the ID physicians in infection control and direct patient care efforts to protect our patients and staff alike. Norovirus outbreaks on campus, while short-lived and rarely fatal, happen at inopportune times in various places in the hospital. Inpatient units have had to be closed to new admissions, and no visitors could come in. In addition, staff potlucks had to be curtailed. These events resulted in lots of infection control work for the ID docs and the infection prevention team.

Surgical site infections (SSIs) have also involved the ID Section in multidisciplinary group work, as we strive to minimize risk factors for SSIs, and reduce infection rates. This group won the 2009 Mary McClinton patient safety award for their work.

More recently, duodenoscope-related infections with resistant gram-negative rods was found to be an issue not only at VM, but nationwide. Chris Baliga and Michael Myint, along with members of the GI Section and microbiologists in the Laboratory (especially Punam Verma, PhD) were instrumental in leading efforts at VM to fix this difficult problem, and disseminate the information to the rest of the world.

Nationwide and worldwide outbreaks of infectious diseases have required inordinate planning efforts by the ID Section and others in determining how to respond to protect our patients and employees. When swine flu (H1N1 influenza) began to sweep the nation in late 2009, efforts at VM switched into high gear to immunize both patients and staff with great success. While other infections such as SARS and ebola have not reached our campus, the ID section members were involved in great efforts, including daily meetings in addition to our clinical responsibilities, to prepare for handling such infections should patients present on our campus. Similarly, when threats of bioterrorism arose in 2001 after the 9/11 terrorist attacks and the Amerithrax episode (sending anthrax spores through the mail) triggered a heightened alert for a variety of potential bioterrorism agents, VM responded. Finding white powder anywhere (would you like some non-dairy sweetener with your coffee?) was cause for panic. Much time and effort by our section went into planning responses for these threats, including a scenario involving smallpox, with plans to immunize if necessary.

Purell! Hard to believe now, when alcohol-based hand gels are ubiquitous in all hospitals, but when these were first promulgated there was tremendous resistance to their use, most notably from the Fire Department. Having a significant amount of alcohol in rooms, and especially in hallways, was suspected to be a huge fire hazard and we were not allowed to install dispensers except in very restricted locations. Of course, this has now been shown to be nonsense, and its benefit for hand-hygiene and reducing nosocomial transmissions is universally accepted. This was another collaborative effort by the ID Section and Infection Prevention Committee, as well as others (such as Central Supply) at VM.

Immunization efforts: Over the years, the ID Section had been at the forefront of efforts to improve immunization rates, particularly for influenza in our population of vulnerable patients. Coordinated rapid process improvement workshops (RPIWs) that included the ID team took place in 2004 with resulting proposals for a variety of measures to increase influenza vaccination. One idea that came out of the workshops was a drive-through flu vaccination station, so that patients wouldn't have to park, come inside, stand in line, etc. to get their vaccination. This innovative delivery system was one of the first of its kind in the nation.

More notably, one of the nurses in an RPIW came up with the idea of mandatory flu vaccination for healthcare workers. The team jumped at the opportunity, and with a tremendous amount of work this came into being in 2005. Healthcare worker immunization rates skyrocketed – from 54% prior to the requirement up to 99% afterwards. This approach also progressed throughout the nation, and rates even in institutions that did not require vaccination jumped upward in response. VM was recognized nationally (and internationally) as the leader, and a paper documenting this was eventually published (after Bob left VM and thus had time to write it up - Rakita RM, Hagar BA, Crome P, and Lammert JK. Mandatory influenza vaccination of healthcare workers: a 5-year study. *Infect Control Hosp Epidemiol* 2010; 31:881-8).

However, there was a downside to this – the Washington State Nursing Association sued VM, claiming that any mandatory vaccine requirement had to be negotiated in a contract. Much time, effort, and money for legal services were expended, and an arbitrator found in favor of the union. Despite this, a very, very high percentage of the unionized nurses at VM still got their flu vaccine, attesting to the validity of the idea.

Influenza has not been the only immunization focus of the VM ID Section. Recent updates (some confusing to implement) in pneumococcal, meningococcal and varicella immunization have required great time and effort on the part of the ID section members. In addition, recent vaccine shortages, such as the yellow fever vaccine, required our section to step up to provide a similar vaccine available only by expanded access, with the help of the Institutional Review Board, Benaroya Research Center, and ID Section staff, to provide seamless travel services.

Teaching has always played a significant role in the ID section's activities. We almost always have a resident on rotation with us, which we greatly enjoy, and the residents have thought highly of the rotation. We also participated in the resident HIV clinic, run through General Internal Medicine, and taught there on a regular basis for many years. The VM ID group eventually took a regular turn in the rotation at the weekly Harborview citywide ID conference. Every 6 weeks or so we present cases, usually as unknowns, and invite discussion from mostly academic ID docs throughout the city. Often, we hear feedback that "VM has the best cases!" Rob Barnes began the tradition of ID Jeopardy, where he created a game show of unusual and esoteric ID information, which he would present at the conference at the end of each academic year. This has continued in his absence, with one of the Veteran's Administration ID docs taking it over.

As in most institutions, the **Clinical Microbiology Laboratory** is critical to the work that ID providers do. This was no less true at VM. Under the able leadership of Stan Sumida, PhD, and Punam Verma, PhD (with the assistance of many talented microbiologists and micro technologists), the Micro laboratory does a terrific job. ID section members routinely visit the lab on a daily basis to interact with laboratory staff and review positive blood cultures and other interesting culture results, ensuring the best outcomes for our patients by getting the most out of our microbiology results. Most recently, Shingo Chihara became the Associate Director of Microbiology.

For many years, the Infectious Disease Section had provided mostly **post-travel care**, but after the retirement of Susan Holt in June 2016, and the departure of Christian Herter, we are now the only section that provides pre-travel counseling in the downtown VM location. Shingo Chihara is the medical director of Travel Health and organizes the Travel Health collaborative every 3 or 4 months to discuss topics in travel medicine. He has been working to standardize care among providers across the institution, and implemented the use of Travax software at all VM sites.

For many years, the ID Section shared the Buck 7 hallway with the pulmonary team. What a lovely, non-air-conditioned spot, where temperatures in the relatively hot days of summer occasionally topped 100 degrees F! On some of those days, VM administrators could be spotted delivering popsicles and water to patients and staff. When the Urology team expanded and needed more space on Buck 7, and Pulmonary moved to their current location near the hyperbaric chamber, the ID team moved over to HRB2, where we shared space with Employee Health, and later Outpatient Infusion Clinic nurses. In January of 2017, the ID team moved to the hospital - Central Pavilion level 7 - in the old Intensive Care Unit North space. This has been a great transition for our section, moving us closer to the hospital, and providing more space for our patients and staff.

Physician Biographies
Bob Rakita, MD (1999 – 2009)
Bob Rakita was born and raised in Cleveland, OH, went to college at

Swarthmore, and then returned to Cleveland for medical school at Case Western Reserve University. He did his residency and fellowship at the University of Washington. His first position was at the University of Texas-Houston where he ran a lab and did basic science research for many years before returning to Seattle and joining VM in 1999. He left VM in 2009 to take a position at the University of Washington. He was known at VM as an outstanding clinician and teacher, serving as the first ID Section Head, and on many committees, including Infection Control, AURG, Surgical Site Infections, Pharmacy &Therapeutics, and the Residency Advisory Committee (RAC). Bob won the John Huff/Robert Hegstrom teaching award in both 2002-3 and 2005-6. Dr. Rakita has been recognized as a "Top Doctor" by his peers in the *Seattle Magazine* and *Seattle Met* surveys.

Margot Schwartz, MD, MPH (2000 – present)

Margot Schwartz was raised in Chappaqua, NY, before leaving in 11th grade to finish high school at Phillips Exeter Academy in New Hampshire. She attended college at Wesleyan University in Connecticut, and medical school at Johns Hopkins University in Baltimore. She then headed west for internship and residency in internal medicine at the University of Washington.

After completing residency, she spent a year doing primary care internal medicine at the East Austin (TX) Public Health Clinic. During that year she also worked at a clinic for the homeless at the Salvation Army in Austin. Dr. Schwartz then returned to Seattle for a fellowship in infectious diseases at the University of Washington. Her research focused on sexually-transmitted infections, specifically looking at the epidemiology and causative pathogens of nongonococcal urethritis. During her fellowship, she also earned a Masters in Public Health in epidemiology at the University of Washington.

After fellowship, Dr. Schwartz stayed on at the University of Washington as an Acting Instructor in the Department of Medicine (Infectious Diseases), working at Harborview's AIDS Clinical Trials Unit (ACTU), Madison Clinic (HIV Clinic), and attending in internal medicine and infectious disease services at Harborview. While there, it became obvious that she loved her time doing clinical medicine more than her time doing research, and decided to pursue other options, which led to taking a job at VM in the year 2000.

Dr. Schwartz has interests in general infectious diseases, HIV medicine, sexually-transmitted diseases (STDs), *Clostridium difficile* infections, travel medicine and prevention of infectious diseases with immunizations. With the arrival of the bad strains of *C. difficile* in 2005 or 2006, Dr. Schwartz became frustrated with the number of patients who developed recurrent *C. difficile* and were running out of treatment options. With Drs. Michael Gluck, Otto Lin, and Myint, and Mike Haas in Microbiology, Dr. Schwartz helped to start the fecal transplant program at VM for patients with recurrent *C. difficile* infection. Of three accomplishments at VM of which Dr. Schwartz is most proud, in no particular order, she would say that building a successful inpatient consultative ID service, treating many HIV patients over the years, and taking a part in building the *C. difficile* stool transplant service have been the most gratifying.

At VM Dr. Schwartz has been fortunate to work with several talented colleagues as the ID Section has grown. She has served as Section Head and Employee Health Co-medical Director, and served on committees including Infection Prevention, Antimicrobial Stewardship, and Immunization. She has been recognized as a top-50 teacher at VM, and has been recognized as a "Top Doctor" by her peers in the *Seattle Magazine* and *Seattle Met* surveys. Dr. Schwartz is proud of her consistently high patient satisfaction scores.

Robert Barnes, MD (2001 – 2007)

Rob Barnes joined Drs. Rakita and Schwartz in 2001, and worked at Virginia Mason until 2007. He did his infectious disease fellowship at the University of Washington, followed by training in the Epidemiology Intelligence Service (EIS) at the Center for Disease Control (CDC) from 1985-1987. He worked at the CDC as the Chlamydia/Mycoplasma Section Head in the STD Prevention Branch. After four years at CDC, he moved to Bellingham, where he worked in private practice infectious disease for the next 12 years. He was encouraged to join the ID Section at Virginia Mason by Dr. Rakita. The section did not have a full-time position at the time, so Dr. Barnes pursued additional training in hyperbaric medicine, eventually becoming board-certified. He thus provided VM with consultative services in both ID and hyperbaric medicine. In February of 2003, he was recalled to active duty for Operation Iraqi Freedom, and spent four months as Internal Medicine Department Head at the Naval Hospital Bremerton. He retired from the Navy and returned to VM in July of 2003. He provided HIV care, general infectious disease and hyperbaric consultations at Virginia Mason, and served as Medical Director of Employee Health until 2007 when he moved to Eugene, Oregon to finish his career at Peace Health.

Chia Wang, MD, MS (2007 – present)

Chia Wang was raised in the suburbs of New Jersey by parents who emigrated from China in the late 1950s. She attended college and medical school at Northwestern University in Chicago. After medical school she and her husband moved to Portland, Oregon for her internal medicine internship and residency at Oregon Health Sciences (OHSU). While she was a resident, she took a 6-month leave to volunteer in a remote region of Kenya, where she saw firsthand the tremendous negative health impacts that infectious diseases such as malaria, tuberculosis, and infectious diarrhea have on the world's population. After that experience she decided to specialize in infectious diseases, and was accepted to the infectious diseases fellowship at the University of Washington, where she also earned a Master's of Science in epidemiology. During her fellowship, she traveled back to Kenya, where she spent 18 months in Mombasa studying the heterosexual transmission of HIV. After being promoted to Assistant Professor of Medicine at the University of Washington, she co-founded the Hepatitis and Liver clinic at Harborview Medical Center and focused her research on viral hepatitis, obtaining several NIH grants to support her research. She stayed on the faculty at the University of Washington for nine years before joining VM's Infectious Disease Section in 2007. While a fellow and faculty member at UW, she authored more than 20 papers in peer-reviewed medical journals on HIV and viral hepatitis.

Since joining Virginia Mason, Dr. Wang has continued her commitment to treating patients with HIV, hepatitis B and C, and HIV/hepatitis B and C co-infection, working in both the Infectious Diseases and the Gastroenterology Sections seeing patients with these infections. She continues to be active in viral hepatitis research, serving as investigator on two NIH-funded studies on Hepatitis B, and has continued to publish in medical journals such as the *Journal of the American Medical Association* and *Hepatology*. In addition to her research and clinical responsibilities, Dr. Wang spends a substantial amount of her time working as the Medical Director of the Antimicrobial Stewardship Program, which she has headed since 2013. She truly enjoys this work, in part driven by a passion for optimizing antibiotic use to improve patient safety and outcomes, and in part because it allows her to collaborate with colleagues throughout the institution on projects to reduce *Clostridium difficile* infections or to update hospital order sets and guidelines to be in line with current medical literature. She has also served on other committees including the Institutional Review Board for Human Subjects Research and the Wilske Committee for Translational Research. She has been recognized as a top-50 teacher at VM, and also as a "Top Doctor" by her peers in the *Seattle Magazine* and *Seattle Met* surveys.

Dr. Wang enjoys being active in the community. She has been a member of the Hepatitis B Coalition of Washington since 1999, a collaboration of community-based organizations, community clinics, health-care facilities, and health departments to foster hepatitis B-related care through educational outreach, testing, and improved linkage to care services. Since 1999, she has also worked as a consulting physician at the International Community Health Services clinic in Seattle's International District, a nonprofit community health center that offers affordable health care services to Seattle and King County's medically-underserved community. Finally, Dr. Wang finds time to volunteer at Seattle public schools and sits on the board of Seattle Central Little League, hoping to improve our children's chances for success in life by giving them a solid education during the elementary and middle school years, and involving them in sports that are fun and foster teamwork and physical activity.

Uma Malhotra, MD (2008 – present)

Uma Malhotra has been a member in the section since 2008, although her history with the institution, as detailed below, began in 1988. She is active in both the clinical and research arenas, and has served as Medical Director for Employee Health. She is also faculty at the UW, serving as Clinical Associate Professor in the Department of Medicine.

She was born in New Delhi and received her MD from the All India Institute of Medical Sciences, the premier institution for medical training and research in the country. She then pursued a postdoctoral fellowship in T-cell immunology at the Benaroya Research Institute (1988 - 91), following which she completed her internship in internal medicine at Oregon Health Sciences University and residency at the California Pacific Medical Center in San Francisco (1991- 94). She returned to Seattle for a fellowship in infectious diseases at the UW (1995 - 98) and then assumed a faculty position at the UW/Fred Hutchinson until her move to VM in 2008.

Through her research at Fred Hutch she helped clarify barriers to the generation and maintenance of effective CD4+ T-cell help in HIV-1 infection. She played a lead role in developing a UW International AIDS Research and training Program (IARTP) site in New Delhi with independent and sustainable research capacities for the prevention and control of HIV. She took on an advisory role for graduate students in the immunology programs and continues to maintain active collaborations with physicians and scientists in India. She remains a regular invited speaker at the annual AIDS Society of India Conferences as well as the National Meeting of the HIV Congress in India, and has served on the organizing committees for these conferences.

After moving to VM in 2008 she continued studies of T-helper responses in collaboration with researchers at the Benaroya Research Institute (BRI), shifting her focus from HIV to influenza and flavivirus infections. In 2009 she was awarded a $7.5 million 5 year NIH contract with

Dr. Bill Kwok at the BRI to "Identify epitopes recognized by Influenza and Flavivirus responsive CD4+ T-cells following vaccination or natural infection." With the funding of this contract, infectious diseases became a major focus of research at BRI for the first time. She now serves as the Clinical Primary Investigator for the Infectious Diseases and Vaccine Registry at BRI. She has 35 publications in peer-reviewed journals and three book chapters.

Dr. Malhotra is a strong clinician and enthusiastic teacher. She has been voted among the top teachers as evaluated by the medicine residents, as well as "Top Doctor" in Seattle by peers in surveys conducted by both the *Seattle Weekly* and *the Seattle Met.* Her specific clinical interests include care of the immunocompromised host and she leads the transplant ID program at VM. Additionally she recently joined the care team at the newly opened wound clinic at VM downtown where she is able to bridge her interests in wound care and ID.

In 2013 she assumed the Medical Directorship for Employee Health (EH), sharing this position with Dr. Schwartz for the first two years and then assuming full responsibility for the role. She also serves on the Institutional Biosafety Committee at BRI, working closely with other members and the Occupational Health & Safety Specialist to develop protocols to ensure the safety of employees who work with biohazardous infectious agents and vectors in the laboratory. In 2016 she began serving as a liaison to support the Children's Hospital Employee and Occupational Health programs, helping them develop protocols to ensure the safety of employees and researchers at their institution as well.

Dr. Malhotra is particularly active in the community, first serving as a member of the Washington Governor's Advisory Council on HIV/AIDS in 2010-11. She then served as a member on the Research and Ethics Committee (REC) for PATH, an international organization driving transformative innovation to save lives and improve health, especially among women and children, working alongside countries in Africa and Asia; the REC members are charged with protecting the rights, safety, and welfare of human research participants (2013-16). Since 2015 she has served as a

Member of the One Health Antimicrobial Stewardship (AMS) Workgroup and the AMS Advisory Committee for the Department of Health (DOH), WA. The former is tasked with providing a comprehensive review of current state efforts, gaps, and needs to promote and implement AMS across human, animal, and environmental health in Washington State, while the latter focuses on activities pertaining specifically to human health care.

Michael Myint, MD, MBA, FACP, FIDSA (2009 – 2013)

Michael Myint was raised in Los Angeles, CA, and attended college at UCLA and medical school at Jefferson Medical College in Philadelphia. He did his internal medicine residency at the University of Wisconsin, Madison, and then moved to Seattle for his infectious disease Fellowship at the University of Washington. His research interest as a fellow was bacterial pathogenesis. After his fellowship, Dr. Myint joined the Polyclinic as an infectious disease consultant. While there, he also did work in hospital epidemiology and infection prevention at Swedish Hospital. After several years there, he joined Virginia Mason in late 2009. While at VM, in addition to providing consultative care in general infectious diseases and HIV care, he also served as Section Head of ID, Medical Director of Employee Health, Medical Director of Infection Prevention, and was a leader in antimicrobial stewardship. Dr. Myint has served as the President of the Infectious Disease Society of Washington. While working at VM, he went on to get his MBA at the University of Washington. He received awards for patient satisfaction at VM, being in the top 5% of Virginia Mason physicians. Dr. Myint left Virginia Mason in 2013 to become the Director of Quality and Safety at Swedish Hospital.

Harold Martin, MD (2011 – 2013)

Hal Martin was born and raised in North Carolina, where he attended Davidson College and the University of North Carolina Medical School. He moved to Seattle for his internal medicine residency, and stayed on to complete his infectious disease fellowship at the University of Washington. He has a clinical and research interest in HIV. After fellowship, Dr. Martin worked at Park Nicollet Clinic in Minnesota for over ten years before being recruited back to Seattle in 2011 to work at VM. After two years of providing excellent HIV and general infectious disease consultative care, Dr. Martin made a career move to the pharmaceutical industry. He now works for Gilead, a maker of HIV medications in San Francisco.

Christopher Baliga, MD (2013 – present)

Dr. Baliga was raised in Virginia and India. He attended college at the University of Virginia, and then medical school at Kasturba Medical College in India. He returned to the US for internship and residency in Internal Medicine at Case Western in Cleveland. He did a postdoctoral research fellowship at Baylor College of Medicine in Houston, and a fellowship in infectious diseases at the University of Washington. His research interests included HIV vaccine design. Before joining the VM Infectious Disease Section in 2013, he had previously worked at VM as a locums hospitalist and also did a 3-month stint as an infectious disease locums physician. Between his locums work at VM and joining the ID Section, Dr. Baliga worked in the Infectious Disease Section at Methodist Hospital in Houston, affiliated with Cornell Medical School, and then at Intermountain Healthcare in Utah. While there, Dr. Baliga developed an interest and expertise in infection prevention and antimicrobial stewardship, which was the perfect segue to taking on the role of Medical Director of Infection Prevention at VM when he joined VM in 2013. He hit the ground running, taking on this position while the story of infected endoscopes used for endoscopic retrograde cholangiopancreatography (ERCP) was unfolding. It was a daunting task, shared with the GI Section, Microbiology Laboratory and King County Public Health, which has led to important work in the area of reporting such infections, doing surveillance for resistant infections related to endoscopes, and designing protocols for endoscope cleaning, testing and "time outs" before they are put into use again.

In addition to his leadership role in infection prevention & control, Dr. Baliga took on the role of Section Head of Infectious Diseases in the fall of 2015. He has served on multiple additional committees at VM including the Residency Advisory Committee, Quality Assessment Committee, and the Hospital Acquired-Infection guiding team among many others. More recently, he has added Employee Health Medical Director to his responsibilities. He has been recognized as a top-50 teacher at VM, and as a "Top Doctor" by his peers in the *Seattle Magazine* and *Seattle Met* surveys.

Shingo Chihara, MD (2014 – present)

Dr. Chihara was born in Japan, and spent his childhood there, as well as in Puerto Rico and New Jersey. He attended Yamanashi Medical University in Japan, followed by a primary care internal medicine residency at the University of Connecticut, and an ID fellowship at Rush University Medical Center and John H Stroger Jr. Hospital of Cook County in Chicago. He did further training in medical microbiology at the University of Utah. In addition to being board-certified in internal medicine, infectious diseases, and medical microbiology, Dr. Chihara has done additional training in travel medicine and wound care. These skills have been put to good use as the Medical Director of Travel Medicine at Virginia Mason, and more recently in the newly established Wound Care Clinic at the VM Main Campus. He also became Associate Director of Microbiology to assist with duties in the microbiology laboratory.

Sophie Woolston, MD (2016 – 2019)

In 2016, Dr. Woolston joined the ID Section at Virginia Mason. Born and raised in Connecticut, she attended college at Wesleyan University, and then medical school and internal medicine residency at the University of Pennsylvania. She migrated west for an infectious disease fellowship at the University of Washington. There, her research and clinical interests were in general infectious diseases, Hepatitis C infection, HIV and telemedicine. She enjoyed her time with this enthusiastic group of colleagues, but moved to Portland, Maine in 2019 to be closer to family.

Robert E Geise MD, MPH (2019 – present)

Bob Geise joined Virginia Mason in the summer of 2019 after 12 years at EvergreenHealth in Kirkland, Washington. He was raised in Western New York and graduated from Cornell University, followed by an MBA in Finance at the University of Wisconsin. He spent 5 years as a financial consultant, specializing in the evaluation of failed financial institutions. He then returned to school and graduated in 1996 from the Virginia Commonwealth University (Medical College of Virginia) School of Medicine. He did his internal medicine internship, residency and chief residency at The George Washington University. He then made the move to the West Coast and Seattle for a fellowship in Infectious Diseases at the University of Washington. His research focused on acute HIV infection and the effects of early intervention. During his fellowship, he also earned a Master's in Public Health in Epidemiology at the University of Washington.

After fellowship, Dr. Geise worked for a year as an adult hospitalist for Group Health Cooperative before moving to California to work as an infectious disease physician in Monterey and Salinas, California. After 5 years, and with a toddler and new baby on the way, Dr. Geise returned to Seattle to be closer to family. He spent one year doing HIV vaccine research at the Fred Hutchinson Cancer Research Center through the HIV Vaccine Trial Network, as well as doing clinical care at the University of Washington Hospital and the Madison HIV clinic at Harborview Medical Center.

Dr. Geise then returned to private practice at EvergreenHealth in Kirkland, Washington. In addition to clinical care, he founded the hospital's wound clinic, growing it from three part-time nurses with no providers to a clinic with eight providers and ten nurses. He was also involved in medical staff leadership and was Medical Staff president from 2016 through 2018. He was recognized by his peers in 2019 with the EvergreenHealth Medical Staff Leadership and Innovation Award. He has been repeatedly recognized as a "Top Doctor" by peers in the *Seattle Met* surveys. Dr. Geise is a Fellow of the Infectious Disease Society of America.

Rebecca Maxim, RN (2016 – present)

Rebecca Maxim was born in Southern California and grew up in Arizona.

She moved to Seattle in 1977. She graduated from The Evergreen State College in 1982 with a liberal arts degree with emphasis on macroeconomics and French. She spent 1981 in France finishing her studies for Evergreen. She graduated from nursing school at Shoreline Community College in 1992, and worked at Harborview for a few years before taking a position in 1995 at Bailey Boushay House where she worked for 16 years. While at Bailey Boushay, she was one of the first five nurses in Washington State to take the AIDS-certified RN exam. She worked at Virginia Mason Employee Health before joining the Infectious Disease Clinic in 2016 as the first RN to work in the ID Clinic.

In 2004, Rebecca graduated from the Northwest Institute of Acupuncture and Oriental Medicine, and maintains her acupuncture license. After graduating from NIAOM, she went to India to volunteer in a Tibetan refugee clinic providing both acupuncture and nursing care. She taught a basic acupuncture class at the Tibetan school of Medicine in McCleod Ganj, India. In 2008 she went to Dhangadi, Nepal with Family Health International to work with providers and nurses to help establish local HIV clinics.

Lisa Roberts, PA-C (2018 – present)

Lisa was born and raised in Albuquerque, New Mexico. She attended college at the University of New Mexico where she studied Biology, Chemistry and Mathematics. While in college she worked in the LTER (long term ecological research) program and at the UNM Hospital in the Cardiology department.

Lisa attended PA school at Northeastern University in Boston and is certified in both primary care and surgery. She then pursued a career in critical care and surgery, where she spent much of the first half of her 22 years as a PA. Since then, she has been faculty at the University of Washington's PA program and has worked in Urgent Care and the Emergency Department. After seeing returning travelers with various concerns, she found she wanted to pursue a career in travel medicine and joined Virginia Mason's Travel Clinic in January 2018.

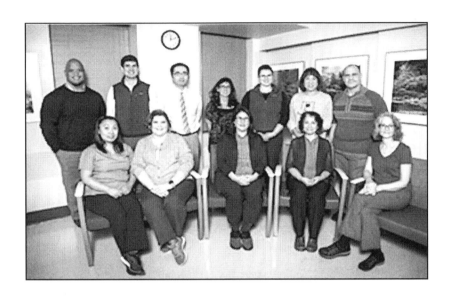

Infectious Disease Team 2019
Standing L to R: Fred DeLeon, clinic manager; Chris Baliga, MD;
Shingo Chihara, MD; Margot Schwartz, MD; Samantha Delmer, MA;
Chia Wang, MD; Bob Geise, MD
Seated, left to right: Venus Facun, MA; Inez Stone, MA;
Lisa Roberts, PA-C; Uma Malhotra, MD; Rebecca Maxim, RN

10

International Medical Services, 1970 –2010

by John Kirkpatrick, MD

Randolph Pillow, MD, who was recruited to The Mason Clinic in 1949 as an internist with a special interest in hematology, had a passion for travel, especially to the Pacific Rim. After his retirement in 1986, Dr. Pillow championed the concept of establishing relationships with physicians and hospitals in this region and in 1989, "VM launched its Center for Asian and International Medical Affairs (CAIMA), which later became known as the Department of International Medical Services." [1] These contacts "took on more formality with signed medical affiliation agreements" with Hong Kong Adventist, Samitivej Regional Hospital in Bangkok, Subang Jaya Medical Center in Malaysia, and Mt. St Elizabeth Hospital in Singapore. Dr. Pillow, the ultimate "VM ambassador", made frequent visits to key Asian physicians and was instrumental in bringing prominent patients to Seattle for care, as well as prominent physicians to VM for weeks of education with VM faculty. Internists were welcomed in VM's Diabetes "School", and foreign surgeons spent time in cardiac surgery and general surgery. Grateful patients supported VM's Foundation and referred friends and relatives, who in turn supported other humanitarian programs helped by VM physicians. All of this would not have happened without the individual efforts of Dr. Pillow. Dr. Pillow was also the official physician of the Seattle Seafair hydroplane races, and a benefactor of the Washington Athletic Club, where, while serving as its president, he personally financed the acquisition of a much-needed downtown parking lot when their balance sheet didn't have sufficient funds. He was truly a remarkable civic-minded and internationally-focused man. (See the history of the Hematology/Oncology Section in this volume for more details).

Ty Hongladarom, MD, was also instrumental in developing relationships with Thai physicians who came to Virginia Mason for training in surgery and internal medical specialties such as diabetes care, oncology and pulmonary medicine. Drs. **Steve Kirtland** and **Albert Einstein** traveled to Thailand to provide consultations in pulmonary medicine and oncology respectively.

Relationships in Tokyo included the Tokyo Medical-Surgical Clinic in partnership with Dr. Kenji Fujii. Japanese interpreter **Suzy Martin** headed interpretation services and physical exams were done for the many Japanese companies who had offices here in Seattle. **Dan Berge** was hired to be Director of International Medical Services – his bilingual capability in Japanese was very helpful. **Keith Lundberg,** administrator extraordinaire, took on administrative responsibility in addition to his duties in Regional Medical Services and the Hospital Consortium. Under his leadership and with the contacts established by Dr. Pillow, VMMC was selected to be the medical provider for the Asia-Pacific Economic Cooperation forum (APEC) meeting held in Seattle in 1994. Whenever the world leaders were together, VM provided an emergency room physician and a surgeon on site to respond directly should any medical situation arise. VM worked closely with the U.S. State Department and then the White House staff as the World and President Bill Clinton came to Seattle. A clinic was staffed in the Westin for the delegates and managed a number of medical issues that arose over the 5 days of the meeting. Numerous stories are still told, including the difficulty of finding a tube of ChapStick® (it had to be black) for the Sultan of Brunei at the retreat on Blake Island (thank goodness for the Boeing yacht!), and the challenge of finding a physician to give a flu shot to the Secretary of State of Mexico - a nurse just wasn't good enough for him!

Virginia Mason physicians joined many international organizations including the Japan America Society, World Affairs Council, the Washington State China Relations Council and the Korean American Society. Further involvement was assured with the formation of the Asian American Clinical Program when internal medicine residents **Karen Ting, MD** (Malaysia); **Leslie Lu, MD** (Taiwan); **Yoo Jin Chong, MD** (Korea); and **Maribeth Chong, MD** (Philippines) formed a subsection in General Internal Medicine headed by the Medical Director of International Medical Services, **John Kirkpatrick, MD.** They hired bilingual staff in Mandarin Chinese, Vietnamese, Cantonese Chinese, Japanese, Korean and Pilipino Tagalog, Laotian and Thai. Each of the providers became heavily involved in their ethnic community and bilingual pre-history forms were developed and utilized widely.

In 1997, Dr. John Kirkpatrick was invited to go on Washington Governor Gary Locke's first trade mission to China – he was the lone physician in the 70-member delegation that visited Beijing, Shanghai and Chengdu. Further involvement in the China Relations Council ensued and Dr. Kirkpatrick was subsequently invited to go on the Governor's second trade mission in 2003. This trip was slated to go to Guangzhou, where SARS (Severe Acute Respiratory Syndrome) had started less than one year before. The world had been stunned by the sudden appearance of this rapidly fatal disease that often affected the caregivers (doctors and nurses) who had treated those afflicted with it. Preparing for the worst, contact was made with the CDC in Atlanta, as well as their representatives in Beijing, Shanghai and Guangzhou. Fortunately SARS did not reappear after 2002, as the source was determined to be the wild animal markets and appropriate measures were taken. Meanwhile, Keith Lundberg went on a trade mission to Korea and many physicians continued to come to VM from multiple countries including mainland China - heart surgeon Dr. Frank Hsu spent an entire year with Drs. **Richard Anderson** and **Dan Paull** in cardiac surgery. Dr. Kirkpatrick was able to visit Dr. Hsu in the Shanghai Chest Hospital where he very eagerly showed what he had learned with his successful outcomes in ICU patients (still very primitive by American standards with no curtains between patients in a 12-bed ward). During this period, **Mark Wen** (native of Harbin, China) became Director, and involvement with China expanded with visits to Hong Kong and Taiwan to recruit patients for VM's bilingual Chinese doctors.

The Russian Far East

In the mid-90s, VMMC Chairman **Roger Lindeman, MD**, was invited to a meeting in the Russian Far East city of Khabarovsk. At that time, Alaska Airlines was flying to Khabarovsk, Sakhalin Island and Vladivostok. He was impressed with the medical needs of the area and a several year humanitarian effort was launched involving about 20 Virginia Mason doctors and staff. Early visitors included endocrinologist **Paul Fredlund, MD**; nephrologist **Bob Wilburn, MD**; urologist **Tom Hefty, MD**, and orthopaedist **Tom Green, MD**. About 25 Russian physicians in many specialties came to Seattle over several years of cooperative efforts led by Keith Lundberg, Mark Wen and Russian native and chief interpreter, **Polina Roytberg**. A particularly arduous task involved hosting the team assembled to learn how to do kidney transplants. Keith and Polina had interpreters for the paired transplant surgeons, nephrologists, anesthesiologists, scrub nurses and recovery room nurses. Tom Hefty and Bob Wilburn with their Russian counterparts performed and managed several kidney transplants over a three-week period while they stayed in Seattle (housed at the Cassel Crag apartments) and also went to Khabarovsk to see how this procedure was going to work there. **Ken Freeman** from materials management assembled all of the necessary instruments and was subsequently involved in helping them purchase other much needed medical equipment. The Russian physicians also willingly and graciously accepted any outmoded equipment, including cardiac monitoring devices, as they were replaced at Virginia Mason by newer technology. Although considered outmoded, everything was 10 years newer than what they had. **Brad Schmidt** from our engineering department was sent to teach them how to fix and service anything that had been donated. The motto was always, "Help them to help themselves" and it guided everything that was done – there were too many examples of used equipment donated (or dumped) from other institutions just sitting idle in the corner, having broken down with no one knowing anything about repair.

Dr. Tom Green set a wonderful example of the strategy as he sought to teach a young Russian orthopaedist Vladimir Sapezhnikov how to do arthroscopy. He convinced an arthroscopy equipment company Linvatec to donate TWO complete sets of equipment and brought the company representative with him to Khabarovsk to teach them not only how to use the devices, but also how to repair them if they broke down. Vladimir made several trips to Seattle and stayed with Dr. Green. Tom also made several trips to Khabarovsk to mentor his prized pupil. The result was not only a new procedure becoming available to the people of the Russian Far East, but also a lifelong friendship for these doctors and their associates. Of course, Dr. Sapezhnikov is now teaching the techniques to young orthopaedists there.

Other VM physicians who traveled to Russia included gastroenterologists **Jim Bredfeldt, MD**, and **Jack Brandabur, MD,** and orthopaedist **Lyle Sorensen, MD**. All were impressed with the basic medical knowledge of the Russian physicians, but their woeful facilities hampered their development. They warmly received our donations of time, experience and supplies and made the VM visitors feel most welcome in their homes and hospitals. All learned some incredible life lessons and virtually every VM person who traveled there came back humbled by the experience, in awe of the efforts of the dedicated Russian physicians who were forced to treat very sick people with extremely limited resources.

At about this same time, a very forward-thinking young Russian psychiatrist, Anatoly Chubakov, made contact with Keith Lundberg and **John Eusek** (radiology director). Dr. Chubakov had obtained an MRI scanner, the first in the Russian Far East, through a deal with India. It was his idea that he could take brain MRI's, make digital images of them, and send them over the internet to physicians in the US, who could comment on them and help their counterparts in Sakhalin. John Eusek took it upon himself to build the website to do this. Keith got a $12,000 digital camera donated by the Soros Foundation and traveled with John Kirkpatrick and Eusek to Sakhalin to help launch this technology. Images of brain tumors on MRI's were beamed through a server set up in Sakhalin to VM's **Charlie Nussbaum, MD**, in neurosurgery and **John Rieke, MD**, in radiation oncology, and pictures of ECG tracings were sent for interpretation to **Chris Fellows. MD.** These physicians sent their diagnoses and suggestions back to Russia by email – an innovation from Team Medicine at VMMC in the early days of telemedicine. The people of Sakahlin benefited greatly from the generosity of VMMC physicians and staff.

These are just a few examples of international medical cooperation sponsored by VM. In addition, individual physicians have given their personal time and skills to help the less fortunate in many areas around the world. A few examples include cleft palate surgery utilizing the talents of plastic surgeons **Dave Zehring, MD**, and **Craig Murakami, MD** (Cambodia), and anesthesiologists **Mani Batra, MD**, and **Brian Owens, MD**. Tom Green has long supported an orphanage in Honduras and formed a team to help with the orthopaedic injuries in the earthquake in Haiti – anesthesiologist **Peter Ackerman, MD**; orthopaedist Lyle Sorenson, MD; **Derek Gallichotte, PA-C** and **Merry O'Barr, RN** were on this team that performed over 300 operations in 3 weeks on the casualties (see the Orthopaedic chapter for more information in volume 2). Cytopathologists **Nick Agoff, MD,** and **Katherine Galagan, MD**, both spent time evaluating Pap smears at a cervical cancer screening clinic in Cuzco, Peru, and there are many other examples, some known and probably many more that are unknown. These "volunteers" have not sought recognition or remuneration, using their own vacation time to answer the call for help and receiving in return the gratification that comes with assisting those in need with the talents (and educational advantages) that one has been given.

References:

1. Ross A. *The First 75 Years, Virginia Mason Medical Center, 1920-1995*. Seattle, WA: Virginia Mason Medical Center; 1995.

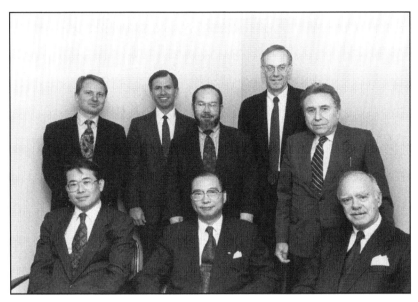

International Medical Group 1993
Standing L to R: Dan Berge, International Medical Services Director, Keith
Lundberg, David Dreis, John Kirkpatrick, Randy Pillow
Seated L to R: Consul Chul Kang, Consul General Hae-Soon Lee,
Robert Buck, Chairman, VMMC Board of Governors (PH 6758, VMHA)

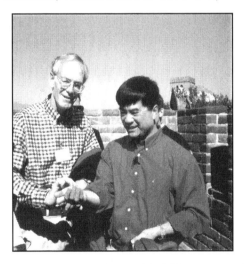

"Virginia Mason physician John Kirkpatrick, MD, accompanied Gov. Gary
Locke on his trade mission to promote Washington state business interests in
China. In the above photo, Dr. Kirkpatrick takes the governor's pulse after
climbing to the top of the Great Wall."
Virginia Mason Magazine, Winter 1998 (PH 9135, VMHA)

11

Nephrology and
Renal Transplantation

by Robert Wilburn, MD, and Cyrus Cryst, MD

Nephrology at Virginia Mason Medical Center (VMMC), like most areas of medicine and surgery, developed progressively from a concatenation of medical and surgical advances with adaptation to those advances.

Nephrology at VMMC was originally part of Endocrinology. **Richard Paton, MD**, was the first nephrologist and came to the clinic in 1960, having been part of the University of Washington's first medical school class. He then did his residency at Massachusetts General, Harborview and the Seattle Veteran's Administration Hospital. He brought with him expertise in fluid balance and electrolytes (especially potassium, which had been a hard-to-measure intracellular ion), and hypertension.

Robert Hegstrom, MD, came to The Mason Clinic in 1964. He had gone to medical school and residency at the University of Washington (UW) and then joined their nephrology faculty, working with Belding Scribner, MD, on the further development of chronic dialysis, which had begun at the UW in the 1960s. It was at the time of Dr. Hegstrom's arrival that Nephrology was split off as a separate section from Endocrinology.

The field of nephrology was changing rapidly in the Seattle area and nationally with development of acute dialysis, peritoneal dialysis, and the Scribner shunt allowing chronic dialysis, followed by living-related and cadaveric renal transplantation. With these changes came a series of technical, surgical and medical advances.

Burton Orme, MD, joined the staff of VMMC in 1969 after medical school at Washington University in St. Louis, followed by internship and residency at Emory University Hospitals and a two-year fellowship in nephrology at the University of Washington.

Dr. Orme, along with Dr. Hegstrom, established acute and chronic dialysis at Virginia Mason. This was not an easy task, but they were aided by tremendous teamwork and talented help. Medicare coverage of the End-Stage Renal Disease Program in 1972 was a tremendous boost to the development of this program. Peritoneal dialysis had already been instituted at Virginia Mason by Drs. Paton and Hegstrom, and was performed by the intensive care unit (ICU) nursing staff. By 1970, it was obvious that Virginia Mason needed acute hemodialysis for patients in renal failure. Initially, ICU nurses were sent to the Northwest Kidney Center (NWKC) for training and twin-coil disposable dialysis machines were used, but it became obvious that to maintain proficiency, a dedicated team was necessary. An Army nurse with dialysis experience, **Sukie**, and an orderly with previous experience as a dialysis technician at the NWKC, **Tom Strang,** provided tremendous esprit de corps and entrepreneurship, which allowed us to develop into a functional unit. **Patricia Paton, RN** had previously run a dialysis unit and brought professional and efficient management skills. With a tremendously devoted staff, we provided inpatient dialysis care and hemofiltration for Virginia Mason patients for many years. This service was later taken over by staff from the NWKC, who continue to provide inpatient dialysis in VMMC. Chronic outpatient dialysis, both in-center and at home, is now provided by the NWKC. Virginia Mason nephrologists continue to manage the nephrology and dialysis care of patients being dialyzed in NWKC units.

As the care of end-stage renal disease developed, transplantation became the preferred treatment for many patients. Tremendous advances in tissue typing, immunosuppression therapy, and our understanding of immunology hastened this treatment option. The Sections of Nephrology and Urology, along with the nursing staff, became a team to provide this service to patients. Drs. **Robert Gibbons** and Burton Orme, along with Pat Paton, worked together to write the first orders for transplant patients when it was realized that a standardized order set was required. This was developed with input from not only physicians and surgeons but also from the laboratory, nursing and pharmacy. With the development of transplant registries, tissue typing, antibody sensitization etc., came the realization that a computer database was necessary to keep track of all the necessary information. This lead to the first rudimentary transplant database developed by **Miriam Cressman, RN** and Dr. Orme. Miriam became the first transplant coordinator. Gradually, this evolved into a coordinated electronic record with modem, and then internet access.

Robert Wilburn, MD, joined Virginia Mason in 1975 having gone to medical school at the University of Nebraska, followed by an internal medicine residency at Virginia Mason, and then a nephrology and transplantation fellowship at Harbor General/UCLA in Los Angeles from 1973 - 1975. Dr. Wilburn became medical cirector of the renal and pancreatic transplant service.

Catherine Thompson, MD, joined Virginia Mason in 1992 after receiving her medical degree – followed by an internal medicine internship and residency along with a nephrology fellowship – at University of Texas Medical School in Houston. She worked in all areas of nephrology, serving as medical director of peritoneal dialysis for many years for NWKC, and starting the section's clinical presence in Federal Way. She retired from nephrology in 2018.

Over the years, the section has established a referral base from Alaska, Montana and Washington, initially using site visits by Drs. Wilburn and **George Brannon, MD**, transplant surgeon, and Miriam Cressman, RN, transplant coordinator. The site visits allowed team members to meet with referring nephrologists, office and dialysis-unit nurse teams, and potential transplant patients and their families. We established methods to share post-transplant care with their referring nephrologist, which minimized required follow-up visits in Seattle each year.

In the 1980s, Virginia Mason had become the largest transplant center in Washington state and among the 25 largest in the United States. We were the first Seattle transplant center to perform 1,000 renal transplants. Our patient and graft survival data exceeded national risk-adjusted results. Our average length of stay was the shortest in Washington state and charges per transplant admit were the lowest. None of this would have been possible without a team of transplant nurse coordinators who were on the front line working with patients and families to coordinate care. (The transplant surgeons are discussed in more depth in the Urology chapter in Volume 2.)

After approximately 20 years as medical director of the transplant service, Dr. Wilburn passed his transplant leadership role first to **Cyrus Cryst, MD**, then to **Andrew Weiss, MD**, who continues as medical director of the renal and pancreas transplant service along with transplant surgeon **Christian Kuhr, MD.** The program has an in-office staff of 25 with eight nurse transplant coordinators, in addition to managers, social workers, dieticians, pharmacists and support staff.

In the 1990s, Virginia Mason, along with UW and Swedish, was selected as one of seven international teams to perform pancreatic islet cell transplants. This involved isolating the islets and then infusing them into the liver along with a standardized immunosuppressant protocol. Preliminary trials had been hopeful that the islets would produce insulin and respond to blood-sugar levels like native islet cells and control insulin-dependent diabetes. Unfortunately, the longevity of functional islets was short and the study was declared a failure and sent back to bench research for further study.

Dr. Wilburn started our section presence in Port Angeles in the late 1990s as medical director of the NWKC Port Angeles dialysis unit, and started doing consultations and follow-up with the growing number of renal transplant patients in the Port Angeles area, which he continued for nearly 15 years. When Dr. Wilburn retired in 2011, Cyrus Cryst, MD (see below), in addition to serving as Section Head, took over in Port Angeles, greatly expanding the work done there. He now travels two days per week both to see consults and follow the growing number of Virginia Mason dialysis and transplant recipient patients in his capacity as medical director of the NWKC dialysis unit.

In the last 15 years, the section has continued to grow. Members now provide nephrology care in the regional medical centers, including **Maria Salazar, MD**, and **Dona Wu, MD, PhD**, at Virginia Mason Federal Way; **Michael Sutters, MD**, at Virginia Mason Edmonds Family Medicine; and **Ahmad Mahallati, MD**, at Virginia Mason Bellevue (see below).

A review of the history of nephrology and transplantation at Virginia Mason over the past 59 years would not be complete without some reflection on how the life of nephrologist at VM has changed and evolved.

In the 1960s and early 1970s, all of our practice was in the downtown clinic and hospital. There were no "regional medical centers". All records were paper. There was no digital record. A clinic or hospital note might be a few handwritten lines limited to information relevant to care of the patient. There were no pagers or cell phones. If on call, one had to be sure to have a pocket of quarters and know where the nearest phone booth was located. How quaint.

Lunch hour was often a walk down to the waterfront for fish and chips at Ivars or a bag lunch in Freeway Park to visit and listen to music. All of which are admittedly selective nostalgic memories. Suffice it to say, it was a different world in which we practiced.

Fast Forward to 2020

Our section now has six nephrologists, two allied health professionals, one full-time pharmacist and many others:

Cyrus Cryst, MD, FASN, Section Head, joined Virginia Mason in 1992 after medical school at the University of Chicago Pritzkar School of medicine, an internal medicine residency at Virginia Mason, and a fellowship in nephrology at Tufts Medical Center in Boston.

Ahmad Mahallati, MD, joined Virginia Mason in 2011 after medical school at the Shiraz University of Medical Sciences, in Shiraz, Iran, followed by residencies in internal medicine at Harbor Hospital, Baltimore and as a transplant hospitalist at University of Maryland Medical Center, and a fellowship in nephrology at University of Michigan, Ann Arbor.

Maria Nieva Salazar, MD, joined Virginia Mason in 2016 following medical school in the Philippines and then an internal medical residency at the University of Connecticut and nephrology fellowship at the Medical University of South Carolina, Charleston, SC.

Michael Sutters, MD, MRCP, joined Virginia Mason in 2008 after earning his medical degree from the Imperial College, St Mary's Hospital, London, England; a bachelor's in physiology from St. Peter's College, Oxford University, England; an internship at St. Mary's hospital, London; residencies in internal medicine, Kansas University Medical Center, Kansas City; cardiology, internal medicine and nephrology at Addenbrook's and Papworth Hospitals, Cambridge, UK; and neurology and nephrology at St. Mary's Hospital, London UK. He then entered fellowships in the United States, including nephrology at Kansas University Medical Center and nephrology at Oregon Health Sciences, Portland, OR, and worked as a visiting scientist at Yale University School of Medicine.

Andrew Weiss, MD, joined Virginia Mason in 2009 after receiving his medical degree from the University of Virginia, followed by an internal medicine residency at the University of Colorado (UC), and fellowships in nephrology and AST/ASN (American Society of Transplantation/American Society of Nephrology) renal transplantation, also at UC.

Dona Tsihwa Wu, MD, PhD, joined VM in 2017 after receiving her MD/PhD, from Albert Einstein Medical College in New York and attending Harvard College. She did her renal transplant training at Emory University before joining our section.

Amy Lavaveshkul, PA-C, keeps our hospital service humming.

Sarah Lai, ARNP, sees our dialysis patients in the units and helps out in the hospital as well.

Rachel Waite, PharmD, is our full-time clinical pharmacist who reviews drug levels, refills and does teaching, injections, and prescription authorizations.

Karlie Wipperling, MBA, FACMPE, has been Director of Transplant and Nephrology now for over 10 years and is the steady hand handling the business and regulation challenges.

In addition, we have many indispensable staff in transplant and in our nephrology clinic. We hold nephrology/transplant clinics at the main campus, and in Federal Way, Lynnwood, Bellevue and Port Angeles as we have expanded north, south, east and west, with the largest presence in Federal Way.

The electronic medical record (EMR) is now fully integrated and all messaging, ordering, scheduling, charting, patient follow-up notes, and most of the MD-to-MD, communication occurs in the EMR. The expectation of rapid email communication with patients adds hours to every day's work. The speed of communication and interdependence of specialists and primary providers to provide care to patients with ESRD and transplants has increased the pace of our practice tremendously compared to the previous description of the early days of Virginia Mason nephrology.

Now, in addition to other activities, the nephrologist spends seven to eight discontinuous hours each day in front of dual flat-screens responding to information and inquiries, seeing patients in between. All clinic visits are done with a computer in the room. Space downtown has not increased, so we have up to three physicians shoulder-to-shoulder in one office. We also all work standing up in the hallways at computer stations. One of us has a treadmill desk. Our clinic schedules are always full. The vacation schedule is made 12 months in advance. Email and computerized records review takes 90-120 minutes a day. Covering for an out-of-office physician takes as long as 90 minutes of additional work a day. And some of us have to use multiple medical records to get necessary information and results.

The challenge is how to contain the workday.

We live in interesting times. Stay tuned and hang on.

The one guaranteed constant is that we will never allow ourselves to be distracted from providing the best possible medical care for our patients – which is always given with compassion and respect for the patient and their family, and always includes sharing complete information and decision-making with the patient and family.

This has not changed in the last 59 years and must never be allowed to.

12

The Neuroscience Institute:
Neurology and Neurosurgery

by James MacLean, MD, and Katherine Galagan, MD
with contributions from Farrokh Farrokhi, MD, and Sally Cramer, RN
(Note: This chapter appears in Vol. 2 as well)

The Beginnings: 1934 - 1964

The Neuroscience Institute at Virginia Mason Medical Center began as the Section of Neurosurgery with a conversation in Chicago in 1934 between James Tate Mason, MD, one of the original founders of The Mason Clinic in 1920, and Hale Haven, MD, PhD, who at that time was a senior resident in neurosurgery studying with Loyal Davis, MD, in Chicago, Illinois. Dr. Haven had been recommended by Dr. Davis, who was the head of Neurosurgery at Northwestern University and was regarded as a national leader in Neurosurgery.

Hale Haven became the original physician in Neurosurgery at The Mason Clinic in 1934, and was the only member of the section until 1958 when he was joined by John Tytus, MD, also a neurosurgeon. Dr. Haven practiced both Neurology and Neurosurgery and founded the electroencephalography (EEG) laboratory. The Section of Neurology began when Paul Altrocchi, MD, joined Haven and Tytus in 1962, specializing in Neurology. He was at the clinic only one year and left because of a "preference for academic medicine" in September 1963, assuming an academic position in Neurology at Stanford University. The position in Neurology was quickly filled, however, when Dr. Tytus reached out to his close colleague at the University of Washington, Dr. Arthur Ward, who was Chief of Neurosurgery at the time. This led to the recruitment of Richard Birchfield, MD, an academic neurologist on the University staff, who joined the Clinic in 1964. Ed Reifel, MD, was recruited to the section of Neurosurgery in the same year. With these additions, the two sections worked as a team to provide the full spectrum of neurological care at the clinic, eventually formally joining to become the Department of Neurosciences.

It was also in this year that Dr. Haven tragically died of pancreatic cancer at the age of 61. Dr. Tytus took over as section head and worked with Dr. Birchfield, who had become Section Head of Neurology when he was hired. The two clinical sections began an expansion strategy (that continues to this day), of recruiting high quality clinicians, often with academic medical backgrounds, to provide the full spectrum of neurologic and neurosurgical care to VM patients. Dr. Tytus led this effort by melding the two sections into a team with the partnership of Dr. Birchfield; the initial plan was to support the three-legged mission of the clinic with high quality medical care, active engagement in research with production of peer-reviewed publications, and the training of young physicians. The strategy also included encouraging participation in regional and national specialty societies. Dr. Tytus, as mentioned, had an especially close relationship with Dr. Arthur Ward, Chief of Neurosurgery at the University, which was primarily responsible for the great collegial relationship with the University's Neuroscience Department that has continued to this day.

Early Growth Years: 1965 - 1970s

Drs. Tytus and Birchfield began a new era by significantly expanding both services in the areas of clinical practice, teaching, participation in national specialty societies and clinical research. Dr. Birchfield recruited Dr. David Fryer in 1965. Dr. Fryer, like Dr. Birchfield, had also served as an instructor in Medicine (Neurology) at the University. James MacLean, MD, also a neurologist, joined the section soon thereafter in 1968. Both Drs. Tytus and Birchfield insisted on open communication between the two sections, using immediate "hallway" consults, formal combined section conferences, partnerships in hospital clinical practice and combined clinical courses in neurosurgery and neurology that were held at the Clinic for our physician referral base as well as our in-house residents. A close partnership was maintained with the divisions of Neurosurgery and Neurology at the University of Washington.

The growth plan also focused on recruitment of companion services vital to the clinical practices of both sections including special expertise in neuroradiology, neurotology, neuropathology, psychiatry, rehabilitation medicine, neuro-ophthalmology, neuro-oncology, and medicine. Conferences were organized so that critical cross communication between all practitioners occurred assuring the maximum quality of individual patient care. Initially, the basic trio of skull films, lumber puncture with cerebrospinal fluid (CSF) analysis and EEGs formed the core laboratory data for both practices, assisted by pneumoencephalography and later, brain scans. In the early days, besides this basic battery of testing, the primary diagnostic tool was the clinical neurological examination at the bedside. This continues to be important but has been greatly assisted by the more recent technological advances in laboratory and radiologic medicine. During this time, the combined sections were on the fourth floor of the Buck Pavilion next to Hematology (with Drs. Pillow, Huff and Ragen).

Era of Enhanced Technologies and Expanded Therapeutic Options: 1970s – 1998

The sections of Neurosurgery and Neurology nearly doubled in size during these years, and as they grew, the focus became more specialized for each group. Still, communication between the two sections was imperative and weekly Neurology/Neurosurgery conferences with complete case presentations were developed coupled with weekly Neuroradiology conferences, where multiple active case studies were reviewed. A separate tumor conference with Oncology was developed to allow review of active patient strategies for therapy and follow-up timing. Supporting specialties that were and continue to be crucial to clinical success in the Neurosciences included Neuroradiology (Ted Margolis, MD, and Burt Crane, MD); Ophthalmology (John Mensher, MD); Otolaryngology (Roger Lindeman, MD; Charles Mangham, MD; Douglas Backous, MD); Neuropathology from the University with monthly conferences (Drs. Alvord, Shaw and Sumi); Oncology (Al Einstein, MD; Bob Rudolph, MD; Vince Picozzi, MD, and David Aboulafia, MD); Vascular Surgery (Jock Beebe, MD; Mondo Raker, MD, and Terry Quigley, MD); Psychiatry (Ted Rynearson, MD; Steve Melson, MD, and Peter Manos, MD); and Physical Medicine and Rehabilitation (Ty Hongladarom, MD; David Fordyce, PhD, etc.).

Outside conferences, including neurology/neurosurgery courses, were expanded and attracted multiple referral physicians from the community as well as our own house staff officers. There was also development of a regional clinical Neuroradiology Conference at Virginia Mason, which was attended by neurologists and neurosurgeons from all over the region, including the University, Swedish Hospital, Everett, Mt. Vernon, Olympia, etc. These physicians would bring their own cases and films for all to review under the leadership of Drs. Ted Margolis and Burt Crane in Neuroradiology. There were also two annual meetings of the National Walsh Society Neuro-ophthalmology Symposium at The Mason Clinic in partnership with physicians from the University of Washington, which included several days of case presentations with clinical input from multiple neuro-ophthalmologists from all over the US.

During this time, numerous advancements in multiple technologies were introduced to the sections, including diagnostic tools allowing quicker and more precise information about the location and nature of the pathological process, as well as multiple new surgical techniques and medication developments, allowing for greatly expanded therapeutic options. The practice model that the two sections had developed was a core asset: a detailed clinical history followed by a highly focused bedside neurology examination resulting in an evaluation plan (including the use and design of important investigational studies) coupled with an immediate exchange of ideas between the members of both sections. This approach led to efficient and complete assessments, which remain the key to high quality neurology and neurosurgery care at VMMC to this day.

In 1990, the sections moved from a less than adequate space on the 4th floor of the Buck Pavilion to the 7th floor of the Lindeman Pavilion, which provided a much more efficient work environment, and accommodated the growth that both sections were experiencing. The original location was especially a concern in the early days, as many trips a day were necessary to review neuroradiology studies with radiologists during a busy day seeing clinic patients. With the modern availability of radiologic imaging on clinic computer desktops, this became less of a concern. The digital age also greatly accelerated clinical assessments with the ability to rapidly review all of the prior clinical data on the computer record, thus eliminating the often frustratingly slow delivery of a large chart coming from some remote area of the clinic with both the patient and physician waiting.

The new location was also important for quick access to the hospital from the clinic during emergency situations with a full clinic schedule. This evolved over the years from having one physician at a time focusing on the urgent hospital needs, then to the concept of one neurologist devoted full-time to hospital neurology, and finally to the development of a neuro-hospitalist subspecialty position.

The separate support staffs were always essential to both sections with great assistance not only from nurses and eventually ARNPs and PA-Cs, but also from the multiple laboratory staff assisting in electroencephalography, vestibular studies, electromyography, and radiology. The office assistant was crucial to success as they were the "face" of the clinic to all patients, in addition to their importance in assisting each of the physicians with their hour-by-hour needs during a busy clinical day, and of course, scheduling, which was a major driver of the day. Annual joint Christmas parties were a time to express how important all of the support staff were to the overall success of both sections throughout the year.

The two sections were also extensively involved in the teaching mission of the clinic with daily contact with Virginia Mason interns and residents, as well as rotating house officers from the University of Washington. Many of the physicians also participated with the University department and had attending assignments at University Hospital, Harborview Hospital,

Children's Orthopedic Hospital and the Veteran's Administration Hospital, all in Seattle. In addition, with the development of numerous clinic satellites in the region, consultations, frequently in person, were given on subspecialty clinical cases in Port Angeles, Kirkland, and Federal Way.

Developments in the Section of Neurosurgery

As mentioned, the Neurosurgery Section grew during these years, going from 2 to 3 physicians. Jim Raisis, MD, was hired in 1976, anticipating the retirement of Dr. Tytus in 1978. When Dr. Raisis left in 1989, Leroy Dart, MD, an established neurosurgeon, replaced him for 2 years. Paul Maurer, MD, was hired in 1990 as the new section head, but was delayed a year because of a military commitment. However, he had insisted that Charles Nussbaum, MD, his chief resident, also be hired, and so Dr. Nussbaum joined the group in 1990 ahead of Dr. Maurer's arrival, eventually becoming section head himself in 1994. Dr. Maurer ended up staying less than 2 years, resulting in Stephen Klein, MD, joining the department in 1993. He stayed for 3 years; John Hsiang, MD, and Peter Nora, MD, replaced him and Dr. Reifel in 1997 and 1998 respectively, when Dr. Reifel retired in 1998.

Although spine surgery remained the most frequent procedure in neurosurgery, therapeutic advances in neurosurgery were extensive during this period of time with the development of transsphenoidal pituitary surgery and movement disorder surgery. Extrapyramidal surgery was greatly enhanced with the use of subcortical electrodes coupled with more precise neuroimaging techniques in order to perform selective therapy for movement disorders. The introduction of surgical magnification scopes improved aneurysm surgery and cerebral tumor removal. Clivus entry for certain posterior fossa lesions became a new avenue for surgical approach to the brain stem and cerebellar lesions. Improvements and specialization in neurosurgical anesthesia were essential for safer surgical therapies as well. Even the area of spine surgery saw advances in hardware, and new techniques and approaches developed around spinal instrumentation.

Also of critical importance was the development of the CT scanner.

173

John Walker, MD, who was Chairman of the Clinic at the time, went to a meeting of the International Society of Radiology in 1973 where they were unveiling the EMI head computed tomography (CT) scanner. Dr. Tytus "polled members of the Clinic while (he) was en route" and then called him there, "urging him to put in an order if possible", which he did (see Radiology chapter in volume 2). As a result, in 1974, The Mason Clinic had the first CT scanner in the Northwest. They would have another first in 1983, when they installed the first MRI scanner on the west coast.

Developments in the Section of Neurology

The Section of Neurology continued to grow with the recruitment of Jim Coatsworth, MD (1973 – 1998) and Laird Patterson, MD (1976 – 2004). For a time, pediatric neurology was also part of the section with the addition of Stephen Glass, MD (1982 – 1989) and Brien Vlcek, MD (1984 – 1989). John Ravits joined the section in 1986 and Lynne Taylor, MD, arrived in 1988. During this time, it was decided that it was not only crucial for all physicians in the section to be able to provide all of the general services in their specialty, but that sub-specialization should be encouraged to provide cutting-edge clinical neuroscience expertise. This would allow these physicians to couple subspecialty training during their residencies with ever-expanding clinical experience in their specific areas of focus. In Neurology, the originating members all provided general services but each developed special areas of expertise over the years and became the go-to person for specific sub-specialty problems. Dr. Birchfield developed a special interest in extrapyramidal disorders along with epilepsy and multiple sclerosis. He also developed a neurological examination-training manual that was very helpful in the teaching mission of the section. Dr. Fryer was a very knowledgeable clinical neurologist and had special expertise is psychiatric conditions impacting the neurological examination and masquerading as a primary neurological disorder, along with a vast understanding of historical neurology. Dr. Coatsworth was especially proficient in epilepsy diagnosis and management, having acquired special experience at the University of Washington before coming to The Mason Clinic. He also was a great teacher and served as Director of the Clinic's residency programs for many years. Dr. Patterson had the most expansive knowledge in the section, having come from a great residency training program with the ability to provide crucial interdivisional input to complex neurological cases, which was especially important in case review conferences. Dr. MacLean had a special interest in the vestibular system and the clinical problems of hearing loss, imbalance and vertigo, along with a subspecialty interest in the field of neuro-ophthalmology and multiple sclerosis. Dr. Ravits had subspecialty training in neuromuscular disease during his residency and thus became the go-to person for complicated neuromuscular problems. He developed special techniques in electromyography and nerve conduction studies, leading to a clinical focus on amyotrophic lateral sclerosis, which he coupled with an important pathological research project completed in the Benaroya Research Center of Virginia Mason. Dr. Taylor had special neuro-oncology subspecialty training during her residency and became the neuro-oncologist at the clinic working with both Neurosurgery and Oncology. Dr. Glass was trained as a pediatric neurologist at Children's Orthopedic Hospital in Seattle, a part of the University of Washington training program, and had a special interest in early childhood cognitive issues. Dr. Vlcek also was a specialist in pediatric neurology and had a subspecialty focus on movement disorders in children.

The major advancements in diagnostic technology were primarily in the Neuroradiology arena, allowing earlier and more precise diagnostic data to be obtained in both the clinic and hospital setting, as mentioned above with the advent of the CT and MRI scanners. Initially, the brain Echo for midline metrics and the radioisotope brain scan provided much clearer radiological demonstrations of pathology beyond the time-honored set of skull films, electroencephalography and lumbar puncture with CSF analysis. Pneumoencephalography, cerebral angiography via carotid or femoral artery entry, and myelography remained as diagnostic tools but were invasive with clinical risks. After the installation of the first MRI scanner in the mid 1980s, vascular MRI studies eventually became available, which allowed clear definition of carotid and cerebral pathology without a need for the more invasive carotid or femoral artery punctures. Carotid ultrasound became quite useful as a bedside technique to define the patency or degree of stenosis of the carotid artery and its branches, and was very helpful in clinical management of cerebral vascular disease. Posterior fossa myelograms were developed, which were crucial in identifying early cerebellar pontine angle tumors assisted by posterior fossa tomograms through the base of the skull. Positron emission tomography (PET) scans followed, allowing for critical data to be obtained in identifying metabolic changes in the brain, which is helpful in the early diagnosis of multiple cerebral pathologies.

There also were great technological advances in other clinical fields supporting the neurosciences including neuropathology, radiation therapy, neuro-ophthalmology, and laboratory medicine. Electromyography with peripheral nerve conduction studies was useful not only for diagnosis but also for monitoring therapeutic measures. Neurotology technologies expanded as well, with the development of acceleration electronystagmograms (AENGs), more sophisticated caloric examinations, bilateral audio evoked responses (BAERs), and more precise audiogram data, and clinical balance metrics.

Therapeutic advances in neurology were also quite dramatic during this period of time with the development of medication for cerebral vasospasm, which was particularly helpful for aneurysmal subarachnoid hemorrhage, multiple new targeted anti-seizure medications, new medications for multiple sclerosis, acute medical therapies for cerebral ischemia that became available in most emergency rooms, new medication strategies for serious headache disorders including migraine, carotid endarterectomies to prevent stroke complicating transient ischemic attacks (TIAs), and medications for extrapyramidal disorders like Parkinson's disease and other movement disorders such as essential tremor.

During this time, a gradual changing of the guard occurred in Neurology, as well as a decrease in the size of the section. The pediatric neurologists, Drs. Glass and Vlcek, both left in 1989, followed by the retirement of Dr. Birchfield in 1990. Dr. Fryer retired in 1994, and both Jim MacLean and Jim Coatsworth retired in 1998. In 1988, the section had 9 neurologists; by 1999, there were 5, including the newly arrived members, Michael Elliott, MD, and Monique L Giroux, MD, in 1998.

Transition Years: 1999 – 2005

The early years of the twenty-first century initiated a new era for neuroscience at VMMC. The traditions for both sections were well engrained since their beginnings in 1934 and the staff, including physicians, nursing and administrative personnel, continued the core values that had long been overall goals of both sections.

Section of Neurosurgery

By 1999, there were 3 practicing neurosurgeons in the section – Drs. Nussbaum, Hsiang and Nora. Their practice consisted of bread-and-butter neurosurgical cases along with an emphasis on spine surgery, including moderately complex cases. Dr. Nussbaum developed a significant neurovascular surgery practice and was one of the busiest aneurysm surgeons in the Seattle area for years. The computer began to be more important in terms of managing patients and information, and the role of the nurses in the section began to change as a result, as noted by Sally Cramer, RN, who had joined the section in 1986 (personal recollections).

Drs. Nora and Hsiang both left Virginia Mason in 2005, and were replaced by David Primrose, MD, that same year, and Farrokh Farrokhi, MD, one year later.

Section of Neurology

Meanwhile, the neurology section was understaffed and Dr. Giroux departed after only 2 years, resulting in the hiring of Mariko Kita, MD, and John Roberts, MD, in 2000. Since joining VM, Dr. Kita has served as director of the Virginia Mason Multiple Sclerosis Center and as the interim medical director for the hospital stroke service. Dr. Roberts has a special interest in movement disorders. During this time, Drs. Elliott, Ravits and Taylor all participated in the overall administrative leadership of the section. Dr. Patterson retired in 2004 and was replaced by Justin Stahl, MD, who joined the group in 2005 and practices general neurology with an emphasis on epilepsy and seizure disorders both downtown and in Bellevue. By that point, the neurology section had grown to 6 members.

Setting the Stage with Growth and Innovation: 2006 – 2013
Section of Neurosurgery

During this period, Drs. Nussbaum, Primrose and Farrokhi continued to see classic neurosurgical cases, with the help of Darlene Downey, ARNP. Changes in the workflow in both the clinic and hospital were notable as on-line ordering in the hospital became available, which had previously been done by hand by Lianne Shea, RN. Physician assistants were hired to perform this function – Maria Marsans, PA-C, MCMS, was one of the first, hired in 2005, and still works in the section. Dr. Nussbaum began doing stereotactic radiosurgery for brain tumors and pushed unsuccessfully for a gamma knife, which was becoming available at other institutions. Dr. Farrokhi, along with Movement Disorders Neurologist partner Dr. John Roberts, developed a regional Deep Brain Stimulation program. This program grew to one of the three major DBS centers in the region with the help of Maria Marsans, PAC, and Sindhu Srivatsal, MD. Complex spine cases continued especially with then Group Health surgeons, Rajiv Sethi, MD, and JC Leveque, MD. Their innovative work of applying a team based approach and pre-operative multidisciplinary case conferences helped build the critical support necessary for these challenging cases.

Dr. Primrose retired from surgical practice and transitioned to a resident teaching position at Harborview Medical Center. Joe Serrone, MD, replaced him in 2014, our first endovascular-trained neurosurgeon. Dr. Serrone and the newly formed Neurohospitalist team started what would become the successful build of a Comprehensive Stroke Center at VM.

Section of Neurology

The neurology section continued to grow to meet patient demand, both downtown in clinic and hospital, as well as in the satellites. Zornitza Stoilova, MD, joined the group in 2008, practicing general neurology downtown and in Lynnwood. Nancy Isenberg, MD, MPH, was hired in 2011 and practices at Bainbridge as well as downtown; Sarah Hermanson, DNP, ARNP, FNP, practices with her in those 2 locations as well. Allen Scott Nielsen, MD, also was hired in 2011; Dr. Ravits left that same year to pursue his interests in ALS at the University of California, San Diego. James F. Bartscher, MD, and Emma R. Burbank, MD, joined the group in 2012; Dr. Bartscher is a neurohospitalist and Dr. Burbank is a general neurologist, practicing in the Federal Way and downtown clinics. Sindhu Srivatsal, MD, arrived in 2013 and has a special interest in movement disorders, practicing both downtown and at Issaquah. Natalie M. Hendon, MD, also joined the section in 2013, practicing general neurology and sleep medicine.

By the end of 2013, the section had expanded to include 11 physician members and 2 ARNPs working downtown, at the satellites and in a hospital-based practice.

2014 – present: Centers of Excellence and other Innovations
Section of Neurosurgery

In 2014, Dr. Farrokhi became Section Head. In 2014, the "Seattle Spine Team approach" was published by Rajiv Sethi and colleagues [1] with significant improvement in early outcomes and most importantly elucidating a new paradigm for identifying patients for surgery using a very different method where all team members are given an equal voice. Based on this, new innovations were put in place under Dr. Farrokhi's leadership with many patients coming to the section through a program known as "Centers of Excellence". In this program, the Neurosurgery group was strongly integrated with PM&R, Neuropsychology, and Anesthesia Pain team members. The multidisciplinary teams include physicians, nurses, PAs, ARNPs, technicians and others who work together, across hospital and clinic, to give the patient a high quality, safe, and streamlined result. Using robust and excellent outcome data (for example, hip/knee replacement surgical results showing 0% complications and readmissions), the Centers have contracted with various companies around the country to provide reliable, high quality care for their workers, especially related to spinal problems and knee/hip replacement surgery. These Centers include VM, the Geisinger Clinic and Mayo Clinic. In these unique shifts in employer lead healthcare delivery, the companies send patients out of their local communities and to a Center of Excellence, paying all travel and medical expenses of both the patient and their companion. Prior to patient arrival, charts are reviewed and all required imaging and consultations arranged. When the patient arrives, they meet with Neurosurgery, PM&R and Anesthesia Pain teams. Their case is then reviewed at the multidisciplinary conference and a recommendation made for surgery or alternative therapies. If warranted, surgery is often coordinated during the same visit. About half of the patients are able to avoid surgery (which may have been recommended elsewhere) and receive solely rehabilitative care. Overall, the companies see improvements in outcomes and overall costs for their patient employees.

Leading the complex spine and center of excellence programs to great international acclaim, Drs. Rajiv Sethi and JC Leveque joined Virginia Mason in 2014 and 2015. They brought their academic and surgical expertise from the Group Health Cooperative and the University of Washington and established the first Complex Spine Fellowship in Neurosurgery. Dr. Vijay Yanamadala was the first fellow, taking a year off from his neurosurgery residency program at Harvard to build his surgical and academic skills. Under the leadership of Dr. Sethi as Director of the Neuroscience institute, a robust research and publication program was developed. This program built on the leadership talents of Anna Wright, PhD, and the NSI's first two Visiting Scholars, Quinlan Buchlack, MPsych, MBIS, and Galit Almosnino, MD. Quin went on to medical school back home in Australia and Galit to pursue an otolaryngology residency. Over the ensuing years, other great fellows trained at the NSI including Dr. Louis Nkrumah from Emory and Dr. Michael Bohl from the Barrow Neurological Institute. A visiting professorship program was established in partnership with the Washington State Association of Neurological Surgeons, where Dr. Farrokhi and Dr. Leveque each served a term as President. The program brought world-renowned experts in the field to Virginia Mason to teach our team and take-home lessons learned at VM. The complex spine team was expanded in 2019 by the fortunate recruitment of Venu Nemani, MD. Research initiatives in spine have led to over 40 original scientific publications in major scientific journals and has resulted in Dr. Sethi being nominated as the first board member of the Scoliosis Research Society from the Pacific Northwest.

Other areas of neurosurgical expertise have been enhanced as well. Joe Serrone, MD, joined the group in 2014, bringing endovascular expertise in the treatment of aneurysms, vascular malformations and stroke. He transitioned to a purely academic career after two years with the department. Robert Ryan, MD, M.Sc., took up the build of the neurovascular program in 2017, leading us to an accredited Comprehensive Stroke Center (CSC) that year. Rene O. Sanchez-Mejia, MD, joined the section in 2018, and also specializes in neurovascular disease, endovascular neurosurgery, cerebral aneurysms and malformations and brain tumor surgery. Together, Dr. Ryan, Dr. Sanchez-Mejia and David Robinson, MD (Radiology) partnered with the Neurohospitalist team, led by Fatimah Milfred, MD, to develop one of only three CSC-certified stroke and neurovascular programs in the region.

Dr. Farrokhi has also expanded his expertise into deep brain stimulation (DBS) procedures for Parkinson's and related disease. An academic program was developed to support research focused on safety and efficiency in DBS surgery. In partnerships with Dr. Jonathan Carlson of Sacred Heart Hospital in Spokane, the first multi-institutional DBS Database was developed in the state and innovative research started in the application of artificial intelligence and machine learning to surgical risk prediction.

The skull base surgery program was enhanced in cooperation with otolaryngologist Seth Schwartz, MD, leading to standardization of joint surgical procedures for acoustic neuromas. This program was further expanded with the recruitment of Daniel Zeitler, MD, to Neuro-otology, and Dr. Sanchez-Mejia to Neurosurgery. Anterior skull base surgery at Virginia Mason was revolutionized with the arrival of Amy Anstead, MD, an otolaryngologist with specialty training in endoscopic rhinology and skull base surgery. Partnering with Dr. Farrokhi, and later with Drs. Nussbaum and Leveque, the endoscopic endonasal approach for resection of pituitary and anterior skull base tumors eliminated the need for large complicated craniotomies in many patients.

To effectively manage such complex diseases and increasing clinical loads (surgical volumes in neurosurgery doubled from 2014 to 2019) required a strong team. The section used an evidence-based approach to build programs, involving all members of the care team – physicians, PAs, ARNPs and nurses – to not only care for patients, but to build high quality care systems and spread these learnings through research and publication. Over these years, the neurosurgery team produced about a dozen peer-reviewed publications per year, again with great leadership and work by Anna Wright and Matt Sikora. In nursing, the team includes Naomi Highland, Elizabeth Krout, and manager Karen McHenry; Sally Cramer, RN, retired in April 2019 after a 33-year career at VM.

With the increase in clinical volumes and complexity came the rapid growth of the Physician Assistant team in neurosurgery. Michelle Gilbert, PA-C, served as the first Lead PA with senior PA team members Maria Marsans, PA-C; Catherine Jackson, PA-C, and Kellen Nold, PA-C, recruiting and training new members, which expanded the team to ten by 2019. Rapidly gaining expertise in clinic, hospital and operating room management of neurosurgical patients, the PA team serves a critical role in high quality neurosurgical care that is sure to expand more rapidly to all areas in the years to come.

As of June 2019, the Section of Neurosurgery has 6 members: Drs. Farrokhi, Sethi, Leveque, Ryan, Sanchez-Majia, and Nemani, two of whom have Orthopaedic surgery board certification (Drs. Sethi and Nemani), and 8 PAs (Devin R. Dickson, PA-C; Philip D. Downey, PA-C; Nicholas I. Eley, MSPA, PA-C; Michelle Gilbert, PA-C; Catherine M. Jackson, PA-C; Olga Klachkovich, PA-C, who works in the Issaquah satellite; Maria Marsans, PA-C, MCMS, and Kellen Nold, PA-C). Other PAs who have served in the section, but are no longer at VM, include Brandon R. Wilson, MPAS, PA-C; Martha Short, PA-C, and Grant Geiger, PA-C. With this approach, the section is fulfilling the medical center's mission of using evidence-based, team-based care to transform health care.

Section of Neurology

The Neurology Section has expanded to meet the needs of patients in many clinical settings – outpatient clinic, both downtown and in some of the satellites, and hospital. Aleksander Tkach, MD (2014 – 2015) and Wendy E. Brown, MD (2015 - 2017) joined the neurohospitalist team briefly. Currently, Kelvin K. Ma, MD, and Fatima E. Mildred, MD, who joined the team in 2016, serve as the neurohospitalists for the section. Justin Stahl, MD, has served as Section Head for the past 2 years.

Drs. Bartscher, Hendon and Nielsen left VM in 2015; Richard A. Mesher, MD, previous Chief of Neurology at GHC, joined the section the same year. The following year, Lucas McCarthy, MD, and Anik J. Amin, MD, were hired to work both downtown and at the Federal Way satellite. Xuan S. Wu, MD, PhD, joined the team in 2017 and works both downtown and in Bellevue. Ye Hu, MD, joined the section in 2019 and works both downtown and in Lynnwood. Dr. Amin left to return to University of Texas, Southwestern to be closer to family in October 2019, although he continues to read EEGs for the section as a 0.1 FTE. Dr. Isenberg will be leaving in February 2020, and nurse practitioner Sarah Hermanson will transition to Neurosurgery in January 2020.

Physician Biographies
Hale Haven, MD, PhD (1934 - 1964): Neurosurgery and Neurology

Hale Haven was born in Waterloo, Iowa on 8/31/1902. He attended Northwestern University School of Medicine and obtained his M.D. in 1928, his M.S. in 1930 and his Ph.D. in 1933. While in medical school, at the beginning of his junior year, he married Mildred Snapp, who was doing some special duty nursing at the time. During his last two years in medical school, Hale and his wife Mildred ran a small industrial hospital, he as house physician and she as the nursing supervisor, x-ray technician and anesthetist. His internship was at Wesley Memorial Hospital from 1927-1928, his residency in surgery was at Northwestern from 1928 to 1931 as the Elizabeth J. Ward Fellow along with a part-time residency at Passavant Memorial from 1929 to 1931, which was followed by a fellowship in neurosurgery at Northwestern, 1931–1934 under the guidance of Loyal Davis, M.D. During these residency years he was an attending surgeon at Cook County Hospital, consultant in Neurological surgery at the Edward Hines, Jr. Hospital and part of the adjunct staff at the Michael Reese Hospital.

He became Section Head of Neurological Surgery at The Mason Clinic in 1934 at the invitation of James Tate Mason and remained head of the section until 1964. While at The Mason Clinic he was on the attending staffs of Virginia Mason Hospital, King County Hospital, the V.A. Hospital, Children's Orthopedic Hospital and Seattle General Hospital along with being a senior consultant at the University of Washington Hospital. He also served as consultant in neurosurgery for the U.S. Naval Hospital in Bremerton and consultant for electroencephalography at the USPHS Hospital in Seattle. He was in the U.S. Navy beginning in 1942 and retiring in 1961 as a Commander. He also served as the Chief of Neurological Surgery at Oakland Naval Hospital in the year 1946.

Dr. Haven belonged to numerous professional societies and had multiple fraternal affiliations along with participating in various administrative positions at the Virginia Mason Hospital and the Virginia Mason Foundation. Over his career, he wrote twenty-four articles ranging from his initial study on the effects of iodized oil in the spinal subarachnoid space published in *JAMA* in 1930, to his presidential address at the ninth annual meeting of the Western Neurosurgical Society meeting in October 1963, published in The *Mason Clinic Bulletin*. His major clinical interests included trigeminal neuralgia, causalgia, and angina pectoris. In 1939, he studied the relationship between the scalenus anticus syndrome and the anomalous first rib and was the first to postulate compression of the subclavian artery rather than the brachial plexus by the scalenus muscles - "Haven's Syndrome."

On March 25, 1964, Hale Haven died of carcinoma of the pancreas after being plagued for several years by multiple infirmities.

John S. Tytus, MD (1958 - 1978): Neurosurgery and Neurology

John Sutphin Tytus was born August 1, 1921 in Columbus, Ohio, obtained his premedical education at Princeton University, graduating in 1943, and then moved on to Ohio State University from 1944 to 1947 to obtain his M.D. He interned at the University of Michigan at Ann Arbor from 1947 to 1948 followed by a surgical residency, neurology residency and finally a neurosurgical residency, completed in 1955. During this time period, he served in the U.S. Army as a general surgeon at Sandia Base in Albuquerque, NM from 1951 to 1953. He attended Radcliffe Infirmary in Oxford, England for a neurosurgical fellowship from 1955 to 1956. His wife Gina was his constant companion throughout his career in surgery. They had three children and multiple grandchildren, most of whom continue to live in the greater Northwest.

His career at The Mason Clinic began in July 1958 when he joined Hale Haven in Neurosurgery after a year as an Assistant Professor of Neurosurgery at the University of Michigan. He was on the active staff of the Virginia Mason Hospital, Children's Orthopedic Hospital, and King County Hospital in Seattle. He was appointed clinical Associate Professor in Neurosurgery at the University of Washington in 1965. He was Section Head of Neurosurgery at the Clinic from 1964 to 1978, Chief of Surgery in 1974 and 1975, Chief of Staff for the Medical Center in 1972 and 1973, and President of the Virginia Mason Research Center.

Dr. Tytus had twelve articles published over his career on a variety of neurosurgical topics including cavernous sinus thrombosis, glioma ossification, extradural hemorrhage, gliomatosis cerebri, and posterior third ventricular tumors. Dr. Tytus joined Dr. David Fryer of the Neurology section to develop a television program on "The Management Decisions in Stroke", which won first place in the 40th annual National Exhibition of Medical Education Programs.

Dr. Tytus and his wife Gina were very interested in the Virginia Mason Research Center and helped administratively in its development as well as with financial support. He also was the primary leader for both Sections of Neurology and Neurosurgery in setting quality goals and fostering the working relationships between them, along with incentivizing the pursuit of clinical research, which enhanced the overall clinical practice.

Dr. Tytus, along with Dr. Haven, was responsible for laying the groundwork for the Department of Neuroscience at VMMC by establishing the essential core standards so crucial to the overall success of the two sections.

He was responsible for developing the Neurology Section after Dr. Altrocchi left for Stanford, with the recruitment and hiring of Dr. Birchfield. He knew and insisted on open communication between Neurology and Neurosurgery, which was the core behavior essential to the overall success of high quality clinical care, which continues to this day.

His great sense of humor and overall wisdom was important to all of us during our many years of partnership. He was a great leader of professional staff, was very good with his patients, had great neurosurgical skill and was responsible for the initiation of open communication with multiple other sections in the clinic. He resigned from The Mason Clinic on July 1, 1978, after leading the Section of Neurosurgery for 20 years. After his retirement from medicine, he owned a sheep ranch up near Arlington, WA for several years. He died peacefully at home on May 31, 2011. [2]

Richard I. Birchfield, MD (1964 - 1990): Neurology

Richard Birchfield attended the University of Washington School of Medicine, receiving his M.D. in 1953; he then did an internship at St. Luke's Hospital in Spokane, Washington from 1953 to 1954. This was followed by residencies in medicine and neurology from 1954 to 1959 at Duke Medical Center. He then completed his neurology residency at the University of Washington Hospital from 1959 to 1960. He was trained in neurology by Dr. Fred Plum, who was Chief of Neurology at the University until he moved to Cornell Medical Center in New York. Dr. Birchfield was then asked to be the interim Chief of Neurology at the University with Dr. Plum's move to New York. He was an instructor in Medicine (Neurology) at the University of Washington from 1960 to 1964 and became a clinical assistant professor of Medicine (Neurology) at the University of Washington Medical Center as well as King County Hospital in Seattle in 1964.

Dr. Birchfield had great residency training at Duke and at the University of Washington with Drs. Plum and Posner, with whom he stayed in close contact for many years even after their departure to Cornell.

Dr. Birchfield completed his Board certification examinations and began his neurology practice at The Mason Clinic in 1964. He was very knowledgeable in general neurology and published ten peer-reviewed papers on topics including narcolepsy, disease of the sino-atrial node, respiratory center function, EEG studies with cerebral vascular disease, Guillain-Barré syndrome, Wernicke's syndrome, and porphyria. His major research interests were blood pressure control, epilepsy and labyrinthine function. He had a keen interest in teaching young physicians in neurology, having learned effective teaching techniques from Dr. Plum. He was actively engaged in the teaching program for medical students and residents both at Virginia Mason and the University of Washington. He also helped develop a handbook for evaluation of patients with neurological disease for house staff officers.

Dr. Birchfield led the Section of Neurology from 1964 until 1982 and remained very active in the section with an emphasis on clinical practice in his areas of interest: epilepsy, extra-pyramidal disease and respiratory disorders. He belonged to numerous medical societies including the American Academy of Neurology, American Federation for Clinical Research and the King County Medical Society. He also was President of the University of Washington Medical Alumni Association.

He and his wife Shirley participated in multiple clinic activities. Dr. Birchfield remained at Virginia Mason until his retirement in 1990. He died July 2, 2000. [3]

Edward Reifel, MD (1964 -1998): Neurosurgery

Ed Reifel was born on September 6, 1929 in Gallipolis, Ohio [4] and began his higher education at the University of Michigan with a degree in sociology in 1951 and an M.D. degree from the University of Michigan in 1956. His internship was at the University of Michigan Hospital at Ann Arbor, followed by residencies there in general surgery and neurosurgery/

neurology from 1956 to 1962. He and his family moved to Pueblo, Colorado where he practiced neurosurgery for 2 years.

Dr. Reifel started his career at The Mason Clinic in 1964 and became Head of the Section of Neurosurgery in 1974. He had an additional year of training in both neuropathology and neurosurgery at the University of Washington in 1967 and became board-certified in Neurosurgery the same year. He held teaching positions both at the University of Washington and its affiliated hospitals, as well as at the Virginia Mason Medical Center. He belonged to twelve surgical societies including the Congress of Neurological Surgeons, the American Association of Neurological Surgeons, the Western Neurosurgical Society and the American College of Surgeons. He was involved with numerous committees in these organizations as well as being a guest examiner for the American Board of Neurological Surgery. He also was extensively involved at Virginia Mason, including serving as the long-time chairman of the professional liability committee, as a key participant on the critical care committee, as chairman of the professional liability committee, as chairman of The Mason Clinic Day committee, and on the insurance committee and the bioethics committee. He had twelve publications ranging from neurological injuries related to football, cerebral blood flow, Cruetzfeldt-Jacob disease, neoplasms of the brachial plexus and Chiari type I malformations. In addition, he had multiple papers and exhibits at local, regional and national meetings during the years that he practiced at the Clinic.

He developed and retained a large practice in neurosurgery while at the Clinic despite the numerous administrative positions that he held over the years. He was respected by all of his professional colleagues and was very supportive in interdepartmental communication so important for the high quality of care for all neurosurgery and neurology patients. Dr. Reifel was always known as an excellent neurosurgeon, being cautious and appropriately conservative in all of his clinical judgments. He was always firm with the clinical directions he chose both diagnostically and surgically but also respectful of clinical differences of opinion from his colleagues.

Dr. Reifel retired from active practice in 1998; he died Dec. 1, 2017.

David G. Fryer, MD (1965 - 1994): Neurology

Dr. Fryer was born on September 20, 1928 in Portsmouth, England. He completed his basic medical training in 1953 at the University Of Leeds School Of Medicine in Leeds, England. His internship was at St. James Hospital in Leeds from 1953 to 1954. He was then a house officer in Pediatrics at the Seacroft Hospital in Leeds from 1954 to 1955. He served as a general practitioner in Portsmouth, England from 1955 to 1956 and as a ship's surgeon on the Orient line S.S. Oronsay out of London for six months in 1956. He had a rotating internship at Vancouver General Hospital in Vancouver, B.C. 1956 to 1957, and was a resident in psychiatry at the Crease Clinic in Vancouver from 1957 to 1959. He then became chief resident in psychiatry at Boston City Hospital from 1959 to 1960, followed by a year of residency in neurology at Lemuel Shattuck Hospital in Boston from 1960 to 1961; another year of neurology at Tufts Medical School from 1961 to 1962; and then a year of neuropathology residency at Boston City Hospital from1962 to 1963. In 1964, he came to the University of Washington as a special fellow and became an instructor in Neurology.

Dr. Fryer joined The Mason Clinic in 1965. He had a wealth of knowledge and experience in neurology, which was easily apparent in joint conferences concerning patient care as well as "hallway" second opinions with his colleagues. This special training and experience in multiple high-profile settings including psychiatric training, was greatly honored by his colleagues and eagerly sought out. He was also known for his wit and wonderful stories, which were thoroughly enjoyed by all and which added some much needed lighter moments during clinical discussions. He was a member of the British Medical Association, the American Psychiatric Association and the American Academy of Neurology. His bibliography includes twelve publications on topics such as clinical cerebral vascular disease, Creutzfeldt-Jacob disease, the effect of alcohol on the nervous system, management decisions in stroke, and Refsum disease. He also developed a series of videotapes on the management of stroke, and the bedside diagnosis of stroke. He held multiple teaching positions both during his training and while in practice in Seattle.

Dr. Fryer remained in the Neurology Section of The Mason Clinic until 1994, when he retired from practice. He passed away on January 8, 2001 after a six-month struggle with cancer.

James B. MacLean, MD (1968 - 1998): Neurology

Jim MacLean was born on March 27, 1937 in Spokane, Washington. He earned his B.A. degree at the University of Washington in 1958, and his M.D. degree at UW in 1962. He did his medical internship at Bellevue Hospital in New York City from 1962 to 1963, and completed his neurology residency at the University of Washington from 1963 to 1966. He joined the U.S. Navy Medical Service for two years from 1966 to 1968. He participated in neurophysiology research at the Veterans' Administration Hospital in Seattle from 1965 to 1966 and had some additional subspecialty training in neuro-ophthalmology with Dr. William Hoyt at the University of California in San Francisco in 1980.

Dr. MacLean joined The Mason Clinic in 1968 as a clinical neurologist. His Boards in neurology were completed in 1969 and he became a fellow in the American Academy of Neurology in 1983. His subspecialty interests were in neuro-ophthalmology and neurotology and he was Section head from 1982 to 1997. He had an academic appointment as Clinical Associate Professor of Neurology at the University of Washington and his research interests included neurophysiology, clinical neuro-ophthalmology, neurotology and higher cognitive functioning. Hospital appointments included Virginia Mason, the Veterans Administration Hospital and Harborview Medical Center, all in Seattle.

Over his career, he gave thirty-four presentations and wrote fifteen peer-reviewed publications focusing on neuro-ophthalmology, vestibular dysfunction and various general neurological issues. He served as a board examiner for the American Academy of Neurology. Teaching was a major emphasis with participation in many Mason Clinic CME programs in Neurology as well as hosting two Frank Walsh Neuro-Ophthalmology symposiums in Seattle.

He coupled his active clinical practice in neurology with multiple ad-

190

ministrative assignments and participated extensively in numerous national professional conferences. He promoted teaching and open communication between all staff members in Neurology and Neurosurgery as well as with his colleagues throughout the clinic. Maintaining a large referral base of referring physicians was always a high priority, as was one-on-one physician-patient communication.

Dr. MacLean retired in 1998. He and his wife Anne have three children.

James J. Coatsworth, MD (1973 - 1998): Neurology

Jim Coatsworth was born on April 15, 1937 in Denver, Colorado and received his B.A. in Biology at Cornell University in 1959, and his M.D. at Cornell University Medical College in 1963. His medical internship was at King County Hospital (now Harborview) in Seattle from 1963 to 1964, and his residency in neurology was at the University of Washington affiliated program from 1967 to 1970. He became a Clinical Associate Professor of Medicine at the University along with holding a consultant position at the NIH on epilepsy. He held many hospital-consulting positions in neurology including the University Hospital, the Veterans' Administration Hospital and Harborview, in addition to Virginia Mason. He belonged to numerous neurology societies including the American Academy of Neurology, American Epilepsy Society and the American Medical Association. His publications included papers on epilepsy, delirium, carotid artery pressure and EEG-monitoring during carotid artery surgery, and GI motility dysfunction in patients with diabetes.

Dr. Coatsworth was a faculty member at UW for 2 years before joining The Mason Clinic, where he worked for the remaining 27 years of his career. He had wonderful skills in both professional and patient communication and built a large practice in seizure management. He was also very important to the clinic in his role as director of medical education for many years as well as serving as chairman of the important clinic compensation committee. He and his wife, Joan and their family lived a number of years both on the Eastside as well as in West Seattle. Dr. Coatsworth retired in 1998 at the age of 60; Jim had a lifelong passion for learning, and in retirement pursued studies in botany, archeology, art history and astronomy, as well as traveling extensively with his wife. He died on March 4, 2018. [5]

Laird Patterson, MD (1976 – 2004): Neurology

Laird Patterson was born on July 18, 1941 in Little Rock, Arkansas. He obtained his A.B., Cum Laude at the University of Kansas, was a Summerfield Scholar and was admitted to the Phi Beta Kappa honorary in 1963. His majors in college were German and chemistry. He was appointed a Fulbright scholar and went to Munich, Germany to focus on the study of German literature from 1963 to 1964. He received his M.D. at Harvard Medical School and graduated cum laude. His internship in medicine was at the Moffitt University of California Hospital in San Francisco, California from 1968 to 1969. He did one year of residency at Moffitt before serving in the military from 1970 to 1972. He became a Major in the U.S. Army Medical Corps. He had a second year of residency at Moffitt in medicine from 1972 to 1973 followed by a neurology residency at Harvard from 1973 through 1976. He obtained board certification in both medicine in 1973 and neurology in 1978.

Dr. Patterson had excellent training both in medicine and neurology, leading to a wonderful recommendation from Dr. Richard Tyler at Harvard to The Mason Clinic in support of his application for a position in the neurology section. He proved to be a very valuable addition to the Neurology staff as he was an outstanding clinical neurologist with great communication skills with patients as well as his colleagues in and out of the section. He always contributed significantly to discussions of complex neurological problems in differential diagnosis. He was capable of handling all of the general neurology challenges and was particularly keen on difficult complex neurological problems. He enjoyed teaching and was an excellent communicator with the house staff during his years at the Clinic, as well as being a big supporter of the University Neurology program. He was also a major contributor to our conference discussions and enjoyed the give and take where we all learned from each other. He retired from the Clinic in 2004.

James Emanuel Raisis, MD (1976 - 1989): Neurosurgery

Jim Raisis was born in Pittsburgh, Pennsylvania on August 27, 1941. His initial education was at Penn Hills High School in Penn Hills, Pennsylvania with graduation in 1959, followed by a B.A. from the University of Colorado in Boulder in 1964 and an M.D. degree from the University of Colorado Medical Center in 1970. He completed his surgical internship at Barnes Hospital in St. Louis in 1971, followed by a neurological surgical residency at the University of Michigan in Ann Arbor, Michigan. He had an athletic scholarship for his undergraduate studies at the University of Colorado, as well as a Boettcher Foundation Scholarship and a National Health Scholarship. Prior to coming to the clinic, he had seven publications generated during his training years covering topics including hydrocephalus, cerebral venous pressure, cerebral hypoxia, and the effects of hypothermia on cerebral metabolism and hemodynamics. He assisted in the production of a movie titled, "First Aid in Football-Associated Head and Neck Injuries" during his residency years at the University of Michigan. He also developed a display on "Football-induced Head and Neck Injuries" that was presented both at the American Association of Neurological Surgeons' Annual Meeting and the American College of Surgeons' Meeting, both in 1975. He had numerous invitations to present the data from his publications.

He joined Drs. Tytus and Reifel when he came to the clinic in 1976, and these three remained the core of the neurosurgical division for many years from the early 1970s until 1989. During this time, there was marked advancement in technological diagnostic tools as well as medical and surgical therapeutic options.

He added a new dimension to our neurosurgery practice, having participated in a great preparatory residency program at the University of Michigan where he developed keen surgical skills. He always was a joy to be around and great fun, armed with a wonderful sense of humor and clear opinions on many matters. He left Virginia Mason in 1989 and currently practices at Northwest Hospital and Medical Center (as of Fall 2018).

Stephen T. Glass, MD (1982 - 1989): Pediatric Neurology

Stephen Glass was born on January 30, 1948. His early education was at Harvard College, from which he graduated in 1970. He received his medical school training at the University of Vermont, receiving his MD in 1974. He then served as a pediatric intern at Children's Orthopedic Hospital in Seattle from 1974 to 1975, followed by a residency there from 1975 to 1977. This was followed by a position as senior fellow in medicine, and Assistant Professor in Neurology at the University of Washington Affiliated Hospitals from 1977 to 1979. He was chief resident in child neurology at Children's Hospital from 1979 to 1980.

Academic positions held included Consultant in Pediatrics, City of Seattle Department of Health from 1977 to 1980; Acting Instructor in Pediatrics (Neurology) at Children's Hospital from 1979 to 1980; Clinical instructor in Pediatrics (Neurology) at Children's Hospital from 1980 to 1981; and Clinical Assistant Professor in Pediatrics (Neurology) at Children's Hospital from 1981 to present. He is Board-certified in pediatric neurology, electroencephalography, and in pediatrics (1981). He belongs to the Child Neurology Society and had multiple hospital affiliations including Children's Orthopedic Hospital (1977), Valley General Hospital (1980), Virginia Mason Hospital (1980) and Auburn General Hospital (1980). He was awarded the Ralph D. Sussman Award (pediatrics) in 1974 and the Pediatric House staff Faculty Teaching Award in 1980.

Dr. Glass joined Virginia Mason in 1982. Publications have included articles on "Subclinical status epilepticus following acute cerebral anoxia" and "Congenital interhemispheric cysts: diagnosis by CT and ultrasound." Dr. Glass left Virginia Mason in 1989 and, as of Fall 2018, works in private practice at Northwest Child Neurology in Bothell/Kirkland.

Brien Wayne Vlcek, MD (1984 - 1989): Pediatric Neurology

Brien Vlcek was born on February 12, 1952. His early education included a Bachelor of Science Degree in biology from the University of Wisconsin-Eau Claire in May 1974 and obtainment of 12 graduate credits in neuroscience in 1975 at the University of Wisconsin-Madison. His medical education was at the Medical College of Wisconsin, Milwaukee from 1975 to 1979. He then did his resident training there in pediatrics from 1979 to 1981. This was followed by a three-year fellowship in neurology at the University of Washington with completion in 1984. He has special training in computerized tomography (CT), ultrasound, EEG, evoked potentials and EMG.

Academic honors include elected membership in the American Society for Neurological Investigation. He became quite experienced in neuroscience research during his early years both at the UW-Madison and the University of Washington.

Dr. Vlcek joined Virginia Mason in 1984. He has authored seven publications and has focused his career on serving children with neurologic problems and their families. Dr. Vlcek left Virginia Mason in 1989 and as of fall 2018 is in private practice at the Pediatric Neuroscience Center in Seattle.

John Ravits, MD (1986 - 2011): Neurology

John Ravits was born on April 7, 1953 in St. Paul, Minnesota. He received his B.A. degree from Yale in New Haven, Connecticut in 1975 and attended the Mayo Medical School in Rochester, Minnesota from 1975 to 1979. Internship was at the University of California in San Diego from 1979 to 1980 followed by a residency in neurology from 1980 to 1983. He then became a clinical research fellow in neurophysiology at Harvard Medical School from 1983 to 1984, moving to the National Institute of Health in Bethesda, Maryland as a medical staff fellow from 1984 to 1986. He became board-certified both in Neurology and Electrodiagnostic Medicine in 1986 and 1989 respectively.

Dr. Ravits joined Virginia Mason in 1986. In addition to serving as clinical neurology staff at The Mason Clinic, he held a clinical professorship at the University of Washington, and was associate staff at Harborview Medical Center and the Muscular Dystrophy Association. He was active with administrative affairs at the Clinic as well as the American Association of Electrodiagnostic Medicine, and participated in the American Board of Psychiatry and Neurology as a board examiner for three years in

1989, 1993 and 1996. His research interests were neuromuscular disease, clinical neurophysiology and movement disorders. He gave ten presentations, six abstracts and wrote fifteen peer-reviewed publications along with four book chapters focusing on neuromuscular disease.

Dr. Ravits is a very astute clinical neurologist with a focus on neuromuscular diseases and special abilities in electromyography. He was the go-to neuromuscular neurologist in the region because of both his clinical skills and his skills in the EMG laboratory. He was extensively involved in teaching residents both at The Mason Clinic and the University. He developed a special research interest in amyotrophic lateral sclerosis (ALS) and used neuropathological studies at the Benaroya Research Institute to further knowledge of this devastating disease. In 2011, he accepted a research position in neurology at the University of San Diego, which allowed him to further his neuropathological studies of ALS.

Lynne P. Taylor, MD (1988 – 2011; 2014 – 2017): Neurology

Dr. Taylor was born in Birmingham, England. Her undergraduate education was at Northwestern University in Evanston, Illinois where she received her B.A. in 1974; she received her M.D. in 1982 from Washington University in St Louis, Missouri. Her medical internship was at Barnes-Jewish Hospital in St. Louis from 1982 to 1983 and her neurology residency was at the University of Pennsylvania from 1983 to 1986. She did a fellowship in neuro-oncology at Memorial Sloan-Kettering Cancer Center in New York from 1986 to 1988, with additional training both at Stanford and London, England in palliative care. Academic appointments included Clinical Associate Professor of Neurology at the University of Washington from 2005 to 2011, and Associate Professor of Neurology at Tufts University School of Medicine from 2011 to the present. She was Director of Neuro-oncology and Chair of the Neuro-oncology Tumor Board at The Mason Clinic from 1990 to 2011. She spent two years at the Tufts Medical Center in Boston, MA and then returned to VMMC as the neuro-oncologist in the Oncology Section. She had major teaching roles at the Clinic as well as the University. Dr. Taylor served as faculty at multiple neurology courses for the American Academy of Neurology over the years, primarily in the oncology arena. She was a Board Examiner for the American Board of Neurology and Psychiatry from 1996 to 2004 and served on the committee for recertification in Neurology.

Her major research interests were in the treatment of primary brain tumors, the quality of life for neuro-oncology patients, and palliative care in cancer patients. She had multiple research grants to perform clinical trials in patients with cerebral neoplasms. She was a board member and reviewer for *Continuum* (AAN), *Neurology* and the *Annals of Neurology* along with the *Journal of Neuro-oncology*. She wrote nine paper presentations, gave two invited paper presentations, authored or edited several books, and published ten abstracts.

Dr. Taylor developed a large referral base for neuro-oncology patients at The Mason Clinic along with maintaining her skills in general neurology. She always insisted on the best clinical care possible for all of her patients as reflected in her interest in the importance of palliative care. She was a great teacher as well as a highly skilled neuro-oncologist and always shared vast knowledge with her colleagues during multiple conferences that she attended or led. She returned to VMMC in 2014 from a position at Tufts Medical Center in Boston, to focus on neuro-oncology in the Department of Oncology at VMMC. She left Virginia Mason in 2017 to lead the Section of Neurological Oncology at the University of Washington.

Leroy H. Dart, Jr., MD (1989 - 1991): Neurosurgery

Leroy Dart was born on September 6, 1930 in San Francisco, California. He graduated from the University of California at Berkeley with an A.B. degree in 1951 and obtained an MD degree from the University of California in 1954. He interned in surgery at the University of California from 1954 to 1955 and initially became a resident in pathology at the Walter Reed Hospital in Washington D.C. from 1956 to 1960; he was certified in anatomic pathology by the American Board of Pathology in October, 1960. He attended his neurosurgical residency at the Mayo Clinic in Rochester, MN from 1964 to 1968 and was certified by the American Board of

Neurological Surgery in October 1970. He served in the United States Army and Air Force from 1955 to 1975 and became Chief of Neurological Surgery at Wilford Hall in San Antonio, TX from 1971 to 1975. He retired as Colonel, USAF, MC, in October 1975. He then entered private practice in neurosurgery in Yakima, Washington from 1975 until 1989. He joined the neurosurgical section at the VMMC in 1989.

Dr. Dart belonged to multiple specialty organizations including the American Association of Neurological Surgeons, Washington Association of Neurological Surgeons, and the North Pacific Society of Neurology and Psychiatry. He left Virginia Mason in 1991.

Charles Enzer Nussbaum, MD (1990 - 2019): Neurosurgery

Charlie Nussbaum was born on May 27, 1958. His early education included Bowdoin College in Brunswick, ME, graduating with an A.B. in May 1980. He then obtained his M.D. degree from the University Of Rochester School Of Medicine in May of 1984. Postgraduate medical training was at the University Hospitals of Cleveland with a general surgical internship, 1984 to 1985, followed by a neurosurgical residency at the University of Rochester Medical Center from 1985 to 1990. He joined the Section of Neurosurgery at the Virginia Mason Medical Center in August of 1990 and served as Section Head of Neurosurgery from 1994 to 2014. He was Board-certified in neurological surgery in November 1992 and belongs to many neurosurgical organizations including the American Association of Neurological Surgeons and the Western Neurosurgical Society, holding many committee positions. He has also assisted with many hospital committees including the Critical Care Committee (1995 – 2003), the Quality Assurance Committee (1995 – 2002) and the Professional Liability Committee, 2004 to present.

His publications include the surgical use of Polyglactin 910 mesh as a dural substitute with Dr. Mauer, and a case study of lymphocytic hypophysitis with cavernous sinus and hypothalamic involvement. He has had multiple presentations on numerous neurosurgical issues including sudden back pain with paraparesis, the use of Vicryl Mesh for a dural substitute, aneurysmal subarachnoid hemorrhage, pituitary adenoma, surgical aspects of arteriovenous malformations, spinal angiolipoma, and the intersection between Lean production techniques and medicine. He also has participated in multiple CME presentations for primary care audiences at the Clinic as well as many regional visits to referral centers to give presentations on neurosurgical topics.

Paul Kurt Maurer, MD (1991- 1992): Neurosurgery

Paul Maurer was born on December 20, 1952 in Rochester, New York. His early education was at the University of Rochester where he received a B.A. in biology in 1975. He received his MD from the University of Rochester in 1980. His internship was in surgery at the University of Rochester Medical Center in 1980 followed by his residency in neurosurgery at the same institution with completion in 1986. He then became attending neurosurgeon at the Letterman Army Medical Center in San Francisco, California from 1986 to 1988, followed by an attending position at Walter Reed Army Medical Center in Washington, D.C. from 1988 to 1991. He was elected to Assistant Professor of Surgery for the Uniformed Services University of the Health Sciences in Bethesda, Maryland, a position he held from 1988 to 1991 and was elected Chief of Neurosurgery for the 86th Evacuation Hospital in the Kingdom of Saudi Arabia from 1990 to April 1991. He was chosen "Teacher of the Year" at Letterman in 1987 and 1988.

Dr. Maurer joined Virginia Mason in 1991 and left a year later; despite his short stay, he was awarded the Attending Teacher of the Year from medical and surgical house staff in 1992. As of the Fall of 2018, he serves as Clinical Professor at the University of Rochester in New York and also has a visiting professorship at Walter Reed Army Medical Center in Washington D.C.

Steven Lewis Klein, MD (1993 - 1996): Neurosurgery

Steven Klein was born on June 24, 1958 in Seattle, Washington. He attended Lakeside High School in Seattle and obtained his B.S. degree from the University of Washington in molecular biology in 1980. He then attended Vanderbilt University School of Medicine in Nashville, Tennessee, obtaining his MD in 1984. His internship was at the Vanderbilt University School of Medicine in general surgery from 1984 to 1985. His neurosurgical residency was at the same institution, completing his training in 1990. He then served in the United States Navy in the Division of Neurosurgery at Brooke Army Medical Center in San Antonio, Texas.

Dr. Klein joined Virginia Mason in 1993. He left in 1996 and, as of Fall 2018, works at Northwest Neurosurgery and is Assistant pProfessor of Neurosurgery at the University of Washington.

John K. Hsiang, MD, PhD (1997 - 2005): Neurosurgery

John Hsiang was born on November 15, 1958 in Hong Kong, China. His early education was at the University of Iowa where he received his B.S. degree in 1981; he received his PhD, at the University of Chicago in 1986 and his MD from the University of Chicago in 1988. He then interned in general surgery at the University of California in San Diego, 1988 to 1989, and was a resident in neurosurgery at the University of California in San Diego, 1989 to 1993. He was chief resident in Neurosurgery from 1993 to 1994. He then became Clinical Lecturer in Neurosurgery at the Prince of Wales Hospital at the Chinese University of Hong Kong. He was appointed Associate Professor of Neurosurgery at the Prince of Wales Hospital in 1996.

His major interests are in head trauma, epilepsy, pain management, primary intracranial hemorrhage and multi-monitoring of severe head injury patients in the ICU. Dr. Hsiang joined Virginia Mason in 1997 and left in 2005; he currently practices at the Swedish Neuroscience Institute – Spine Program in Seattle (as of Fall 2018).

Michael Elliott, MD (1998 – 2015): Neurology

Michael Elliott attended George Washington School of Medicine and Health Sciences, graduating in 1990. He did his internship at Letterman Army Medical Center, and his residency at Madigan Army Medical Center, which he completed in 1994. He is Board-certified in neurology with subspecialty certification in Nneuromuscular medicine. He joined Virginia

Mason in 1998 and left in 2015. He currently serves as Executive Medical Director and Chief of Neurology at the Swedish Neuroscience Institute (as of Fall 2018).

Peter C. Nora, MD (1998 - 2005): Neurosurgery

Peter Nora was born in Chicago, Illinois on June 18, 1965. He obtained his B.A. in Biology in June 1987 for Colgate University. He received his MD degree from Tulane University School of Medicine in June 1991, completed his residency in general surgery in June 1992 and his neurosurgical residency in July 1998 from George Washington University. Professional societies include the Congress of Neurological Surgeons, American Association of Neurological Surgeons and the American College of Surgeons. Dr. Nora joined Virginia Mason in 1998. His two areas of major clinical interest at the clinic were cervical cord surgery and subcortical approaches to movement disorder therapy. He left in 2005 and, as of the fall of 2018, practices at the Swedish Neuroscience Institute – Spine Program in Seattle.

Monique L. Giroux, MD (1998 – 2000): Neurology

Monique Giroux received her medical degree from the Ohio State University College of Medicine in 1992. She then did an internship and residency in internal medicine/neurology at Yale New Haven, followed by a 4th year as chief resident. This was followed by a fellowship in movement disorders/functional neuroimaging of movement disorders in the Department of Neurology and Division of Nuclear Medicine at Emory University in Atlanta, Georgia, which she completed in 1998.

Dr. Giroux joined VM in 1998 and stayed for 2 years. In 2009, she did a two-year fellowship in integrative medicine at the University of Arizona. She now serves as medical director and co-founder of the Movement and Neuroperformance Center in Fort Collins, Colorado.

Mariko Kita, MD (2000 - present): Neurology

Mariko Kita is a 1994 graduate of Northwestern University School of Medicine in Chicago. She completed an internship at Northwestern Memorial Hospital in Chicago, followed by a neurology residency at the University of Pennsylvania Hospital in Philadelphia. She then undertook a clinical neurology immunology fellowship as the Sylvia Lawry Post-Doctoral Fellow at the University of California, San Francisco Mt. Zion Multiple Sclerosis Center, which she completed in 2000.

Since joining the Virginia Mason medical staff in 2000, Dr. Kita has served as Director of the Virginia Mason Multiple Sclerosis Center; as interim Medical Director for Hospital Stroke Services; and as Section Head for Neurology. Her specialties include neurology, stroke and multiple sclerosis with a concentration on the design and conduct of clinical trials. She has served as Principal Investigator on multiple clinical trials. In 2017, she was appointed Chief of Medicine, and is serving in that role at the current time (fall 2018).

John W. Roberts, MD (2000 – present): Neurology

John Roberts graduated with a BS in entomology from Oregon State University in 1983 and an MD, from Oregon Health Sciences University School of Medicine in Portland in 1987. He then did an internship at the University of Utah School of Medicine, followed by a neurology residency there, which he completed in 1991. He then took a position as Clinical Associate at the Experimental Therapeutics Branch at the National Institute of Neurological Disorders and Stroke in Washington, DC for 2 years.

In 1994, he took a position as a neurologist at the Veterans Affairs Medical Center in Salt Lake City, and Assistant Professor at the University of Utah School of Medicine. He left that position in 2000 to join Virginia Mason as staff neurologist. Since 2004, he has served as Clinical Associate Professor of Neurology at the University of Washington as well.

Dr. Roberts has a special interest in movement disorders and is a member of the Movement Disorder Society. He has published 29 articles in peer-reviewed journals as well.

Justin H. Stahl, MD (2005 – present): Neurology

Justin Stahl received his BS in cellular and molecular biology from the

University of Michigan in 1996, and his MD from Pennsylvania State University College of Medicine in 2000. He then did a transitional year at Lehigh Valley Hospital, followed by a neurology residency and neurophysiology fellowship at the University of Wisconsin, which he completed in 2005.

Dr. Stahl joined Virginia Mason that same year, and practices general neurology with an emphasis on epilepsy and seizure disorders. He has served as section head for the past 2 years, and as Director of the Clinical Neurophysiology Lab since 2012. He has been principal and sub-investigator on several research projects. He also served as Medical Director of General Neurology at the Evergreen Neuroscience Institute from 2013 to 2016, and currently holds an appointment as Assistant Clinical Professor at the University of Washington.

David Primrose, MD (2005 – 2013): Neurosurgery

David Primrose graduated from the University of Minnesota School of Medicine in 1982. He did his residency in neurosurgery at Upstate Medical Center in Syracuse, NY, which he completed in 1989. This was followed by two fellowships, one at Montreal Neurological Institute and the second at the University of Washington, which he completed in 1990.

Dr. Primrose initially worked at Group Health when starting his practice in Seattle. Later he transitioned to private practice, working at Evergreen and Overlake Hospitals. He joined Virginia Mason in 2005 and retired in 2013. His areas of interest were spine surgery and epilepsy.

Farrokh R. Farrokhi, MD (2006 – present): Neurosurgery

Farrokh Farrokhi attended undergraduate school at Johns Hopkins, where he received a BA in biophysics in 1994. He obtained his medical degree at Baylor College of Medicine, graduating in 1998. This was followed by a year of general surgery residency and four years of neurosurgical residency at the University of Texas Health Sciences Center at San Antonio. He transitioned to Seattle and completed his training as chief resident in neurosurgery at the University of Washington from 2003 to 2005, and fellow in pediatric neurosurgery at Seattle Children's Hospital the following year.

Dr. Farrokhi joined Virginia Mason in 2006 and assumed the role of Section Head of Neurosurgery in 2014. He has served on the Executive Board of the Washington State Association of Neurological Surgeons from 2009 to 2019, serving as President from 2015 to 2017. At Virginia Mason he served as Deputy Director of Quality starting in 2011 and Chairman of the Quality Assurance Committee since 2015. He was an at-large member of the Medical Staff Committee from 2011 to 2014.

Dr. Farrokhi practices general neurosurgery and has special interests in deep brain stimulation, skull base surgery, brain tumors, and minimally invasive and complex spine surgery. His research interests include safety and efficiency in DBS surgery, operating room efficiency through the application of Lean methodology and quality improvement in neurosurgery.

Zornitza Stoilova, MD (2008 – present): Neurology

Zori Stoilova received her BA in biology (2000) and MD (2004) from Northwestern University in Chicago. She then did 2 years of an internal medicine residency followed by 3 years of a neurology residency at the University of Washington, serving as chief resident in 2008, after which she joined Virginia Mason as a staff neurologist and neurohospitalist. Dr. Stoilova practices general neurology.

Nancy B. Isenberg, MD, MPH (2011 – present): Neurology

Nancy Isenberg attended University of California, Berkeley, achieving a BA in biophysics in 1986. She then attended Columbia University in New York, receiving an MD, from the College of Physicians and Surgeons and an MPH from the School of Public Health in 1992. This was followed by a one-year internship in internal medicine at the University of New Mexico, and a neurology residency at Columbia. She then did a two-year fellowship in behavioral neurology and neuropsychiatry at Cornell University in New York, finishing in 1998.

Following completion of her fellowship, Dr. Isenberg took a position as Assistant Professor at Seton Hall University in New Jersey, with a promotion to Associate Professor in 2007. During this time, she was active in research, teaching, and clinical practice, and has authored 21 peer-reviewed publications, 3 book chapters, and 16 abstracts (as of October 2018). She also pursued an interest in Far East religions and mind-body medicine, and was a participant in the Newark Peace Education Summit with HH the Dalai Lama in 2011, and the AVALOKITESHVARA initiation with HH the Dalai Lama in Vancouver, BC in 2014. She completed her Teacher Certification Program at the Center for Compassion and Altruism Research and Education at Stanford University in 2014.

Dr. Isenberg joined Virginia Mason in 2011 as Director of the Memory Wellness Program. She has a special interest in healthy aging, evidence-based holistic treatments of dementia, frontotemporal dementia, Alzheimer disease, and cognitive, behavioral and memory disorders. She is Co-Director of the Wellness Steering Committee at VM and has given many presentations at VM and around the region on topics related to wellness, mindfulness, resilience, compassion and general neurology. She has participated in several TV, documentary and magazine interviews on general neurologic topics as well. She is planning to leave VM in February 2020.

Allen S. Nielsen, MD (2011 – 2015): Neurology

Allen Nielsen graduated from the University of Colorado in Denver, receiving his MD in 2005. He then undertook an internship at the University of Utah School of Medicine, followed by a residency in neurology at the University of Colorado. This was followed by training as a neurocritical care research fellow in neurology at Beth Israel Deaconess Medical Center in Boston, which he completed in 2011. He joined VM in 2011 and worked both downtown and in one of the satellites. He left VM in 2015 and now works for Kaiser Permanente in Fontana, CA.

Emma R. Burbank, MD (2012 - present): Neurology

Emma Burbank attended the University of Massachusetts Medical School, Worcester, graduating in 2007. She then did her internship and neurology residency at Oregon Health Sciences University in Portland, OR, finishing in 2011. This was followed by a one-year fellowship at the University of Utah. Dr. Burbank joined Virginia Mason in 2012 and specializes in neurology, headaches and epilepsy. She practices both downtown and at the Federal Way campus.

Joe Serrone, MD (2014 – 2016): Neurosurgery

Joe Serrone attended the University of Missouri, Kansas City School of Medicine, graduating in 2009. He did a residency in neurologic surgery at the University of Cincinnati, followed by a fellowship there in endovascular neurosurgery and a second fellowship at Helsinki University Central Hospital, Finland, in endovascular and skull-based surgery. He joined Virginia Mason in 2014 but only stayed 2 years; he currently serves as assistant professor at Loyola University Medical Center in Illinois.

Sindhu R. Srivatsal, MD (2013 – present): Neurology

Sindhu Srivatsal received her MBBS (Bachelor of Medicine and Surgery, equivalent to an MD degree) from the Rajiv Gandhi University of Health Sciences in Bangalore, India in 2003. She then came to the US, where she received an MPH from the University of Maryland in 2006. She did a neurology residency at the University of Wisconsin, serving as chief resident her final year. This was followed by a fellowship in movement disorders at the University of Washington, which she completed in 2013.

Dr. Srivatsal joined Virginia Mason in 2013. She practices general neurology with a special emphasis on movement disorders and botulinum toxin administration.

Kelvin K. Ma, MD (2016– present): Neurology, Hospital Medicine

Kelvin Ma received his medical degree from McGill University in Montreal, Canada in 1983. He then did an internship at the Royal Alexandra Hospital in Edmonton, Canada, followed by a neurology residency at the University of Washington, which he completed in 1987.

He joined VM in 2016, first as a locums for hospital-only coverage, and then full-time as a neurohospitalist.

Richard A. Mesher, MD (2015 – present): Neurology

Richard Mesher received a BA in Human Biology from Stanford University in 1975, and his MD from the University of Washington in 1979. He did an internship in internal medicine at the Mt. Zion Hospital and Medical Center in San Francisco, followed by a neurology residency at UW, which he completed in 1983.

Dr. Mesher then took a position at Group Health Cooperative, where he served as a staff neurologist for 31 years. During this time, he also was a visiting attending neurologist at the VA Puget Sound Health System, from 1985 to 1995. He has held an appointment as Associate Clinical Professor of Neurology at UW since 1990.

Dr. Mesher joined Virginia Mason in 2015 and practices general neurology.

Jean-Christophe A. Leveque, MD (2015 – present): Neurosurgery

JC Leveque attended the Amherst College in Amherst, Massachusetts, where he received a BA in neuroscience in 1994. He received his MD from Duke University Medical School in 2001, and then did a residency in neurosurgery at the University of Michigan Medical School with an embedded fellowship in complex spine, all of which he completed in 2008.

Dr. Leveque joined Virginia Mason in 2015, following several years at Group Health Cooperative (GHC). The VM neurosurgeons became acquainted with him and Rajiv Sethi, MD, also a GHC neurosurgeon, as they interacted in the VM Hospital operating rooms. His areas of expertise include complex and minimally invasive spine surgery, pituitary tumors, and peripheral nerve surgery. He is the current President of the Washington State Association of Neurological Surgeons, and has authored 30 peer-reviewed articles and 3 book chapters. He has given numerous invited presentations on a variety of neurosurgical topics. He has also served on several medical missions, including 3 years in Guatemala and a one-week mission to Nairobi, Kenya with the NuVasive Spine Foundation™ in September 2016.

Rajiv K. Sethi, MD (2014 – present): Neurosurgery

Rajiv Sethi attended Brown University in Rhode Island, where he received a BS in neuroscience and a BA in Middle Eastern studies. He then spent a year in Amman, Jordan as a Fulbright Scholar in public health/preventative medicine. He attended medical school at Harvard, from which he graduated in 2001. Dr. Sethi then entered a general surgery internship and orthopedic residency at Harvard, where he served as chief resident the final year and which he completed in 2006. He undertook a one-year fellowship in complex spine surgery/scoliosis and deformity at the University of California, San Francisco, finishing in 2007.

Dr. Sethi took a position at Group Health Cooperative (GHC) in 2007, with a special interest in complex spine surgery; in 2009, he became an investigator at the Group Health Research Institute and the University of Washington where he is still active. He joined Virginia Mason in 2014, having spent many hours in the VM operating rooms as a GHC spine surgeon, and now serves as the Medical Director of the Neuroscience Institute (NSI) as well as Medical Director of Health Economics. Dr. Sethi has been the busiest spinal surgeon at Virginia Mason for the past decade and patients from all over the United States have sought his expertise in recent years for the most complex disorders of the spine. Dr. Sethi's practice focuses on complex adult and pediatric spinal surgery, as well as routine spinal degenerative conditions. To date (as of Fall 2019), Dr. Sethi has given 140 invited presentations regionally, nationally and internationally, and served as chair of multiple summits and courses related to spine deformities and complex spinal reconstruction. This has included visiting professorships in 26 countries. He has produced 47 peer-reviewed articles at Virginia Mason and 17 book chapters, and is associate editor of the *Spine Deformity Journal*. He has edited 2 textbooks on the topics of spine safety and Centers of Excellence and is currently serving on several boards including the Scoliosis Research Society and the Spine Safety Foundation (S3P). Dr. Sethi became a full clinical professor of Health Services Research in the Schools of Public Health and Medicine at the University of Washington in 2018.

He has mentored undergraduate and graduate students from all over the world who come to Virginia Mason for tutelage in the "Seattle Spine Team approach". [1] This also includes fellows and visiting professors, who have visited the NSI from all over the United States, as well as the Netherlands, United Kingdom, India, Japan, Canada, Spain and Brazil.

Fatima E. Mildred, MD (2016 – present): Neurology, Hospital Medicine

Fatima Mildred attended medical school at Universidad Nacional Pedro Henriquez Urena in Santo Domingo, receiving her degree in 1987. This was followed by an internship in internal medicine at the Dispensario Medico La Esperilla in Santo Domingo, and a neurology residency at the University of Aix-Marseille II in Jardin du Pharo, France, which she completed in 1994.

Dr. Mildred then returned to the Dominican Republic, where she took a position as Assistant Professor in the Department of Neurology including the Ramon de Lara Hospital, the Dominican Institute of Cardiology, and the Materno Infantil General Hospital. In 2004, she moved to Jacksonville, Florida, where she worked as a clinic assistant at Nabizadeh Neurology and Neurophysiology for one year. This was followed by an internship in internal medicine at Woodhull Medical Center in New York, a neurology residency at the University of Florida College of Medicine in Jacksonville with her last year as chief resident, and a one-year fellowship in stroke, which she completed in 2010.

Dr. Mildred then took a position as Assistant Professor at the University of Florida, Jacksonville in the Department of Neurology. Two years later, she moved to the Legacy Health System in Jacksonville, where she worked as a neurologist with a focus on vascular issues.

Dr. Mildred joined Virginia Mason in 2016, where she is Attending Neurologist and Director of the Comprehensive Stroke Center. Much of her practice is centered in the hospital, where she specializes in stroke, as well as stroke and heart attack prevention.

Lucas H. McCarthy, MD, M.Sc. (2016 – present): Neurology

Lucas McCarthy studied Neuroscience (BS) and Computer Science (BA) at the University of Rochester, New York, completing his degrees in 2004. He then attended Albert Einstein College of Medicine in the Bronx, NY, where he received his MD as well as a M.Sc. in Clinical Research Methods. Dr. McCarthy then moved across country to undertake a preliminary year internship at California Pacific Medical Center, followed by a neurology residency at Stanford. In 2013, he became an attending neurologist with a focus on multiple sclerosis at the VA Puget Sound Health Care System in Seattle, and started a one-year fellowship in multiple sclerosis at the UW in 2014.

Dr. McCarthy brought these talents to Virginia Mason in 2016. His practice focuses on multiple sclerosis as well as general neurology.

Anik J. Amin, MD (2016 – present): Neurology

Anik Amin attended the Baylor College of Medicine in Houston, graduating in 2011. He did a residency in adult neurology at Rush University Medical Center in Chicago followed by a fellowship in clinical neurophysiology at the University of Washington, which he completed in 2016. Dr. Amin joined Virginia Mason in 2016 and specializes in neurology and epilepsy. He left VM in October 2020 to return to Texas (UT Southwestern) to be closer to family.

Robert Ryan, MD, M.Sc. (2017 – present): Neurosurgery

Robert Ryan received his B.Sc. and M.Sc. in Physiology/Neuroscience from Queen's University in Kingston, Ontario, Canada. He then attended the University of Calgary in Alberta, Canada, where he received his MD degree in 2005. This was followed by a neurosurgical residency at the University of Alberta in Edmonton, Canada, which he completed in 2011. During this time, he did a one-year fellowship at the Barrow Neurological Institute in Phoenix, Arizona, which he completed in 2009. His residency was followed by a two-year fellowship in endovascular neurosurgery at Cedars-Sinai Medical Center in Los Angeles, completed in 2013. At that time, he took a position at the Community Regional Medical Center: UCSF, Fresno. Dr. Ryan joined the Section of Neurosurgery in 2017 and specializes in endovascular and vascular neurosurgery, as well as cranial and general neurosurgery.

Xuan Wu, MD, PhD (2017 – present): Neurology

Xuan Wu attended the Third Military Medical University in Chongqing, China, receiving her MD in 1993 and her PhD in 2001. She entered an internship at Mount Sinai School of Medicine/Queens Hospital in Jamaica, NY in 2009, followed by a neurology residency at Methodist Neurological Institute in Houston, TX, which she completed in 2013. Dr. Wu did a fellowship at the University of Pittsburgh the following year, and then returned to Houston, where she worked as a clinical assistant professor of Neurology at Baylor College of Medicine.

Dr. Wu joined Virginia Mason in 2017 and specializes in neuromuscular disease, amyotrophic lateral sclerosis (ALS) and electromyography (EMG)/nerve conduction studies (NCS).

Rene O. Sanchez-Mejia, MD (2018 – present): Neurosurgery

Rene Sanchez-Mejia attended Harvard Medical School, and graduated in 2002. This was followed by internship and residency in neurosurgery at University of California, San Francisco, and a fellowship at Massachusetts General Hospital and Harvard Medical School, which he completed in 2009. He then took a position with the Scripps Medical Center in La Jolla/San Diego, California. In 2018, he joined the Neurosurgical Section at Virginia Mason, bringing expertise in neurovascular disease, endovascular neurosurgery, cerebral aneurysms and malformations and brain tumor surgery.

Venu M. Nemani, MD, PhD (2019 – present): Neurosurgery

Venu Nemani received a PhD in Neuroscience from the University of California, San Francisco in 2008, and graduated from the UCSF School of Medicine in 2010. He then did a residency in orthopedic surgery at the Hospital for Special Surgery in New York, followed by a fellowship in adult and pediatric spine surgery at Washington University in St. Louis, which he completed in 2016. He then took a position with Raleigh Orthopaedic, a part of University of North Carolina Health Care. During this time, he specialized in cervical and reconstructive spine surgery and also volunteered as a spine surgeon in Ghana, where he surgically treated some of the most rare and complex spinal deformities in both children and adults. [6]

Dr. Nemani joined the Neurosurgical Section at Virginia Mason in May 2019 and will be continuing his practice in complex spine surgery.

Ye Hu, MD (2019- present); Neurology

Ye Hu grew up in Michigan, and attended St George's University School of Medicine in the West Indies, graduating in 2014. She then did a neurology residency, serving as Chief Resident, at the University of Miami, followed by a fellowship in multiple sclerosis at the University of Washington, which she completed in 2019. She joined the Section of Neurology at Virginia Mason shortly thereafter, and has a special interest in multiple sclerosis.

References:

1. Sethi RK, Pong RP, Leveque JC, et al. "The Seattle Spine Team Approach to Adult Deformity Surgery: A Systems-Based Approach to Perioperative Care and Subsequent Reduction in Perioperative Complications." *Spine Deform* 2014; 2(2):95-103.

2. Obituary of John Sutphin Tytus, at: http://www.legacy.com/obituaries/seattletimes/obituary.aspx?n=john-tytus&pid=151462431. Accessed 1 October 2018.

3. Death record, Richard I Birchfield, Department of Health, Death Index, 1907-1960; 1965-2014, Washington State Archives, Digital Archives, http://www.digitalarchives.wa.gov, Accessed 1 October 2018.

4. Obituary of Edward Reifel, at: http://www.legacy.com/obituaries/seattletimes/obituary.aspx?n=edward-reifel&pid=187470622&fhid=11546. Accessed 1 October 2018.

5. Obituary of James Joseph Coatsworth, at: http://www.legacy.com/obituaries/seattletimes/obituary.aspx?n=james-joseph-coatsworth&pid=188423642.Accessed 1 October 2018.

6. "Venu M. Nemani, MD, PhD." at https://findadoc.unchealthcare.org/details/23418/venu-nemani-orthopaedics_and_orthopaedic_surgery-cary-raleigh. Accessed 9 May 2019.

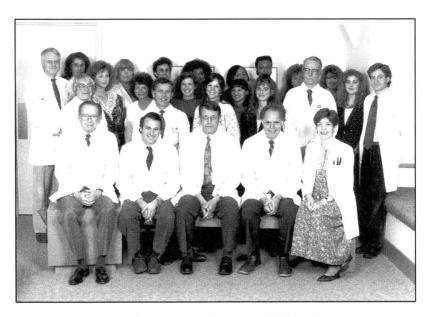

The Neuroscience Team circa 1990 - 1991
Standing, L to R: Laird Patterson, 2 unidentified, Arlene Thomas,
2 unidentified, Sally Cramer, 6 unidentified
Middle row, L to R: Unidentified, Jim MacLean, Leanne Shea,
unidentified, Ed Reifel, unidentified, John Ravits
Front row, seated L to R: Leroy Dart, Charles Nussbaum,
Jim Coatsworth, David Fryer, Lynne Taylor (PH 8317, VMHA)

Farrokh Farrokhi, MD,
Section Head, Neurosurgery

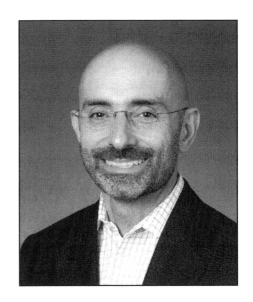

13

Physical Medicine & Rehabilitation

by Dottie Nelson, PT, Michael Weinstein, MD, and Andrew Friedman, MD

Part one: The Early Days of Physiatry at Virginia Mason
by Dottie Nelson, PT

On November 1, 1920, Virginia Mason Hospital admitted its first patient. At that time the hospital had a sixty-bed capacity, laboratory, and x-ray department. A School of Nursing at the hospital was established in 1922. The first dietitian was employed in 1923.

"Treatment of medical ailments and of post-traumatic conditions during World War I brought recognition of the merits of massage, heat, hydrotherapy, electrotherapy, heliotherapy, and diathermy as therapeutic aids." This with the "insistent joint demands of injured workmen and the State Industrial Insurance Commission for the shortest period of disability" [1] led to the opening of a physical therapy department in 1924. It was located on the first floor of the hospital and staffed by Scandinavian-trained **Signe Fossum**, a physiotherapy technician.

In 1927, **Cornelia Newman**, post-graduate of the Harvard Medical School Physical Therapy program, succeeded Signe Fossum. A year later **Dorothy M. Remick**, a qualified therapist, was added to the staff. At this time the first floor department was enlarged to handle an increasing patient load. A 1932 issue of the *Clinics of the Virginia Mason Hospital* describes:

215

"The physiotherapy department, in charge of Miss Cornelia Newman, is equipped with the apparatus necessary for electrotherapy, hydrotherapy, actino-therapy. As much of the equipment as possible is portable so that treatment in the hospital rooms can be given when it is not feasible for patients to be moved. Miss Dorothy M. Remick is associated with Miss Newman in this department. Treatment is available at all times." [2]

In the 1930s the name "physio-therapy technician" was changed nationally to "physical therapist". About this time **Mrs. Madison** took charge of the department. During the years of World War II, the department ran without a qualified therapist as none was available. In 1945, **Vlasta Donahue Guistino** became the chief physical therapist. In 1947, a new and larger one-room department with six treatment booths was opened on the ground floor of the hospital. A second physical therapist was added and the department staff level continued with two therapists until 1957. In that year a full-time aide, **Genevieve Crosby, w**as added to the staff. In 1959, a third therapist was added and staff remained at that level through the 1960s. ·

In 1960, **Ellen Twichell** replaced Vlasta Guistino as head of the department. In 1965, **Jean Unwin**, an English-trained therapist, started a chest therapy program within the department. In 1967, she returned to England but came back in 1969 to form a chest therapy program within the inhalation department. The combination of these two programs, chest and inhalation, were the basis for the hospital's respiratory therapy department.

In 1969, the department expanded to include six treatment booths, two hydrotherapy rooms, a gymnasium, a physician's office for part-time physiatrist **Sherburne Heath, MD**, and a reception area.

In 1970, **William Borba** replaced Ellen Twichell as the head of the department. One of the treatment booths was converted into a combination office-education room to accommodate staff and the new physical therapy students from the University of Washington who began affiliating with VMMC in 1970.

In 1972, the Clinic contracted the half-time services of an occupational therapist, **Mary Ellen Macpherson**. In 1973, **Gayle Green Smith** replaced her as an employee of the Clinic. This was the start of the occupational therapy (OT) department; Gayle was replaced by **Carol Wyble, OTR,** as supervisor in 1979. **Vicki Becker, OTR,** started as supervisor in 1981. By 1985 the department had 10 OT's and 2 COTA's (certified occupational therapy assistants).

In 1974, **Sherwood Young, MD**, joined the staff as full-time physiatrist and head of the Physical Medicine Section. In 1975, a second physiatrist, **Ty Hongladarom, MD,** was added to the staff. Also in 1975, **Dottie Nelson** replaced Bill Borba as supervisor for physical medicine.

Speech pathology was a contracted service in the late 1970s. In 1981, speech pathology was added as a department service when **Marilyn Wyse, MSPA,** became a half-time employee. By 1985, there were four speech pathologists (2.3 FTE's).

There was a major expansion of the department in 1979, which included expansion of the gym, adding an occupational therapy area with a kitchen, and office space for therapists. **Tom Williamson-Kirkland, MD**, joined the staff in 1981, quickly followed by **Steve Fey, PhD,** in 1982. Together they developed the Pain Management Program. **Rita Frangione,** vocational rehabilitation counselor, was added in 1983, thus starting Vocational Rehabilitation Services.

In 1982 Physical Medicine outgrew its space on the ground floor of the hospital, so outpatient services and the clinical psychologist moved to the HRB building. This space was expanded in 1983 to accommodate the Pain Management Program, outpatient occupational therapy, vocational rehabilitation services, and speech pathology services.

As expansion was occurring in the department, a rehabilitation unit was developing in the hospital. This started as 6 beds on 10 East in 1979. In 1985, the rehabilitation unit expanded to 22 beds and moved into remodeled quarters on 5 Main.

In 1981, we established our first PT program in a satellite at the then Phillips Clinic, which was later renamed Mason Clinic Mountlake Terrace. In 1984, we opened an independent satellite PT department one block from Mason Clinic East. This satellite PT department moved into Mason Clinic East in late 1985.

In 1984, Dr. Hongladarom replaced Dr. Young as Section Head of Physical Medicine, and in that same year, **David Fordyce, PhD,** joined the section as the second clinical psychologist. In 1985, Dr. Young resigned and **David Haberman, MD**, joined the staff.

Part two: Remembrances of the PM&R section 1986 - 2011
by Michael Weinstein, MD

Dr. Hongladarom (also known as Dr. Ty) served as section head beginning in 1984 and wanted to build a department of Physical Medicine and Rehabilitation that would rival the UW and provide comprehensive services to the VM patient population. He also encouraged staff parties, which built long-lasting friendships and an esprit de corps in the section.

Not long after the inception of the Pain Management Program, Dr. Ty turned towards developing the Inpatient Rehabilitation Service and outpatient general musculoskeletal and neurological rehabilitation services. In 1986, **Michael Weinstein, MD**, was hired as part of this development (Dr. Weinstein practiced at Virginia Mason for 25 years until his retirement in 2011). His first task was to integrate with the Cardiothoracic and Cardiology sections by establishing cardiac rehabilitation services. Along with **Charlene Tachibana, RN,** (now an administrator), and many dedicated others, both inpatient and outpatient cardiac rehabilitation programs were created. It was not an easy task, as the standard of care at that time was to have patients following surgery or a "heart attack" (myocardial infarction) rest for several weeks prior to resuming activity. During presentations of risk stratification and remobilization, at least one surgeon and cardiologist would pound their fist on the conference table insisting that patients would be harmed through rapid remobilization and targeted exercise. Of course this never occurred, and these approaches remain the "new" standard of care today, improving outcomes and reducing costs of care.

Following the establishment of cardiac rehabilitation services, efforts were untaken by Dr. Weinstein and **Faren Williams, MD** (1990-1998)

218

to create standards, policies and protocols for an Electrophysiology Lab in conjunction with **John Ravits, MD**, of Neurology. This greatly improved the quality of electromyography services for potentially neurologically-impaired individuals. Prior to this time, there were great discrepancies in the performance and interpretation of the studies.

Next, Dr. Weinstein focused on services for brain-injured patients. He worked with David Fordyce, PhD, and **Mary Pepping, PhD**, who were nationally known for their neuropsychology training and skills especially in brain injury. A formal treatment program was created for post-concussion and mild traumatic brain injury. It became the only accredited (Commission on Accreditation of Rehabilitation Facilities, CARF) treatment program in the Pacific Northwest. This was 20 years before the term "chronic traumatic encephalopathy" was coined. Unfortunately, without widespread recognition and acceptance of these conditions, efforts to interface with local sports teams were unsuccessful. Much medical-legal work, especially in British Columbia, arose from this program. Dr. Weinstein and **Rochelle Winnett, PhD** (Dr. Winnett replaced Dr. Pepping, who left to run the Neuro-Rehabilitation Program at the University of Washington) regularly interfaced with the Worker's Compensation System in Washington state and Canada to educate officials in the development of evaluation and treatment protocols. **Maura Grant, SLP,** Director of the VMMC Brain Injury Program, sponsored multiple continuing education courses on brain injury that attracted participants from throughout the USA.

Integration with the section of Neurology remained an important priority for the Rehabilitation section, as so many hospitalized and outpatients shared services and evaluations from both sections. With support from Dr. Ravits of Neurology, Dr. Weinstein, **Cathy Jorg**, and neurological rehabilitation support staff created a template for the treatment of patients with amyotropic lateral sclerosis (ALS), which led to the program becoming the only nationally accredited treatment program in the Pacific Northwest.

Further efforts led to rehabilitation treatment programs for patients with multiple sclerosis and Parkinson's disease. Specialized tools for treatment of neurological complications of these diseases, such as botulinum toxin, deep brain stimulation, and epidural intrathecal pumps, were incorporated into rehabilitation treatment approaches. Protocols and objective measures were frequently shared at regional, national, and international conferences, which are now adopted and incorporated into many other programs outside of Virginia Mason and across the nation.

During this period of program development, a Clinic for Performing Artists was created, which was one of 12 similar clinics in the US. Thousands of amateur and professional musicians, dancers, and vocalists sought evaluation and treatment at VMMC. This program brought national and international attention and recognition to the section.

On the Inpatient Rehabilitation Unit (IRC), many exciting things were also developing. Dr. Ty ceded the Medical Directorship to Dr. Weinstein, as he was preparing to retire. The IRC was the first hospital unit to have its own bladder ultrasound machine. This greatly simplified the evaluation and treatment of patients with bladder dysfunction. Partnerships were developed with Orthopaedics to further improve their outstanding outcomes through rapid remobilization and early, intensive physical and occupational therapy interventions of patients with bilateral knee replacements. The IRC was CARF-accredited, and outcomes were routinely in the top 10% of all rehab units in the nation. Awards were common from CARF. Physician staffing models for the IRC developed at VMMC are now common throughout the nation.

Dr. Weinstein worked closely with the American Heart Association (AHA) to develop the American Stroke Association (ASA). He was on the board of directors for the Northwest/Western States AHA/ASA affiliate and developed protocols for management along the continuum of stroke care. At VMMC, this led to improved treatment protocols from the emergency department through outpatient rehabilitation. He received an award from the AHA/ASA for this work.

Unfortunately, monies for rehabilitation services, both within the hospital and for outpatient management, gradually became less available. Insurance companies and the Centers for Medicare and Medicaid Services

(CMS) started to shunt hospital patients to skilled nursing facilities and cap reimbursement for outpatient services. This led to the closure of multiple programs, including the inpatient program at VM in 2014.

Nonetheless, the outpatient musculoskeletal and spine programs continue to thrive under the directorship of **Andrew Friedman, MD,** Section Head of Physical Medicine and Rehabilitation …

Part Three: General Considerations and Changes in the Department to Current Times, by Andrew Friedman, MD

Physical Medicine and Rehabilitation (PM&R) became prominent as a field in response to underserved needs in the middle of the 20th century. Advances in diagnosis and management of medical and surgical conditions were remarkable, but required a field of medicine that would help patients overcome the functional disabilities that accompany even the successful management of disease and injury. The field advanced dramatically after WWII when returning soldiers prompted improvements in the management of functional disability.

Seattle was a primary center for the development of PM&R. Justus Lehman, MD, founded the department and training program at the University of Washington, which has remained one of the top four or five departments in the world.

In the 1970s the first physiatrist, Sherwood (Woody) Young, MD, came to Virginia Mason and was soon after joined by Dr. Ty Hongladorum. The initial practice was an outpatient clinic working with a therapy team. Soon after they were able to open a four-bed rehabilitation unit in the hospital.

During the 1980s, both the inpatient and outpatient practices grew significantly. Physical and occupational therapy, rehabilitation nursing and psychology all became part of the rehab team. Dr. Thomas Williamson-Kirkland or "WK" was recruited from the University to develop a multidisciplinary pain management program along with his close working partner Steven Fey, PhD. This program had both inpatient and outpatient arms and grew to be the most respected program of its kind in the state. Dr. Arnel Brion also joined the section during this time.

221

At the same time the rehabilitation unit grew to 18 beds. Dr. Michael Weinstein, **Thomas Curtis, MD,** and **Mary Kay O'Neill, MD**, joined the practice, as did David Fordyce, PhD, Mary Pepping, PhD, and **James Moore, PhD**. Specialized units for neurological rehabilitation, industrial rehab and pain were developed. The section joined forces with neurology to develop the electrodiagnostic laboratory under the leadership of Drs. Michael Weinstein, Faren Williams, and John Ravits.

During the 1990s the practice thrived despite changes in the payment structures for medicine as HMOs developed and Virginia Mason began its own insurance product. The benefits of coordinated outpatient rehabilitation were apparent as studies showed the significant cost savings and quality of life gains that could be realized by early rehabilitation involvement in musculoskeletal and rehabilitation care. **Andrew Friedman, MD**, joined the practice in 1995. The pain program had grown to two full-time physicians and four psychologists as well as a team of ten therapists; the inpatient rehab unit was running a census of 16-18 patients at any one time.

The decade from 2000 - 2010 brought significant change. Virginia Mason leadership introduced Lean principles, which would grow to become the Virginia Mason Production System, and there was a strong interest in the concept of value streams—meeting the needs of patients through integration and efficiency in clinical delivery. This challenged the section, which, at that time, was devoting a large proportion of its energy to treating patients from outside the institution in the pain program. **Dr. Heather Kroll** joined the department in 2002 to work in this program. While this continued to produce excellent results for these patients, the access to physiatric care for the patients treated in other Virginia Mason sections was inadequate. In 2004 a decision was made to close the pain management program and focus exclusively on the internal value streams supporting the integration of rehabilitation with other medical teams in the medical center. The pain program survives today as the Rehabilitation Institute of Washington under the direction of Drs. Kroll and Moore. At the same time the section used the Virginia Mason Production System to develop the Spine Clinic model, which became a primary example of how these methods could transform health care by providing early access to rehabilitation care—fostering appropriate early interventions for patients who might otherwise develop significant disability. This model has become a prototype for appropriate spine care nationally.

Additional physiatrists joining the section during this decade included **Leilei Wang, MD**, in 2000, **Ken Takemura, MD**, and **Jill Williams, MD**, in 2002, and **Antoine Jones, MD,** and **Kurt Graham, MD,** in 2007, each with special areas of interest.

From 2010 forward the section has continued to evolve as trends in health care demand. Changes in reimbursement forced the closure of the inpatient rehabilitation unit in 2014, a phenomenon that has been seen around the country. **Julie Hodapp, MD; James Babington, MD; Matthew Grierson, MD,** and **Kristoffer Rhoads, PhD**, joined the section and brought expertise in neurorehabilitation, interventional spine care, regenerative medicine and image-guided procedures, as well as a focus on the diagnosis and management of cognitive disorders and the disabilities associated with cancer and its consequences. The section became more closely integrated with neurosurgery and neurology in the Neurosciences Institute at Virginia Mason. The strength of this integration has helped Virginia Mason differentiate itself from other organizations by offering truly integrated care and demonstrating a commitment to appropriateness and value in neurological and spine care.

The department currently (as of August 2018) has six physiatrists – Drs. **Andrew Friedman, Julia Carp, Thomas Curtis, Kristen Gage, Atul Gupta** and **David Yu. Jennifer Kelly, PsyD**, is a Rehabilitation Psychologist and Rochelle Winnett, PhD, practices neuropsychology in the department. Their work is supported by a staff of 24 physical therapists, one PA-C (**Taryn Erbe**), two Occupational Therapists, two Speech Pathologists, one Pharmacist, one Naturopathic doctor (**Kevin Connor**), and one COTA, as well as other support staff. Through partnerships with the Virginia Mason Institute and through an increasing emphasis on research and publications, the Virginia Mason PM&R section is now seen as a model for care delivery and has strongly influenced care design and contracting at both the state and national level. As of this time, the pace of change appears to be accelerating with movement towards value-based care and accountable contracting models. The section appears to be in a strong position to help drive adaptive change for the medical center.

References:

1. Palmer LJ, Schultz M, Windom AL. "PM&R at Virginia Mason Medical Center." *Clinics of the Virginia Mason Hospital.* Vol III, number II, page 51, Seattle, WA: August 1, 1924.

2. "The Virginia Mason Hospital." *Clinics of the Virginia Mason Hospital.* Vol X, number III, Seattle, WA: January 1, 1932.

14

Psychiatry and Psychology

by Edward Rynearson, MD; Scott Hansen, MD, and Stephen Melson, MD

with contributions from Peggy Flanagan, LICSW;
Bill Thurman, MFA, MSW; John Adams, MD; Lawrence Rainey, PhD;
Arden Snyder, PhD; Maxine Nelson, MSW, & Steven Juergens, MD

1972 – 1998: The Beginnings and Growth of an Outstanding Psychiatry/Psychology Section
by Ted Rynearson, MD

The section of psychiatry at Virginia Mason began in September of 1972 when I joined Virginia Mason as the 78th physician – and first mental health consultant. I had interned at Virginia Mason in 1965 so I was warmly welcomed by most, though there were several MDs who had little time or respect for Psychiatry.

John Walker, MD, was chief of radiology and Chairman of the clinic when I joined. He welcomed me the first day and while shaking my hand said, *"We know psychiatry is never going to make us much money – don't worry about that. We need your help in developing a service our patients need."*

That WAS a different time.

Trained at the Mayo Clinic, I had a clear idea of the importance of offering prompt consultation service for outpatients and the hospital, and that was my focus for the first two years as the only psychiatrist. I always had time to see patients within 24 hours including a face-to-face conversation with the referring physician so I could develop collaborative relationships. I also spent considerable time visiting surrounding psychiatric hospitals, psychiatric clinics, etc. to establish a network of support, referral and recognition. Herb Ripley, MD, was the first chair of psychiatry at the University of Washington and he arranged a faculty appointment for me and began sending psychiatric residents to work in our section over the next several years.

There were only a handful of administrators and they functioned as allies – their role began to change as their numbers swelled and they became more enforcers than allies – but in those early years they added to our efficiency and assisted us in developing new services.

Steve Melson, MD, also trained at Mayo and joined the section in 1974. We considered opening an inpatient psychiatric unit, but Cabrini Hospital (then situated on Madison and Ninth Avenue) had a 30 bed psychiatric unit, which dampened the possibility of receiving state and federal approval (required in that era) for a new unit. So, we hospitalized patients on the 7th floor with neurology patients – and began using ECT (electroconvulsive therapy - given with anesthesia in the surgical recovery room! – try doing that in 2015).

In 1975, with administrative support, we refurbished the Penthouse at the Inn at Virginia Mason, hired additional staff and opened an intensive day hospital Psychotherapy Unit for patients with non-psychotic disorders, which is discussed in more detail in the following section. For the next 22 years we treated 150-200 patients each year with a program of intense, time-limited psychotherapy and pharmacotherapy. We published several pilot studies documenting improvement with pre/post standardized measures. This unit was closed by administrative fiat in 1997.

During the late 70s we began hiring PhD, psychologists (to provide testing and specialized group and individual therapies) and additional social workers for psychotherapy. This group included **Steve Troner, PhD** (1976); **Arden Snyder, PhD** (1979); **Jan Dortzbach, PhD** (1980); **Peggy Flanagan, LICSW**; **Susanne James, MSW,** and **Bill Thurman, MFA, MSW.**

Roy D. Clark, Jr, MD, joined the group in 1978, and **Peter Manos, MD**, arrived in 1984 from the University of California, San Diego and soon began working full time in the hospital, meeting the increasing need for comprehensive psychiatric evaluations.

Another important milestone occurred in 1984 with the establishment of the Separation and Loss Service, which continues to this day. The goals of this program include:

1. **Clinical Service** – to provide free consultation and short-term treatment to local community members disabled with grief.

2. **Clinical Training** – to sponsor local, regional and national trainings for clinicians providing clinical intervention(s) for grief.

3. **Clinical Research** – design and fund clinical outcome pilot studies of short-term treatment(s) for grief.

4. **Clinical Networking** – to extend clinical service through trainings and research to a regional and national network of consultants and service providers for grief.

The program is funded partially by Virginia Mason, and partially by grants and gifts. The program has a long record of success and has produced numerous clinical papers and two books clarifying the specific effects of violent dying on bereavement. Most of these studies have been anecdotal – illustrating specific clinical findings with specific case illustrations and treatment strategies (Restorative Retelling). In 1990, a manualized agenda was created for a time-limited group psychotherapy (Restorative Retelling) that could be empirically tested and applied at multiple sites, and this process continues to be used successfully both at VM and other sites.

Lawrence Rainey, PhD, joined the section in 1985 and Roy Clark left in 1987. **Maxine Nelson, MSW,** joined the section the same year. **Dick Gode, MD**, transferred from the University of Washington, Children's Hospital in 1987 to begin our Child Psychiatry Sub-section, quickly adding additional child psychiatrists and pediatric clinical psychologists including **Lee Carlisle, MD** (1995 – 1999); **Deborah L. Thurber, MD** (1997 – 1998); **Jim McKeever, PhD** (1988 – 2003) and **Carol Cole, PhD** (1990 -1999), and supported by social workers **Peggy Diggs, MSW;**

Laura Reilly, MSW, and **Molli Wilson, MSW,** to provide specialized services for comprehensive evaluation and treatment of children and adolescents.

Steve Juergens, MD, left the staff at Mayo to begin the chemical dependency program in 1988 – an outpatient program that ran successfully for the next 12 years – and hired chemical dependency counselors to staff that effort.

It was also at this time that we added two psychiatrists (**Michael Ruthrauff, MD**, and **Jim Houser, MD**) and a social worker (**Duane Prather, MSW**) to provide psychiatric service at the Federal Way Satellite. Several social workers also joined the section downtown in the early 1990s, including **Nancy Mundt, MSW,** and **Mary Hodge-Moen, MSW. Decky Fiedler, PhD**, joined the group a few years later.

In 1988, the Virginia Mason Center for Women's Health opened with **Jennifer D. Bolen, MD**, providing psychiatric staffing; she was joined a few years later by **Patsy Paddison, MD**, in 1991, and **Shubhada K. Kode, MD**, in 1995. Although successful for a few years, the program collapsed in the late 1990s; Dr. Bolen left for private practice shortly thereafter and Drs. Paddison and Kode moved their practices to Adult Psychiatry; Dr. Paddison left the section in 2003.

At that point the number of providers and support staff (including three full-time secretaries to ensure the confidentiality of our records) required a move from the main campus to one of the Metro towers. That move provided a significant upgrade in our physical space, but significant diminishment in our contact with our medical and surgical associates. In retrospect, it was a time that heralded our downward spiral as a section able to provide comprehensive psychiatric evaluation and service to adults and children. Peter Manos's office, however, stayed on the main campus so prompt hospital consultations continued as usual. Eventually he became a member of the Hospitalist Service.

During this time, **Marianne Kampf, ARNP,** was hired as a full-time therapist to run the outpatient day program (Psychotherapy Unit described below). Marianne was an incredible asset, not only prescribing medications

228

but also offering cognitive behavioral therapy with groups both mornings and afternoons. She left a few years later when the outpatient day program closed in 1997.

Psychiatry and psychology practice migrated outward to the satellites in the 1990s as that system grew in prominence within the Medical Center. Drs. Cole and Snyder saw patients at VM East (now Kirkland) with social worker Nancy Mundt; Decky Fielder, PhD, saw patients in the North satellite (now Lynnwood); Drs. Ruthrauff, McKeever, Carlisle and Houser saw patients at VM South (now Federal Way) along with social workers Duane Prather, Molli Wilson and Laura Reilly; and social workers Peggy Flanagan and Bill Thurman saw patients at VM Issaquah.

All of these practices were discontinued in the late 90s, which was a time of increasing austerity and administrative edicts – severe cuts over which we had no control – and when offered an early retirement in 1998, I accepted. It was very painful watching the dismemberment of a section we took such personal and professional pride in creating. There were 24 professional staff members when I retired in 1998 (10 psychiatrists, 4 psychologists, 10 social workers) – by 2015, there were four psychiatrists for adult outpatients and two psychiatrists for hospital consultation, with only one (Dr. Kode) longstanding staff member.

The clinic has continued to be supportive of me since my retirement allowing me to function with the Separation and Loss Service as a locums associate. In retrospect, I feel very fortunate to have been associated with Virginia Mason at a time that was so creative and comparatively uncomplicated for all of us "old timers".

The Psychotherapy Unit at Virginia Mason Medical Center (1975 - 1997)

This is written more as a remembrance than a report about the Virginia Mason Psychotherapy Unit. The intensive day treatment program at Virginia Mason ran for over 20 years from 1975 to 1997. It is a psychiatric "Dodo" in contemporary times and terms, but worked for many patients and was a great place to practice and learn for staff. And it was a professionally inspiring place for me.

At the Mayo Clinic in 1966 (over 50 years ago), Loren Pilling, MD, a new member of the psychiatric staff, began an all-day, 3-week group therapy program for Mayo Clinic outpatients for $25 per day/patient with a break-even point at 20 patients. At that time and place there were abundant patients seen as outpatient consults willing to remain for focused therapy for reactive disorders and stressors and resonant conflicts.

Roy MacKenzie, MD, was a chief resident who staffed the unit with Loren, and they both left the Mayo Clinic in 1968 (Pilling to Minneapolis and MacKenzie back to Canada where he pioneered work in group therapy teaching and research). I arrived in 1968 for my three years of residency just as they left.

The three months I spent in that unit were pivotal experiences in my training, and I hoped to replicate a similar program and research its effectiveness in Seattle, where I eventually settled. There was no rigorous demand or interest in psychotherapy research at Mayo. Despite a large number of patients (400-500 per year?), treatment studies of the day hospital unit offered little beyond pre/post-MMPI measures to document good outcomes with no control or comparison treatment cohort.

H.R. Martin, MD, and Gerry Peterson, MD (a fellow resident who joined the Mayo staff) continued running the day hospital program at the Mayo. I think it closed down in the late 1990s when they each retired, but by that time they must have treated several thousand patients.

When I left Mayo in 1968 I made a search to find and review other day treatment programs. Community mental health centers were new and abundant with day treatment facilities but were focused on patients disabled with chronic psychotic disorders (their focus has not changed). The only existent program with a psycho-dynamic model that I was able to find was in Vancouver, B.C.

Ferdinand Knobloch, MD, a Czechoslovakian psychiatrist, immigrated to British Columbia after surviving the Holocaust. Before the Holocaust, he had been an early innovator of community psychiatry. In an affiliation with the University of British Columbia section of Psychiatry, he embedded the principles of community in an intensive outpatient psychodynamic treatment center. Patients remained in an all-day treatment format (multiple insight-oriented group and individual modalities) for 3 or 4 months during which they not only focused on their personal difficulties, but were "forced" to meet the social and political demands of the community government. Dr. Knobloch published several books describing his treatment model and center, but with little empirical confirmation.

I was very impressed, but after visiting him and spending a day observing the program, I found him to be overly absolute and patriarchal. I knew 3 or 4 months in a rigid community would not fit the attitudes of our patients and staff in Seattle and thought comparable improvement might occur in a looser structure over a shorter period of time. He was dismissive then, and later, when we presented a thoughtful outcome study with standardized pre/post measures - his response was: "I don't believe it."

When I first settled in Seattle in 1972, I was the first and only psychiatrist at VM until Steve Melson, MD, arrived in 1974. Steve also trained in psychiatry at Mayo as did Roy Clark, MD, and Steve Juergens, MD, who joined us later. We all had rotated through the Mayo Day Treatment program.

In 1974, opening an in-patient psychiatry unit was limited by Washington State statutory regulation. Because Cabrini hospital had a 30-bed inpatient psychiatric ward, we could not apply for approval. Steve and I were allowed to hospitalize psychiatric patients on the neurology floor at Virginia Mason for short-term stabilization and electroconvulsive therapy (ECT - we performed ECT with anesthesia in a corner of the recovery room!) However, this was far from ideal, and without nursing support staff and room for programmatic expansion, we decided to develop a more intensive program for outpatients.

At the time we were seeing enough out-of-town, outpatient and inpatient consults to open a day hospital program for 8 to 12 patients, so we met with George Auld (one of only FOUR full time administrators at The Mason Clinic); over a hand shake approval, and, to the best of my recollection, we charged $100 per day or $500 per week for the program, which was often covered by outpatient insurance benefits. George also approved a generous budget to remodel the Penthouse Suite at the Inn at Virginia Mason as a therapy space – particularly handy for out-of-town patients who could rent a room in the same building at a nominal fee.

A consultant from Miller/Pollard (a local furniture store) helped to design the space and select furniture, drapes, and kitchen equipment, and we equipped a group therapy room with AV cameras, monitor and tape recorder so we could tape groups for replay.

Our first hire was Peggy Flanagan, LICSW, who was newly hatched from her training at the UW. This rather major decision was decided after one, or possibly two interviews. We immediately liked Peggy, and though she hadn't ever worked in a day hospital setting (there weren't any in the area), Steve and I forged ahead and offered her the job. As I recall, she was somewhat dazed by what we expected from her (spending 8 to 10 hours each day, 5 days a week with 8 to 10 patients) while Steve or I co-led morning and afternoon groups with her and arranged to see each patient for an individual appointment every week.

We also required someone for bare, minimum staffing to serve as a "greeter, organizer" - someone to answer the phone, take messages, arrange tours of the unit for prospective patients … and a host of other chores. **Ruth Hetherington** had moved to Seattle from Alaska where she and her husband had run small businesses. She saw an announcement for the position on a bulletin board as she was leaving her cardiologist's office at VM and applied that same afternoon. She and Peggy bonded, and because she was from Alaska, she could deal with "almost anything without claws or fangs" - she was the glue that held us together in the early days.

We opened the unit in late 1975.

I insisted on introducing a "real" artist into the week's agenda rather than an occupational therapist. Patients needed to process dreams, life diagrams and non-verbal images. Making ashtrays and weaving bracelets would not measure up. We found Bill Thurman, MFA, who was teaching at a local art school. Although he hadn't any experience working as a psychotherapist, we admired his art, his eagerness and his wicked sense of humor. That was enough. We piled our patients into one or two cabs and trans-

232

ported them to the art school (imagine doing that now!) to paint and draw, and Bill would lead a group in the unit to review the art with group members and staff. Eventually Bill earned an MSW to complement his MFA.

Each of the group therapy sessions was taped.

Some years later, another social worker and artist from our staff, Maxine Nelson, MSW, began sharing in some of the unit rotations and was particularly interested in audio-visual techniques (including profile self-confrontation) that she developed with patients.

Soon we also included our PhD, psychologists in the mix as they joined our section staff – Arden Snyder, PhD, and Larry Rainey, PhD, who alternated in leading cognitive and anxiety management skill enhancement groups in the afternoons. We invited them to join in staffing the unit despite their extensive training and sophistication compared with most staff members.

I started a projective group once a week. Initially Peggy and I would take the group to a matinee movie feature with a discussion to follow. Several patients had panic attacks while viewing *The Taxi Driver* at a local theater, so it became obvious that we had to be more selective. I developed a library of emotionally evocative, short tapes. After viewing a 20 or 30-minute tape and enacting psychological crises and family issues, group discussion would follow, highlighting variance in group members' sensitivity and/or avoidance of themes.

Another valuable non-VM addition was **Gerry Olch, MD,** a child therapist and psychoanalyst, who met with unit staff members once a month over a group lunch as an outside consultant reviewing problem cases and staff challenges. Including an outside consultant was clarifying for the program.

There were additional opportunities for teaching and research:

• Several members of the Virginia Mason house staff were interested in psychiatry and spent elective rotations in the unit with us during their internships and residencies. I remember 4 or 5, one of whom went back to the East Coast for her psychiatric residency.

• In the 1980s and 90s, the UW Department of Psychiatry allowed their psychiatry residents to electively rotate through the unit.

- Sometime in the 1980s, a PhD student spent considerable time with us developing an extra-mural research evaluation of our program through pre/post audiovisual patient monologues. Each patient completed a monologue on the first and last day of therapy while looking at a card that read, "What change or changes do I anticipate with psychotherapy?" and these comparative tapes were reviewed by outside graders following an evaluative protocol. Of greater importance than the study, however, was our continuous use of pre/post monologues and our viewing them at the beginning of each patient's treatment.
- We completed an outcome study on a sizable group of patients with standardized measures published in a refereed journal.

Comments from other members of the team:

Steve Melson, MD:

Ted and I considered the nascent Psychiatry Section's clinical needs at The Mason Clinic in the mid-1970s — the predominance of the Department of Medicine's outpatient population (middle-class and working-class individuals and families); referrals from internists and surgeons to psychiatry approaching 80% of new cases; relatively low numbers of chronically mentally ill/psychotic patients; the presence of a competent inpatient psychiatric facility literally across the street from the Medical Center — our experience with the Mayo Clinic program led us to request the opening of a small-group therapy program for individuals and couples, which would be intermediate between low-intensity outpatient weekly or biweekly psychotherapy sessions and inpatient hospitalization.

It is difficult to reconstruct today just how different the world of psychiatry/psychology was then. Psychopharmacology was in its infancy together with neuropsychiatric knowledge of brain chemistry/neurotransmitters/functions of specific clusters of neurons and their connections. Freudian psychoanalysis was in decline, mental health/medical insurance was virtually unknown, and the stigma of seeing a psychiatrist for anything was in full force.

Virginia Mason, in spite of little experience or knowledge of then-current psychiatric practices, had a trusting relationship with the Mayo Clinic and the 2 young psychiatrists they had hired who had been trained there. CEO John Walker, MD, hired me as the second psychiatrist on the staff in the summer of 1974 on a handshake - I never signed a contract of employment in all my years with VM, nor did I feel the need to do so. He and John Allen, MD, Chief of Medicine, were always steadfast supporters of our section.

In 1976, we put out an inquiry to the University of Washington's MSW program for candidates to join the staff of the newly-approved Intensive Psychotherapy Unit (IPU). Peggy Flanagan, LICSW, applied, was interviewed, and joined us for what was to be a 20+ year position as lead psychotherapist, followed over several years (chronologically) by the other members of the IPU staff: Bill Thurman, MFA, MSW, art therapist and psychotherapist; Arden Snyder, PhD, and Larry Rainey PhD, clinical psychologists who added behavioral and anxiety management, important components to the intensive curriculum; Steve Juergens, MD, as the third psychiatrist rotating with Ted and myself in providing direct group and individual therapy plus medical/pharmacologic care to patients; Maxine Nelson, MSW, as a group and individual psychotherapist; and program coordinators Ruth Hetherington and later, **Ruth Lieu.**

What was so unusual about this staff? It was a prescient example of Team Medicine, years before that became Virginia Mason's marketing ad, with Masters' level, PhD, and MD staff functioning as a cohesive, integrated unit in a complex, patient-centered multidisciplinary therapeutic milieu. It is a rare and serendipitous occurrence when such a collection of highly educated, emotionally stable and intellectually astute professionals come together over many years' time to care for a diverse patient population, and to learn from and enjoy each other's respective contributions, in friendship and mutual regard.

Peggy Flanagan, LICSW:
I laughed at your description of my being "dazed" by the expectations and

the experience. I remember sitting in with either you or Steve with your new patients - I was speechless most of the time when one of you would ask for my input. I learned so much more than in graduate school - I was overwhelmed to say the least! I had gone from marrying at 17, starting college when my son started kindergarten and completing an MSW in 6 years. I did volunteer work, worked a summer at the Crisis Clinic, but really, this was my first "real" full time work. Ever! You and Steve really did take a chance on me. To my credit, I had a good 6 years of pretty intensive psychotherapy before starting graduate school.

Ruth was such a mentor and support to all of us. She was gracious to a fault. I, on the other hand, was what Ruth would call "A Little Green Apple". The first in my family to go to college, or have a profession - it was life altering for me.

Those movies were really something as were Thursday lunches to various restaurants in Seattle. What a different city in the 1970s. We saw *Close Encounters of the Third Kind* too, but *Taxi Driver* was the scariest! I remember being frightened myself. Lunches and trips to Pike Place Market were the usual Thursday routine in the early days. It was not quite the same after leaving the Mason House - that Penthouse was special. The elevator would get stuck and we would climb those nine flights of stairs.

Do you remember the man (not in one of the groups) who came up to the Penthouse to commit suicide by jumping from the balcony? The group members saved him! It was quite a dramatic scene. I believe many were helped by knowing how much they could be of help to others. On one grocery-shopping trip to gather food for our infamous Friday lunches that the group prepared, one group member stopped a robbery, I believe. One of my saddest memories is of an elderly Alaskan native gentleman who described his experience in boarding school as a young boy. He was so abused! He told his story with such heart and spoke about "water dropping from my eyes".

It also seemed that we were in the very beginnings of women opening up about sexual abuse. It was a common story for many of the women in the group. I watched one young woman knit hats while in group. She had an expression I've not heard before (or since) but will always remember: "Time Wounds All Heels".

Somehow I think it may have been such a wonderful time for me because I really didn't know what was supposed to happen! So, listening, welcoming, feeding, caring, nurturing, all the stuff that really matters, that's what we did. We created a safe place to be heard.

Bill Thurman, MFA, MSW:

Matisse did not possess an MFA - Henri didn't need it. However for those of us with lesser artistic chops, the attainment of a two-year Master of Fine Arts degree represented a possible stepping-stone toward finding a teaching position in a college or university. Such patronage allows for the continuation of one's artistic pursuits replete with a dental plan. The arrival in my UW studio by a former graduate inquiring whether I might be interested in a part-time teaching position at a local private art college fit in nicely with the above-mentioned design, and I, of course, answered in the affirmative.

The art school I was to apply to was the Factory of Visual Art situated in the former Good Shepard Home in the Wallingford district of Seattle. The Pacific Northwest Ballet was housed within these venerable walls at the time, and I recall those graceful birds as lending a sense of professionalism to the place.

I interviewed with the director, and she hired me after a brief interview and informed me of the responsibilities I would have. In addition to a drawing class, I was to work with a group of individuals who were part of a new psychotherapy program at Virginia Mason Medical Center, something referred to as "art therapy". I had no conception of what that was, but I had ventured into a variety of stranger things over the course of my existence, and I was up for a new adventure.

Three days a week patients were taxied from First Hill for their hour and a half art sessions where they were provided the opportunity to freely paint and draw as part of their treatment. I learned that **Dr. Edward Rynearson**, the head of Virginia Mason's then tiny department of Psychiatry, had trained at the Mayo Clinic in Rochester, Minnesota, where art had been a component within the intensive outpatient treatment program. He chose to continue this interest after moving west.

Over the course of my work as an artist, I have come to appreciate that feeling lost might signal an opportunity for new growth and impending change. I thought it wise in this novel endeavor, however, to investigate what art therapy might entail. This was 1976, a few decades prior to the internet. The local libraries were woefully limited in what I could find, and what I did find was reductionist or projective (draw a person, house, a tree). Ok, I'm an artist, I told myself, just make stuff up, and see what happens.

My first day I was introduced to the once and future Peggy Flanagan, social worker, and the elegant Ruth Hetherington, the program coordinator for the Psychotherapy Unit, a kind of dorm mom with dance moves. Both accompanied the group to the art sessions, and for two years the taxis came and went three times a week until it was decided that enduring these often wild rides was taking time that might be used more effectively. The decision was reached to move the art component closer to the medical campus, and an apartment was found in what then was the Northcliffe apartment building, now the home of the new VM hospital.

With the change in venue it was necessary that I become an employee of Virginia Mason and a grueling gauntlet of interviews was endured. Actually it was a one-hour lunch with Drs. Rynearson and Melson, over glasses of wine at the Sorrento Hotel's Hunt Club across from the Emergency Room. Dr. Rynearson asked what I had in mind regarding the art process, and I uttered spontaneously that I thought mask-making would be an interesting idea. I hadn't noticed that Dr. R. had ordered a Karl Jung salad with anchovies, but his spirit and curiosity rose significantly at that point.

I found myself once again having to invent another unknown process, and again I reminded myself that I was an artist – just make something up.

The mask-making actually turned out over the years to be a fascinating exercise, and a review, coauthored by Dr. Melson and myself, was ultimately published in the *Psychiatric Annals* and partially republished in *Psychology Today*. Apparently using masks as a method to explore personality was at the time a novel concept in psychotherapy.

Gradually the art component of the Psych Unit grew to occupy perhaps 30% of the program, as patients not only created their artifacts but later brought them into the group sessions to present and discuss. Having been through both undergraduate and graduate schools of art, I remain to this day amazed at what was created by individuals who for the most part had not produced a work of art since their 3rd grade teacher informed them that elephants can't be blue.

Along the way I had continued to maintain a studio under the shadow of the Space Needle and work on my art. Gradually I began to realize that a dental plan would not be forthcoming from my efforts, and I had no desire to move to New York. I approached Dr. Melson one day and inquired how I might become a larger part of the program, and he said to go gather another graduate degree, which I did. I was accepted into the University of Washington's School of Social Work. I spent my first year field placement in Harborview's ER and my second at American Lake Medical Center in Tacoma. I became a full-time employee of Virginia Mason in 1982.

As timed passed, unfortunately the luxury of having such a kind and patient three-to-four-week program as the Psychotherapy Unit bumped into new administrative and economic realities. I summarized the arc of the department of Psychiatry recently to one of my physicians as moving from memories, to milligrams to money. As Vonnegut might say, "so it goes". Adios Camelot. It was a great way to spend several decades. The "unit" closed in 1997. I recall thinking at the time I was never fully confident in what I was doing with the art, maybe I should have just made something up.

John Adams, MBChB, FRANZCP:

(In 1983, Dr. John Adams, MBChB, Department of Psychological Medicine, University of Otago, Dunedin, New Zealand, spent six months in the VM section of psychiatry. John was particularly interested in the Psychotherapy Unit and established a similar program when he returned to New Zealand at Ashburn Hall, a private psychiatric hospital. This program blossomed under John's directorship for the next 20 years but closed after John became Dean of the Otago Medical School, a position that required all of his

professional time and energy.)

I got to know Ted during one of his visits to the Psychological Medicine Department in Dunedin. When I was looking to go overseas for 6 months in the final year of my registrar (resident) training, Ted suggested that I come to The Mason Clinic and work partly in the Intensive Group Psychotherapy Unit. My wife Rosie, son James and I were hugely fortunate that Steve Melson decided to come to New Zealand (NZ) at the same time, and we were able to live in his house on Bainbridge, close to Ted's ongoing support and mentoring. Knowing what Steve came to in NZ, I'm very sure that we got the better part of the deal.

We arrived at the beginning of 1983 and stayed 6 months. The time at Virginia Mason, and particularly in the Psychotherapy Unit, was one of the most formative experiences in my development as a psychiatrist. Being able to watch Bill, Peggy, Ruth and Ted work with such expertise with the group, and with people individually, was a huge privilege and an enduring learning experience.

I had come from a working environment at Ashburn Hall in Dunedin where I worked in groups in a therapeutic community setting, but this outpatient group unit treating some of the most psychologically resistant patients was at a different level. I witnessed huge change in patients. I saw how the quiet persistence and skilled delivery of psychotherapy through art, movies, eating together and family work, finally enabled many patients to understand and express the emotional turmoil that had been driving their physical symptoms.

I saw how Ruth's understanding and administration created the foundation of safety for the group participants; how Peggy's great sensitivity and capacity for empathy on the background of her professionalism allowed people to talk about things they previously had been unable to; how Bill's artistic skill and perceptive therapeutic intervention made art such a conduit to patients' inner worlds; and how Ted worked with such clinical knowledge, attunement, and capacity for relationship that groups seemed to move and flow in a way that I had not previously witnessed. It is one of the things I feel most fortunate about in my life - that out of this experience

240

grew an enduring friendship with Ted that I continue to treasure.

There were some interesting cultural differences for me. You would think that New Zealand and the US would be pretty similar culturally, but as I quickly found, and commented to people about, Americans' more verbal way of being made the whole process quite different. In New Zealand I spent most of my time in groups trying to get people to talk; in the US, it was trying to get them to stop talking!

My time at the unit was a part of my training. I wrote a review of short-term group psychotherapy and put that together with five case studies of patients I helped treat at the unit as my final assessment for my training. I kept those for a long time, and re-read them intermittently when I needed to remind myself of the things that I learned. Unfortunately, they eventually got water damaged by a leak, and I had to throw them away – no digital files in those times!

When I returned to Ashburn Hall, I was determined to put in place some of the things that had impressed and enthused me. The first thing that I managed to do was to convince my bosses that we should employ an art therapist. I can remember interviewing and engaging Jill Thompson, an occupational therapist with a keen understanding of art in a therapeutic context. Jill was wonderful, and together we reviewed some of Ted and Steve's writing, as well as my experience, and transposed some things into our context. We started with patients making masks and talking about them; we had patients expressing themselves in art and talking about the meaning of it in groups, and eventually we had people making a tile to go on the wall when they left that expressed their experience and their feelings about leaving. One of the big changes was setting up art rooms and helping people with the technical side of their art. When Jill eventually left Ashburn Hall many years later, she set up an organization in Dunedin called *Artsenta,* a place where patients in the community could go, spend time, talk with others and express themselves through art. They held regular exhibitions of their work. Jill has retired, but *Artsenta* lives on as a really important part of the Dunedin mental health treatment scene.

When the opportunity arose some years after my return, we set up at

Ashburn Hall (now called the Ashburn Clinic) a day group psychotherapy unit, as one of the programs at the hospital. We called it the James Hume Day Psychotherapy Unit, after one of the founders of Ashburn Hall in 1882. It was modeled on The Mason Clinic unit and was highly successful. We were fortunate to have a building that we remodeled to house the unit. Patients lived in a mostly independent living arrangement also on the hospital grounds, and attended the unit daily. Some would transition out into the community and continue to come to the unit as outpatients. Sadly, the unit had to be closed as part of austerity measures at Ashburn Hall when things got very bad financially. I have not given up hope that the unit will open again.

Every day when I walk into my office at the Medical School, I am reminded of the Intensive Group Psychotherapy Unit. On my wall is a piece of art, one of 5 productions that a patient did as her art project while at the James Hume Unit just before I left Ashburn Clinic. She was very clear that she wanted me to put it on the wall in my office so that people could understand how important her experience there had been. On my shelf is a set of three masks, gifted to me in the same way by a woman who was in the James Hume Unit when I left. The masks fit over the top of one another. They represent what she presented to the external world, what was in the first layer behind that, and what lay deeper. I have shared them with medical students, as was her instruction. Again, the work of the Intensive Group Psychotherapy Unit and all its wonderful staff continues a long way away and in a context that you probably never anticipated.

Lawrence Rainey, PhD:

I joined the VM Psychiatry Section as a psychologist in 1985 and participated in the Psychotherapy Unit as a part of my clinical activity until the Unit closed in 1997. My role included both conducting a twice weekly afternoon anxiety and stress management skills group (rotating with Arden Snyder, PhD) and, for a few years, serving on a rotation basis as one of the two clinicians leading the morning, dynamically oriented psychotherapy groups. Part of the morning program was a weekly "family" group (Fridays) to which spouses, adult children and/or close friends of patients were invited. Along with all staff involved in the program, I attended weekly clinical meetings during which patients' histories, clinical status and progress in the program was reviewed. What follows are some thoughts on various aspects of the program, as viewed through the lens of my clinical involvement.

Anxiety and Stress Management Group: This was a cognitive-behavior-oriented, patient education and skills building group (CBT). Meeting twice weekly in the afternoons (as I recall), this group complemented, in some regards, the more dynamic, personal-narrative-focused psychotherapy groups. Dr. Snyder had worked out a basic curriculum for the CBT group prior to my arrival, consisting of elements such as progressive muscle relaxation and guided imagery training for stress/anxiety reduction, basic patient education about cognitive distortions that often contribute to anxiety, assertiveness in interpersonal communication, as well as general stress reduction strategies. Written handouts and self-assessment questionnaires also were used to give patients further input. The somewhat more "structured" feel to this part of the overall program was welcome, and probably quite helpful, for some of the Unit patients who may not have had as much experience with psychotherapy or who were, at least initially, reticent about being in an intensive psychiatric treatment program.

Family Group: This once weekly, end-of-the-week group also was, in my view, a valuable part of the program. My recollection is that participation was quite good, meaning that most of the patients had some member of their family or a close friend/associate attend this group. This served to give significant others in the patient's support network some sense of key issues for the patient (sometimes, of course, directly related to the family) and also afforded patients a sense of emotional support and affirmation during what often was a very difficult or even crisis period in their lives. We, as clinicians, often gleaned new perspectives and clinically valuable information from observations made by family members.

Art Therapy Group: Although I was not directly involved in the art therapy portion of the Unit, I was able to look at what patients had done in the art room and would hear in clinical groups about patients' feelings and insights from their art therapy work. This was, in my view, a very potent and important part of the program, giving participants avenues to express emotion-laden material that they may not have been able or ready to verbalize. A particularly creative and evocative exercise in the art room was the creation of masks—often very elaborately and imaginatively formed—symbolizing "inner" and "outer" self-images. (I am sure that Bill, Peggy, and Maxine can elaborate on this much better than I. The art therapy aspect of the Unit should also be documented with pictures, as well as words, for any historical record.)

Primary, daily psychotherapy group: Here patients would share their histories, formulate their current clinical complaints/problems/foci for the group, and attempt to work through these issues or, at least, achieve an emotional balance and formulation of their issues that allowed a fruitful transition back to outpatient care. Length of treatment in the Unit was variable but usually in the range of 2-4 weeks, I believe. The psychiatrists and other psychotherapists conducting these groups probably have a variety of observations and viewpoints about the groups. The psychodynamic groups were characterized by being emotionally intense, clinically challenging (due to the wide variety of mood, anxiety, psychosomatic, and personality disorders represented in the group), group-dynamic oriented (e.g., encouraging the engagement of patients with each other, as well as attention given to the process of the group as a whole), and intensively staffed (by a psychiatrist or clinical psychologist and a clinical social worker). It should be noted that patients would not have committed to this level of time commitment and intense personal examination if they were not in considerable distress. Though these were non-psychotic patients, they may have been, for instance, in the throes of an acute depressive episode, experiencing panic attacks, having prolonged and intense psychosomatic problems, or experiencing affective dysregulation and significant interpersonal problems related to characterological disorders. I recall, for instance, clinicians in training or other professional visitors who might sit in on a group feeling "exhausted" after just one such group. I also recall a young, visiting psychiatrist from China, wondering out loud after observing a few such group sessions, "why we didn't just tell the patients what they should do!" (or words to that effect), reflecting not only what I took to be a notable cultural difference but also the understandable wish to escape the strain of the psychotherapeutic process. These groups, stressful and confusing as they could be, did allow patients the time, support, and a safe place to explore complex and very difficult issues in a concentrated way (i.e., several hours per day, five days per week).

Impact on staff: As one who worked in the Psychiatry Section both during and for several years after the disbanding of the Psychotherapy Unit, I came to appreciate the positive role the Unit had for professional staff education, cohesion, and morale. Outpatient clinical mental health work can be quite isolating. The Psychotherapy Unit work was something that we did conjointly as a professional staff team. This afforded one of the few times that we actually were able to observe each other working with patients or to reflect and share with colleagues about what had been a joint clinical experience. This was a welcome change from the many hours alone in an office seeing a parade of patients individually. While "staffing" patients in the unit (formally, on a weekly basis, and informally between groups on a daily basis) we also learned much from each other (e.g. about psychiatric medications, varying insights about assessment and diagnosis, a variety of perspectives on psychotherapeutic methods, etc.). The Psychotherapy Unit and the collaborative work it provided for the staff afforded a type of ballast to the Psychiatry Section that, in my opinion, went wanting in years after the Unit's termination.

Importance of the physical space: We were very fortunate to have a separate and well-designed space for the Psychotherapy Unit. Having, for instance, a designated, camera-equipped group therapy room, an art therapy room, and lounging/dining space for patients provided an important "feel" to the program that facilitated the clinical work. This helped facilitate a sense of group cohesion among the patients, I believe, and also helped reinforce the focus of the work (as if to say, "Here is a place, set aside and designed for psychotherapeutic exploration.") One could have put the same therapeutic groups and clinical content in generic office and conference room space and had a quite different impact, I would posit. At the same time, having the program housed as part of the larger medical center (not a set-aside psychiatric facility) gave the program a certain "legitimacy" for some patients and helped them accept such treatment as part of their healthcare. (The white lab coat "vestments" worn religiously by some staff in the early years also helped serve this purpose.)

Role of the coordinator: Others would be much better prepared to elaborate on this, but I think it must be noted that the Unit Coordinators who had daily contact with the patients throughout their entire stay played a very significant role. With regard to orienting new patients, providing informal but important emotional support outside the designated clinical groups, problem solving various logistical issues patients might have had during their stays, and keeping professional staff informed about what might be happening outside the clinical groups, the coordinator functioned as a type of "mortar" for the program.

Observations after the Unit closed: Working for many years as a psychologist in the Psychiatry Section after the closing the closing of the Psychotherapy Unit, I often wished that the Unit were still available—especially when referred patients who were in crisis and/or presented with very intense and complex clinical problems, yet were not acutely suicidal, psychotic or otherwise requiring psychiatric hospitalization. These situations called for a level of care more intense than that which could be provided by outpatient psychotherapy (e.g. weekly sessions) and intermittent medication management visits. The Psychotherapy Unit could have filled this gap. Virginia Mason also treated a number of patients from rural locations throughout the Northwest and Alaska, where outpatient psychiatric services were not available; an in-house intensive outpatient program provided a good option in such cases. A third group that could have benefitted from the Unit was comprised of patients who had gone through extensive medical workups without clear findings and were thought to have significant psychiatric issues contributing to the clinical picture (somatoform disorders of various types). Often referring medical providers would be hoping to find a more intensive mental health treatment intervention to

246

offset a pattern of repeated medical consultations, emergency room visits, or unnecessary medical hospitalizations. There were, at times, other partial hospital programs in the area (e.g., at Overlake Medical Center), but ease of referral and coaxing sometimes reluctant patients into treatment, plus coordination of care and facilitating ongoing follow-up care, became much more cumbersome and less effective as compared to an in-house program.

Closing thoughts: The Psychotherapy Unit was discontinued not because of lack of clinical relevance, nor due to ineffectiveness, but rather, I believe, because its structure and mode of operation were out of step with a then prevailing ethos that prioritized cost containment, short-term treatment and faster patient turnover, increased patient volume per provider, physician extenders, etc. Such steps were sometimes assumed to mean "efficiency," though whether this approach to patient care is truly more efficient in the longer run remains, to my knowledge, an unanswered, empirical question, at least as it pertains to psychotherapy outcomes. I would not be at all surprised if something resembling the Psychotherapy Unit again becomes integrated in medical centers in the future, particularly those trying to provide a full array of mental health care within a comprehensive healthcare system.

Arden Snyder, PhD:
I greatly enjoyed leading the Cognitive Behavior Therapy and Anxiety Management sessions to which the patients were very responsive. Many of us gave several professional presentations on the VM PTU and there were several publications that resulted.

Maxine Nelson, MSW:
In 1987, I became the third social worker to join the staff of the Virginia Mason Psychotherapy Unit. Following a moderately successful but financially uncertain career as a visual artist, I decided to become a psychotherapist. I did my graduate studies in social work at the University of Washington, and after graduation, began reaching out to people I knew for leads about potential jobs. One of these people was Bill Thurman, who

I had become acquainted with in the late 1970s, when both of us were part of the Seattle art scene. Bill invited me to have lunch with the staff of the Psychotherapy Unit and, after an informal interview, I was hired to join the staff. I recall feeling both overjoyed and anxious, as I was such a green therapist and was certain that my academic studies (based on cognitive behavioral approaches) hadn't prepared me for the task at hand. Once I started, I eagerly soaked up all I could from the rest of the staff, particularly Ted Rynearson and Peggy Flanagan, with whom I regularly co-led the different groups that constituted the program.

The program we implemented, originally based on a similar program at the Mayo Clinic, was life saving for many, if not most, of the patients who went through it. Many of them expressed that coming to the Unit was their "last straw," and expressed gratitude to both the program and the staff when they were ready for discharge. I feel that the homey atmosphere, particularly of the Inn at VM penthouse, served as an institutional container and that they were able to explore the origins of their current crises and to explore—both with the staff and with other patients—various approaches or solutions that hadn't been available to them prior to admission. The care they experienced was provided in groups with more or less the same people, 6-8 hours a day, five days a week, for 3-6 weeks. I believe that it was both the intensity of treatment, as well as the consistency of the staff and the program, that allowed so many of them to resolve the initial crisis that had brought them in, and to provide the motivation to continue working through their problems once they were discharged.

Later on, in the spirit of ongoing innovation, I was encouraged by Ted Rynearson to employ my creativity, which I did first by becoming trained in psychodrama in 1990 and later by instituting a split profile video technique, where patients could explore different aspects of themselves through viewing their two profiles simultaneously, in real time, on the video monitor. Psychodrama is a powerful projective technique and, while I believe the experience was helpful for many of the patients who participated in the weekly groups, it was ultimately discontinued when I realized that, for extremely vulnerable patients, the psychodrama experience could produce

248

regressive states that are difficult to contain in a day hospital program. The split profile technique, also projective, was quite fascinating for patients to participate in, and I only regret that I didn't have sufficient psychoanalytic knowledge at the time to make optimal use of it. Despite this, I am grateful to have had the opportunity to co-present this work along with Ted, under the title "Profile Self-Confrontation," at the APA Annual Meeting in New York in May 1990.

My work in the Psychotherapy Unit has influenced my practice in several important ways:

1. Through my experience on the staff of the Psychotherapy Unit from 1987 – 1997, I learned the value of intense, albeit brief, psychodynamic psychotherapy. I realize that being able to have that kind of experience as a patient today is a rarity, as most outpatient and inpatient programs have been modified in response to changes in insurance coverage as well as to the popularity of psychotropic medications. This is indeed unfortunate as I feel that no matter how efficacious psychotropic medications are, they are not a substitute for working through emotional conflicts, which can only occur with long-term psychodynamic psychotherapy or psychoanalysis. In part inspired by my work in the Psychotherapy Unit, I began psychoanalytic training in 2003 and currently have a mostly psychoanalytic practice.

2. Another aspect of my practice that has been influenced by my experience in the Psychotherapy Unit is my interest in psychosomatic disorders. Most of the patients who came to the Unit were referred by Virginia Mason physicians, primarily specialists. Because Virginia Mason functioned as a multi-specialty clinic, modeled after Mayo, I found these physicians to be fairly psychologically minded. Most of them were both interested in and respectful of our psychological assessments, which then enabled the Psychotherapy Unit staff to work collaboratively with the referring physicians. I believe that we helped many of these patients to put their feelings and unresolved conflicts into words, rather than express them somatically. As a result, I have a particular interest and sensitivity to patients who experience psychic conflict somatically and have recently developed this as a sub-specialty.

3. One of the most innovative aspects of the Psychotherapy Unit was its use of short animated films and art to help patients access feelings. In the safety of the group setting, patients were able to draw timelines of their lives, make paper boxes depicting—among other things—discrepancies between the inside and the outside, and make life masks using plaster to depict how they saw themselves. As a result of my experience there, I began showing films to professional and later, to mixed audiences, inviting them to share their responses as a form of "communal dreaming". The first instance was the screening of the Malian film *Brightness* (1987), which was presented in the 1990s. This was followed by two psychoanalytic film festivals I produced at the Seattle Art Museum, one in 2003 and the second in 2005, in which psychoanalysts and film scholars would present brief commentaries on films to a mixed audience. I continue to write and present films today.

Steve Juergens, MD:

I came to Virginia Mason in 1988 and so enjoyed my work in the Psychotherapy Unit. As I am about to retire from private practice, I reflect on my years and see that the times working in the unit were among the most rich, enjoyable and rewarding. Why was that? The three or four-week intensive time frame, the group setting, the time for art and mask making, the milieu giving time for people to do real work. It was creative and not cookbook. There was pain but allayed by humor and perspective. It was gentle and a shelter from the storm. It involved families as well, so there was a fuller view into our patients' lives.

There was an engagement with patients that propelled the therapeutic relationship. I am closing my private practice and saying goodbye after 30 years to patients that I first met in the Unit, and I recall with them our time together and they invariably bring up an experience "in that Unit thing in that weird apartment building" and their memory of what their mask meant, what became clear in family session or how they understood their reactions had to do with their development, "not that their husband was really so bad, just that he was like my father."

It was also a place to develop close collegial relationships. We all knew that foxhole and shared it often together. Ruth was a glue of compassion and patience. It was great to be able to meet together and holistically draw a picture of what to do as best we could. It was a place full of humor. I have never had as much enjoyment or humor or intensity in any other area of my practice.

The Managed Mental Health Program (1991 - 2001)
By Stephen J. Melson MD, Section Head

As Ted Rynearson, founding father of the Section of Psychiatry and Psychology, noted in his excellent chronologic narrative, the section got off to a low-profile start in the Department of Medicine with his arrival in 1972; I joined him in October 1974, freshly minted from my residency in internal medicine (one year) and psychiatry (3 years) at the Mayo Clinic. We quickly became professional colleagues and lifelong friends, building the section over the first 10 years or so into a highly-regarded and referred-to service in the downtown clinic and hospital, with the addition of excellent clinical psychologists, psychiatric social workers/therapists, hospital and outpatient psychiatrists, the innovative Intensive Psychotherapy Unit day hospital, a chemical dependency program ...

It was a true Team Medicine section (well before that became a marketing term) along with many other medical/surgical sections that made Virginia Mason a smaller "Mayo Clinic of the Northwest". Ted Rynearson was a mentor to me and many others, interested in and engaged in direct clinical practice, psychiatric pedagogy and innovation/improvement of psychiatric/psychological therapies. He was not much interested in administration nor attending non-clinical meetings, so we traded off the section head position every couple of years until I agreed to take it longer-term in 1988.

By that time, as Ted noted, we had become a much larger, multidisciplinary, geographically diverse section, and by 1990, like the rest of the medical center's clinical sections, were faced with increasing services in several satellites as well as the burgeoning partnership with Group Health and

251

the Alliant HMO. We were a very large multidisciplinary section at the height of our growth, with 11 Psychiatrists (2 Child/Adolescent, one Consultation-Liaison in the hospital), 5 PhD, Clinical Psychologists, 2 ARNPs, and up to 26 Master's Level Psychotherapists in 7 locations—Downtown, Lynnwood, Federal Way, Port Angeles, Kirkland, Bellevue, Bainbridge Island, and later, (after my time) Issaquah and University Village.

It was around this time that VM Administrator Sarah Patterson asked that I, as section head, get involved in recurring accreditation efforts with JCH Accreditation for our section, and attend a National Committee for Quality Assurance (NCQA) organizational meeting (at that time it was a new quality assurance organization for developing rigorous standards for large medical groups). I then was named Medical Director of the brand new Managed Mental Health (MMH) program, where, with an excellent manager and former clinician staff, we developed a Puget Sound Behavioral Health Referral Network that efficiently evaluated and connected patients with credentialed, certified therapists, inpatient and chemical dependency units — all coordinated with their insurance benefits.

I knew little about this complex work in the beginning; thanks to the manager, Mike, and dedicated MMH staff, mostly from Group Health, I learned a lot and the MMH program was a great success, lasting 10 years until it was summarily disbanded with the collapse of the VM/Alliant HMO contract with Group Health. Sadly, the network, consisting of contracts of considerable value with high-quality, regional therapists, ARNPs, clinical psychologists, psychiatrists, and inpatient units, dissolved in 2001.

At the height of VM's partnership with Group Health, (1991 - 2001) the two very different organizations were cooperating well and integrating several service lines, including our Psychiatry and Psychology section with their much larger Behavioral Health Department—in fact they asked, and I acceded to (with some internal resistance) change our name to the Section of Behavioral Health. Their leaders and I spent many hours over 2 years' time researching and planning for a full integration of our two services, which would have made for the largest integrated Behavioral Health Department on the West coast. As I learned more about their "peculiar" (to a fee-for service practitioner) cooperative, got to know their people and how well they coped with a very limited mental health benefit while thoroughly integrating with Primary Care, and observed the world-class research they were conducting on major depression and anxiety disorders in large primary care populations, I looked forward to more years working with them. Unfortunately, this didn't happen as the collapse of the Alliant contract led to the two organizations mostly parting ways.

Despite these disappointments, my career as a psychiatrist was a satisfying one. I had wonderful training in a medical-science/clinically-focused, patient-centered institution (the Mayo Clinic), which was great preparation for the life's work I found at Virginia Mason—if you like people, growth in knowledge and experience in your (still young) chosen specialty, it's the most interesting, challenging, and often rewarding job in the world.

1999 – 2010: Downsizing and Restructuring

With the closing of the Psychotherapy Unit in 1997, the retirement of Drs. Rynearson in 1998 and Dr. Melson in 2002, the Psychiatry Department underwent a series of changes. It continued to serve the outpatient needs of Virginia Mason patients and providers with an ever-diminishing staff of providers. The Child Psychiatry and Chemical Dependency Programs closed in 2000 as an administrative decision related primarily to cost concerns that were affecting Psychiatry programs nationwide. Stalwarts Patsy Paddison, Steve Juergens and Michael Ruthrauff went into private practice. **Alice Laurens, ARNP,** joined the section in 1999, and **Grzegorz A. Longawa, MD**, arrived in 2002 or 2003, staying only 2 years. Psychiatrists **Marty Hoiness, MD** (who later served as Section Head) and **John Fredericks, MD,** were hired from UW training programs in 2003 and 2007 respectively, and **Joseph Doumit, MD**, joined the group in 2011; meanwhile, Shub Kode continued her practice. Psychologists Lawrence Rainey and Arden Snyder and therapists Susanne James, MSW and Bill Thurman continued to provide much needed clinical support, and Peter Manos managed the inpatient psychiatric service until his retirement in 2010. At that point, first **Karina Uldall, MD, MPH,** and then **Scott**

Hansen, MD, were hired to replace Dr. Manos and manage the expanding inpatient needs.

2011 – present: Focusing on System Changes in Inpatient Psychiatry by Scott Hansen, MD

Since 2011, there has been an increased focus on systemic changes to psychiatric and behavioral health services at Virginia Mason. Areas of emphasis have included delirium prevention and early recognition/intervention, addressing the clinical precipitants to code gray events, management of involuntarily-detained/civilly-committed psychiatric patients in the hospital, improvement of staff de-escalation skills, routine screening and intervention in primary care for depression/anxiety/alcohol use and integration of psychiatric and behavioral health services in primary care.

As these changes have occurred there has been growth in teams that have led the improvement work. After the retirement of Peter Manos in 2011, Karina Uldall joined Virginia Mason and started developing the behavioral health care capabilities of the Emergency Department and the hospital inpatient services. She continued Dr. Manos' role of direct clinical consultation care, while focusing on team education, care quality, and safety for patients with behavioral health conditions in the hospital. Scott Hansen joined the inpatient consultation service in 2012. The growth of the ED social work team, which developed into a cohesive and skilled group under the guidance of **Megan Bott, MSW,** and Karina Uldall, was important to extending the capacity of the hospital psychiatry consult service. The ED social workers and hospital consultant psychiatrists developed an important partnership in evaluation and treatment planning for patients with behavioral health conditions. During the period of time between 2012 and 2019, the volume of patients detained for involuntary psychiatric civil commitment from the Emergency Department or hospital service rose from a handful to hundreds per year. The number of patients who remained at Virginia Mason after detention on Single Bed Certification orders also rose dramatically during this same period. To manage this increase in volume, the psychiatry consult service team increased to in-

254

clude social worker Natalie Anderson, LICSW and Involuntary Treatment coordinator Stacey Bell, who is currently in a MSW program.

Dr. Uldall left Virginia Mason in 2019 and **Jay Owens, MD**, has joined the hospital psychiatric consultant team.

The outpatient group saw many changes during this time. **Maria Yang, MD**, joined the group in 2011, but left only a year later. Drs. Frederick and Doumit left in 2015, and Dr. Hoiness left the following year. Bill Thurman retired in 2013 and began a second career as an artist. **Brian Neal, MD**, began to practice outpatient psychiatry with Dr. Kode, but left two years later.

Today (September 2019), the section includes 3 psychiatrists (including Drs. Kode, Hansen, and Owens), one PhD, psychologist (**Rachel A. Freund, PhD**); an attention deficit disorder specialist in pediatrics (**Jason Law, MSN, ARNP**); 4 social workers (**Adam M. Gleason, MSW, LICSW; Leighanna D. Kilgore, LICSW; Nancy Y. Namkung, MSW, LICSW**, and **Rebecca J. Springer, MSW, LICSW**) and one counselor (**Seiko Y. Ryan, LMHC**), working in various locations, including the downtown campus, Kirkland, Bellevue, Issaquah, Bainbridge Island, and University Village.

Programs And Timeline For Psychiatry/Psychology Staff
Adult Psychiatry/Consultation/Day Hospital Program – Psychotherapy Unit
Edward (Ted) K. Rynearson, MD: first "straight medical intern" at The Mason Clinic in 1965; started section in 1972. retired in 1998; serves as a locums associate in the Loss and Separation Program.
Stephen J. Melson, MD: 1974 – 2002; Section Head from 1988 - 2000
Arden Snyder, PhD: 1979 - 2013
Larry Rainey, PhD: 1985 - 2015
Peggy Flanagan, LICSW: 1975 - 2001
Bill Thurman, MFA, MSW: 1975 – 2013
Maxine Nelson, MSW: 1987 - 1998
Marianne Kampf, ARNP: 1995 - 1997

PhD Psychologists
Steve Troner, PhD: 1976 – 1978
Jan Dortzbach, PhD: 1980 - 1982
Rachel A. Freund, PhD: 2016 - present
Decky Fiedler, PhD: 1990s

Hospital Psychiatry Consultative Service
Peter J. Manos, MD: 1983 – 2010
Susanne James, MSW: 2002 - 2015
Alice Laurens, ARNP
Karina K. Uldall, MD: 2011 – 2019
Scott M. Hansen, MD: 2012 – present; Section Head of Hospital
  Psychiatry Consultative Service
Jay Owens, MD: 2019 - present
Natalie Anderson, LICSW
Stacey Bell (currently obtaining an MSW degree): Involuntary Treatment
  Coordinator

Child Psychiatry
Richard O. Gode, MD: 1987 – 1996
Jim McKeever, PhD: 1988 - 2003
(Lynda) Lee Carlisle, MD: 1995 – 1999
Debra L. Thurber, MD: 1997 – 1998
Carol Cole, PhD: 1990 - 1998
Peggy Diggs, MSW: 1991 - 1998

Chemical Dependency / Adult Psychiatry
Steve M. Juergens, MD: 1988 – 2003; served as Director

Federal Way Satellite Psychiatry
Michael Ruthrauff, MD: 1988 – 2000
Jim Houser, MD: 1998 - 1999
Duane Prather, MSW: 1991 - 1999

(Lynda) Lee Carlisle, MD: 1995 – 1999 (see above; Child Psychiatry)
John T. Frederick, MD: 2007 - 2015

The Virginia Mason Center for Women's Health (1988 – 1999)
Jennifer D. Bolen, MD: 1989 – 1998
Patsy L. Paddison, MD: 1991 – 2003; joined Adult Psychiatry staff when Women's Center closed
Shubhada K. Kode, MD: 1995 – present; joined Adult Psychiatry staff when Women's Center closed and later served as Section Head; currently practices outpatient psychiatry at the Bellevue and Issaquah satellites.

Adult Psychiatry – Outpatient
Marty H. Hoiness, MD: 2003 – 2016; served as Section Head
John T. Frederick, MD: 2007 - 2015
Joseph R. Doumit, MD: 2011 – 2015
Maria Yang, MD: 2011 - 2012
Brian Neal, MD: 2016 - 2018

Current Mental Health Professionals Serving VM Patients (as of September 2019)
Rachel A. Freund, PhD: approximately 2016 – present; Seattle campus
Adam M. Gleason, MSW, LICSW: Seattle campus
Scott Hansen, MD: 2012 – present; inpatient psychiatry
Leighanna D. Kilgore, LICSW: Kirkland satellite
Shubhada Kode, MD: 1995 – present; Bellevue, Issaquah satellites
Jason Law, MSN, ARNP: Attention Deficit Hyperactivity Disorders in children; University Village
Nancy Y. Namkung, MSW, LICSW: University Village
Jay Owens, MD: 2019 – present; inpatient psychiatry
Seiko Y. Ryan, LMHC: Seattle campus
Rebecca J. Springer, MSW, LICSW: Bainbridge Island

15

Pulmonary Medicine

by Steven Kirtland, MD

The Section of Chest Diseases at The Mason Clinic was created by **Edward Morgan, MD**, in 1950. The section has changed its name several times over the ensuing years, and is now known as the Section of Pulmonary Medicine. It has spawned 4 additional department of Medicine (DOM) sections, including Infectious Disease in 2000, the Sleep Disorders Center in 2003, Critical Care Medicine in late 2002/early 2003 (although the final separation in titles was not until 2012), and the Center for Hyperbaric Medicine in 2010. (For more information on these four sections, please see below as well as chapters 9, 18, 30, and 8 respectively in this volume.)

In addition to clinical medicine and research, teaching residents, fellows and colleagues has been a priority of the section since its inception. Over a 20-year span, under the tutelage of **Richard Winterbauer, MD,** the section produced six fellows, three of whom went on to join the staff at Virginia Mason (**David Dreis, MD; Bill DePaso, MD**, and **Steve Kirtland, MD**). Multiple members have received the Department of Medicine "Teacher of the Year" award, led by Dick Winterbauer, who received the award an unprecedented 5 times. Section members have been recognized nationally through hundreds of peer-reviewed publications as well as holding leadership positions in various national and international societies. In addition, the pulmonary section has been active in the Medical Center with several members serving on multiple Medical Center and Research Center boards and committees, as well as holding various leadership positions including Chief of Medicine, Chief of the Research Center and Chief of Staff. Finally, three of our members are **James Tate Mason Award** winners.

In July of 1950, "fresh from completion of a fellowship in internal medicine at the Mayo Clinic, Dr. Morgan's high energy and devotion to research had already produced a bibliography numbering 20 articles at the time of his arrival." [1] He quickly became known as one of the premiere pulmonologists in the Northwest. Patients adored him and he was the primary internist to many. Dr. Morgan was respected throughout the medical center for his astute clinical skills and research prowess. Along with H. Rowland Pearsall, MD, in the Section of Allergy and Immunology, they were the first to describe "Bird Fancier's Disease", a hypersensitivity pneumonitis to avian protein. They arrived at this insight after seeing a patient with an odd "waxing and waning combination of obstructive air flow disease, migratory pneumonitis, and pleural effusion." [1] Through careful questioning, they elicited that the patient had over 400 parakeets in his basement, and then devised a skin test to prove that they were acting as an allergen. They published their findings in the *Bulletin of The Mason Clinic* in 1960. [2] "This scenario typifies an interest and dedication" to clinical research "that has continued in the Section of Pulmonary ... Medicine." [1] Dr. Morgan became the first board-certified pulmonologist at Virginia Mason, and served as Section Head for many years. He also was involved with the residency program and was always asked to perform the "mouse trick" at every resident graduation celebration. Dr. Morgan retired in 1982 and died in 1996.

John D. Allen, MD, joined the Section of Chest Diseases in 1961. Known for his direct approach and dry humor, not to mention his flashy bow ties, he gained respect throughout the institution. He provided leadership as the Chief of Medicine from 1970 to 1990. During his tenure a Satellite system was established and he was paramount in the creation of the first VM-based health care plan and served as its Medical Director. He served in many leadership capacities including President of the Washington Thoracic Society and the American Lung Association. Dr. Allen retired in 1997 and passed away December 7, 2012.

Eugene "Neely" Pardee, MD, joined the section in 1967. He had previously established himself as an expert in tuberculosis as the director of the Firland sanitorium. Dr. Pardee championed the art of the physical exam and would teach residents and fellows alike the variances of different breath sounds. His clinical wisdom was invaluable. Dr. Pardee introduced fiberoptic bronchoscopy to Virginia Mason, and was the first to treat endobronchial disease with laser bronchoscopy. In 1992, during the last third of his career, he introduced sleep medicine to Virginia Mason along with **Kenneth Casey, MD** (who joined Virginia Mason in 1987) and became the inaugural medical director of the first sleep lab at VM, as well as Virginia Mason's first board-certified sleep medicine physician (For more information on sleep medicine, please see chapter 18 in this volume: "The Virginia Mason Sleep Disorders Center".) Dr. Pardee retired in 1999.

The most historic and influential member of the pulmonary medicine section, **Richard Winterbauer, MD**, joined the section in 1969. He had trained at Johns Hopkins Medical Center in both pulmonary medicine as well as infectious disease (having worked for a year at the CDC). He became section head in 1970, a position he held until his retirement in 1999. Under his leadership the section became known as the Section of Chest and Infectious Diseases. He was widely known throughout the institution as "the Buddha" - the physician to go to with all of the difficult cases. During his tenure he created and led the pulmonary medicine fellowship. Residents clamored to rotate with him just to glean a morsel of his knowledge. Dr. Winterbauer was known throughout the Northwest as the most astute clinical pulmonary physician in the region, and he was regularly referred a variety of difficult cases from outside physicians. He was especially sought after for his expertise in sarcoidosis and interstitial pulmonary fibrosis. In 1973, he developed and published "guidelines for a clinical interpretation of bilateral hilar adenopathy", which has been "widely used in the diagnosis of sarcoidosis both in the USA and internationally". [1] He also did extensive work with **Steven Springmeyer, MD** (who joined the section in 1984) and Sam Hammar, MD, a member of the Pathology Department, on the use of bronchoalveolar lavage in various clinical situations. Dick authored hundreds of peer-reviewed articles and numerous chapters throughout his career. Over his 20-plus-year span as section head, he hired 7 additional members. He received multiple "Teacher of the Year" awards as well as the **James Tate Mason Award** in 1994 and retired in 1999.

C. James Martin, MD, was also hired in 1968 as Director of the Institute of Cardiopulmonary Research at the VM Research Center. He divided his time between this position and a position at Firland Sanatorium where he continued his clinical research as Director of their cardiopulmonary laboratory. [4] He was replaced by **Dan E. Olson, MD, PhD,** in 1977. Dr. Olson only stayed a few years. **John W. Little, MD**, joined the section in 1980, but only stayed for 3 years.

David F. Dreis, MD, was the first homegrown member of the section, having completed his pulmonary fellowship and medical residency at Virginia Mason. He joined the section in 1983 after the retirement of Ed Morgan. Dave was a master clinician and loved by patients, staff and colleagues. He was a learned teacher and rose to become Chief of Medicine for 9 years (1991 – 1999). He was also a recipient of the "Teacher of the Year" award. Dreis left clinical practice and worked solely in Administration for several years before retiring in the fall of 2014. He died January 26, 2015.

Steve Springmeyer, MD, joined the group in 1984. He grew up in Utah, and attended medical school there before coming to Seattle for internship, residency and fellowship at the University of Washington. He was working at Fred Hutchinson Cancer Center as Director of Pulmonary Services when he accepted the position at Virginia Mason. He brought his knowledge of bronchoalveolar lavage and created a laboratory with Dr. Hammar in Pathology that served many outside pulmonologists. Steve, along with Don Low, MD, introduced lung volume reduction surgery to Virginia Mason. He also was the first in the Northwest to utilize fluorescent bronchoscopy. Dr. Springmeyer left Virginia Mason in 2001.

Kenneth Casey, MD, joined the section in 1987. He was recruited from Henry Ford Medical Center where he directed their interventional bronchoscopy program. Ken brought these talents to the section and made Virginia Mason the referral site for complex airway disease. He later became interested in sleep medicine and helped create the sleep disorder clinic with Dr. Pardee. He left the institution in 1999 to return to his home state of Utah to practice full-time sleep medicine.

Neil Hampson, MD, was born in Seattle, WA. He attended the University of Washington School of Medicine. He left the state to go to the University of Iowa for residency and then Duke University for his pulmonary fellowship. He was recruited back and joined Virginia Mason in 1988. Neil was the consummate clinical researcher. His approach was to ask the question and then scientifically prove the answer. His data was precise. In 1989 he was "asked" to direct and develop the hyperbaric medicine program. Neil took on this task with great energy and wisdom and eventually created one of the premiere Hyperbaric Medicine Centers in the world. He went on to write hundreds of research papers on the science of hyperbaric medicine and its use for radiation tissue injury and carbon monoxide (CO) poisoning. To this day he is one of the world's experts on CO poisoning. In 2005, the largest chamber the Northwest was built under his directorship accommodating up to 16 seated patients plus 2 attendants. Neil was a recipient of the "Teacher of the Year" award in 1991, and received the **James Tate Mason Award** in 2007. He retired in 2010, at which time the subsection became a separate section under the leadership of James Holm, MD, who was recruited to VM in 2009 to become section head and Medical Director of the program. (For more information on the section of Hyperbaric Medicine, please see Chapter 8 in this volume.)

Steve Kirtland, MD, did his pulmonary fellowship at Virginia Mason from 1991 - 1994. Upon completion, he took up practice in Eugene, Oregon until 1995 when he returned to join the section. Dr. Kirtland authored many publications on various topics including chronic pneumonia, ventilator-associated pneumonia, sarcoidosis, and idiopathic pulmonary fibrosis. Boarded in Internal Medicine, Pulmonary Medicine, Critical Care Medicine, Sleep Medicine, and Undersea and Hyperbaric Medicine, Steve has a very diverse practice. He served as ICU and Respiratory Care Medical Director prior to his current 12-year tenure as Chief of Staff (COS). In addition to COS, Dr. Kirtland has been director of the Cancer Institute, and currently serves as Medical Director of Thoracic Oncology, Director of Bronchoscopy Services and as Section Head of Pulmonary Medicine. His major interest at VM has been interventional bronchoscopy and he has brought various technologies to the section including endobronchial ultrasound, percutaneous tracheostomy, and electromagnetic navigation bronchoscopy. Dr. Kirtland received the "Teacher of the Year" award in 1998 and the **James Tate Mason Award** in 2016. One of VM's professional couples, Steve's wife Cynthia has served as Director of Spiritual Care since the year 2000.

Bruce Davidson, MD, joined the group in 1999, and served in the section almost 3 years. Bruce's work during his years at VM focused on venous thromboembolic disease, where he was involved in a number of various anticoagulant investigations.

Dan Loube, MD, also joined the section in 1999 and succeeded Gene Pardee as director of the Sleep Lab at Virginia Mason in 1999. His tenure was short, however, as he left in 2001. He was replaced by **Bill DePaso, MD,** who had been the third pulmonary fellow at VM from 1988-1991. He attended the University of Chicago Medical School before completing his medicine residency at VM. Bill's area of study was interstitial pulmonary fibrosis and dyspnea. After completing his fellowship he joined a practice at Valley Medical Center in Renton and started the fourth clinical sleep center in western Washington there. A natural leader, he soon became director of the multidisciplinary group practice. He became interested in sleep medicine under the tutelage of Carla Hellekson, MD, and after obtaining his boards in sleep medicine, returned to Virginia Mason to lead the Sleep Medicine division from 2001 to 2013, retiring in 2015.

During his tenure, the subsection became a section of its own in 2003 with Dr. DePaso as section head. He also served as deputy Chief of Medicine for many years.

In the summer of 2001 the section suffered significant attrition, with the retirement of Dr. Dreis from clinical practice and the departures of Drs. Davidson, Loube and Springmeyer, creating a 3-month period where the Section of Pulmonary Medicine was composed of only Drs. Hampson and Kirtland. In the fall of 2001, **Tony Gerbino, MD**, joined the group after completing his pulmonary fellowship at the UW. Previously he had attended Harvard Medical School and done his residency at UCLA. His tremendous research acumen along with leadership qualities catapulted him to Section Head of the Pulmonary Section from 2006 - 2017. He continues as the only physician in the pulmonary section who still practices critical care medicine. Tony is married to Ingrid Gerbino, MD, the current Chief of Primary Care. Outside of medicine, he is an award-winning tri-athlete.

Dave Kregenow, MD, joined the section in 2002. He was recognized by the residents as an accomplished educator as he was awarded the "Teacher of the Year" multiple years in a row. Dave eventually became boarded in Palliative Care Medicine and left VM in 2014 to serve as Director of Palliative Care Medicine at Evergreen hospital.

Critical Care Medicine, which was part of the section of Pulmonary Medicine for many years, was included in the "Hospital Services" group in late 2002/early 2003, along with Emergency Medicine, Hospital Medicine, and Infectious Disease initially. In 2012, the title of the section, "Pulmonary and Critical Care Medicine" became "Pulmonary Medicine" only. In 2019, a formal "Department of Hospital Care Services" was formed, of which Critical Care Medicine is a part (for more information on Critical Care Medicine and the formation of the Department of Hospital Services, see chapters 30 and 27 respectively in this volume)

Several physicians have served in the critical care section since its formation, including Drs. Gerbino, Kregenow and Kirtland; **Michael Westley, MD** (2002 – 2014), who served as the first Medical Director of the

264

newly constituted critical care program in late 2002 until 2011; **Anne Mahoney, MD,** and **Kathleen Horan, MD** (see below); **David Hotchkin, MD** (2005 – 2009); **Ian Smith, MD** (see below); **Ann Chen, MD** (2006 – 2010); **Amy Morris, MD** (2006 – 2008); **Christopher Slatore, MD** (2006 – 2009); **Eric Walter, MD** (2007 – 2009); **Philip Royal, MD** (initially hired as a hospitalist in 2000, but practicing in critical care since at least 2007); **Martha Billings, MD** (2007 – 2008); **Soumya Parimi, MD** (2008 – 2012) and **Blake Mann, MD** (2012 - 2019). Current members of the section include Dr. Royal; **Aneal S. Gadgil, MD** (2008 – present); **Hashim Mehter, MD** (2014 – present) and two anesthesiologists, **Robert Hsiung, MD** (2008 – present) and **Eliot Fagley, MD** (2013 – present, also serves as Section Head), who also include critical care medicine as part of their practices.

Anne Mahoney, MD, the first female pulmonary medicine physician in the history of VM, joined the section in 2004. Anne matriculated at Stanford University where she was a champion swimmer—just missing qualifying for the Olympics. Subsequently she completed her residency at Parkland Hospital in Dallas, Texas and then did a pulmonary fellowship at the University of Washington prior to joining VM, where she directs the Pulmonary Function Lab as well as serving as the pulmonary resident advisor.

Katherine Horan, MD, met Anne Mahoney at Parkland. An accomplished swimmer as well, they became close friends and Anne advised her to attend the University of Washington for fellowship and then follow her to VM after graduation. Katy brought special expertise in non-tuberculous mycobacteria to the section, having been the co-director of the King County Public Health Clinic. Katy became the first pulmonary physician to have a steady regional medical center practice in Federal Way. Now all of the physicians in the section split their time between downtown and a regional medical center, including Federal Way, Issaquah and Edmonds.

Drs. Kirtland, Gerbino, Mahoney and Horan have all achieved their boards in Undersea and Hyperbaric Medicine and actively practice this specialty in addition to their pulmonary practice under the leadership of

James Holm, MD, current Medical Director of the Center of Hyperbaric Medicine.

Ian Smith, MD, joined VM in 2006 solely as a Critical Care Physician. He became director of the CCU in 2011. After serving 4 years as director, he transitioned to part-time and joined the pulmonary section, practicing half-time for a short time before leaving VM in 2017. In 2011, he won the "Teacher of the Year" award from Graduate Medical Education, "and led a number of quality improvement efforts including delirium detection and management in the critically ill, standardizing family care conferences, and implementation of a safety checklist during multidisciplinary rounds. He also chaired the Code Blue Committee among other formal and informal leadership roles." [5]

Three new pulmonary physicians have joined the section in the past year, building the section back to its maximal number of 7. **Yunhee Im, MD**, joined in 2018 after completing her fellowship at Baylor University. Dr Im brings great energy and passion to her practice. She has already built a large Korean patient group in the North Seattle area. **Catherine Miele, MD**, joined in 2019. Boarded in adult internal medicine and pediatrics as well as pulmonary and critical care, she returns home after completing her pulmonary fellowship at Johns Hopkins University. She continues research on the cardiopulmonary effects of indoor and outdoor air pollution. Lastly, **Luke Seaburg, MD**, recently joined the group this past fall (2019) after completing an interventional bronchoscopy fellowship at Duke University. Dr Seaburg plans to introduce a host of interventional techniques and procedures to the pulmonary section including pleuroscopy, endobronchial valve lung volume reduction and endobronchial lung cancer ablation.

The pulmonary section since its inception 70 years ago at Virginia Mason has always been a leader in the field. From sarcoid to idiopathic pulmonary fibrosis, pneumonia to endobronchial treatment of lung cancer, VM pulmonary physicians have provided many firsts in the region. They were the first to describe many clinical conditions including hypersensitivity pneumonitis, CREST syndrome, and chronic pneumonia. VM was the first to utilize bronchoalveolar lavage (BAL) in clinical practice, the first to treat endobronchial disease with laser therapy, and the first to introduce navigational bronchoscopy to the Northwest. The future of pulmonary medicine at Virginia Mason is bright as we embark on the next 100 years, building on the foundation created by so many giants who came before, blending pragmatic objective pulmonary research with the art of personal clinical care.

References:

1. Winterbauer RH, Hampson NB, Kirtland SH, et al: "Clinicians Performing Research: A Brief Synopsis of One Section's 45-Year Tradition." *The Virginia Mason Medical Center Bulletin*, Spring 1996; 50:29-37.

2. Pearsall HR, Morgan EH, Tesluk H, et al: "Parakeet dander pneumonitis. Acute psittacokerato-peumoconiosis." Report of a case. *Bulletin of The Mason Clinic*, 1960; 14:127-137.

3. Lindeman R. "Chairman's Report: 1997." Virginia Mason Archives.

4. "Carroll J. Martin, MD." *Pulse* newsletter; April 1968.

5. "Ian Smith, MD." Vnet announcement, 2017.

16

Radiation Oncology

by Mark Hafermann, MD, and Kasra R. Badiozamani, MD
with contributions from Huong Pham, MD

Part I: 1920 – 2000

Virginia Mason has been a leader in cancer care in Seattle and the state of Washington since the 1920s, modeling collegiality and multidisciplinary care. The Mason Clinic was the first in the region to use superficial x-rays to treat skin cancers in 1923, under the leadership of Maurice Dwyer, MD, who was one of the founding fathers of The Mason Clinic, having met James Tate Mason, MD, as a house officer at Providence Hospital from 1914-1915. He joined him in practice the following year, and thus was part of the early plans for the clinic, which was initially called the Mason-Blackford-Dwyer Clinic (see Radiology chapter in volume 2). Dr. Dwyer became interested in radiology around 1915, both as a diagnostic and therapeutic tool, and was listed as "Director, Virginia Mason Hospital X-ray Laboratory, Diagnosis and Therapy" in the first issue of the *Clinics of the Virginia Mason Hospital*, dated May 1, 1922.

The therapeutic use of external radiation was just beginning in the 1920s. X-ray units at the time were able to deliver radiations in the 200-500 KV range (deep x-rays). These energies are above the typical energy range used for diagnostic purposes, but are useful to treat skin cancer and other superficial neoplasms including metastases to superficial lymph nodes. The first radiation therapy equipment was a superficial unit, but in 1923, a 280 kV Victor orthovoltage "deep x-ray" unit was acquired (see Radiology chapter).

In 1937, the first 400 kV deep therapy unit in Seattle, and possibly in the Pacific Northwest, was added. In 1941, Virginia Mason established the first multidisciplinary cancer program in the Pacific Northwest, with repeated accreditation by the American College of Surgeons thereafter. That same year, recognizing the importance of basic research, the Virginia Mason Research Center was established. In 1942, The Mason Clinic began the first Radiology residency program in the Northwest. Radiologist training included the medical indications, techniques, and underlying physics of both the diagnostic and therapeutic modalities.

Thomas Carlile, MD, came to The Mason Clinic in June of 1939 for his internship, and stayed on as a medical resident. He spent much of his time helping Dr. Dwyer in Radiology, and decided to do a radiology residency at the Mayo Clinic, which he began in 1941. Due to the declining health of Dr. Dwyer (who retired in November of 1943 and died 3 months later), Dr. Carlile was recalled to The Mason Clinic and completed his residency with radiologists in Seattle. He became Chief of Radiology while still a resident, and was joined by John Hunter Walker, MD, who first provided locums coverage at VM in the early 1940s, and then joined the clinic in 1947, the first in the department to complete a formal residency program. Dr. Walker would serve as Clinic Chairman from 1964 to 1976.

Dr. Carlile became interested in nuclear medicine during its early days and "traveled to the University of California at San Francisco in 1947 to explore the potential use of radioisotopes in clinical medicine" (from Radiology chapter). He acquired an early license for the use of radioactive phosphorus and iodine, and developed the first nuclear medicine department in the Northwest in 1948; by 1953, he and Dr. Walker were founding members of the Society of Nuclear Medicine, with Dr. Carlile serving as their first president.

Kenneth D. Moores, MD, joined the department in 1956, following his radiology residency at the Mayo Clinic. As he noted in a personal communication: "We all did radiation therapy and diagnostic radiology about equally at that time, but soon after I arrived I started doing most of the nuclear medicine, and then headed up the nuclear medicine department until the arrival of Frank Allen." (from Radiology chapter). Meanwhile, Willis J. Taylor, MD, was completing his radiology residency at VM and joined the department in 1957, which was also the year when the department acquired the first Cobalt-60 radiation unit in the Northwest. It was Dr. Taylor who would form the core of the radiation oncology section that eventually was formed in 1968, and he would serve as its section head until 1983 when he became national president of the American Cancer Society. Dr. Carlile had also served as national president from 1961 – 1962.

The Radiology department gave an annual cancer conference starting in the 1960s, supported by the American Cancer Society. These conferences would have VM faculty, with invited nationally or internationally known guest speakers.

Participation with multiple national cooperative groups for clinical research in cancer and radiation therapy also began in the early 70s, and in 1972, Mark D. Hafermann, MD, joined Dr. Taylor in the radiation oncology section. One year later, Frank H. Allen, MD, was hired to work in the new section of Nuclear Medicine. This subsection was dissolved by 1981 with his departure.

Meanwhile, cobalt treatments fell out of favor, and in 1976, the section installed the first linear accelerator in the Northwest, a Varian Clinac 8 (10 meV). The section also had a Varian Clinac 4 (4 meV). Garratt Richardson, MD, had joined the section the previous year, bringing the number of radiation oncologists to 3. "VM's Radiation Oncology staff were also instrumental in getting clinical radiation physics to the NW. Peter Wooten, PhD, of Swedish Hospital was probably the first physicist in Seattle. There were no other qualified individuals in Seattle, until Doug Jones, PhD, was hired by a consortium of radiology groups including VM, Robert Parker of the UW, and Pat Lynch of Yakima." (from Radiology chapter).

In 1984, the section began relationships with other regional hospitals that continue to the present day. The first affiliation was with Valley Medical Center in that year, when Dr. Hafermann began providing coverage there. Eric W. Taylor, MD, Will Taylor's son, joined the section in 1983, and moved his practice to Evergreen Hospital in 1986 when an affiliation with that hospital was begun. He was a member of the section between 1986 – 1999, and 2003 – 2007 when the partnership was briefly reignited. Dr. Taylor continues to work at Evergreen.

John J. Travaglini, MD, joined the section in 1986 – he would practice at Valley Medical Center for his career, resigning from the section to take a position there when the affiliation ended in 2000.

In 1990, an affiliation with Sequim and Olympic Memorial Hospital on the peninsula was begun, and the position was staffed by Heath Foxlee, MD, who practiced at the Sequim location until the affiliation was ended, and briefly downtown from 1990 – 2002.

The late 1980s also saw the arrival of John W. Rieke, MD (1988 – 2002) and Sandra S. Vermeulen, MD (1987 – 1991). It was during this time that the cancer center program was organized to further foster multi-disciplinary coordinated care. A breast cancer task force in the mid-to-late 1990s set out to specifically develop an integrated practice model for breast cancer. Deborah Wechter, MD, a breast surgeon, was appointed to lead this multidisciplinary team, which included representatives from radiation oncology, medical oncology and radiology. Subsequently, these earlier organizational efforts culminated in the formation of the Cancer Institute.

Other additions to the department included; Michael A. Hunter, MD, who practiced with Dr. Travaglini at Valley Medicine Center from 1993 – 1997 and with Dr. Taylor at Evergreen Hospital from 2003 - 2007; Berit L. Madsen, MD (1993 – 2009); Christine M. Cha, MD (1998 – 2003); and R. Alex Hsi, MD (1999 – 2009).

Part II: 2000 - 2020

At the turn of the millennium, the Section of Radiation Oncology at Virginia Mason continued to build upon a tradition of patient-centered innovation. The section became the first in Seattle to utilize Intensity Modulated Radiation Therapy (IMRT) following the installation of the Varian

EX linear accelerator. Using Pinnacle treatment planning and the new treatment delivery platform, radiation oncologists were able to tailor doses more carefully to tumors, resulting in a significant improvement for patients, particularly those with head and neck, and prostate cancers.

Dr. Madsen led this effort to bring IMRT to Virginia Mason's patients, while also developing a novel short course, highly focused treatment for prostate cancer patients. The "SHARP" protocol (Stereotactic Hypofractionated Accelerated Radiotherapy for the Prostate) allowed prostate cancer patients to receive external beam radiation treatments in a matter of a few days, compared to the standard courses of daily therapy that lasted over seven weeks. Created with the technical skill of physicist Doug Jones, PhD, this treatment became the foundation for subsequent trials and pioneering techniques such as CyberKnife SBRT for early stage prostate cancer.

Alongside these developments in external beam radiotherapy, prostate brachytherapy continued to develop. Dr. Hsi brought his expertise in Real-Time Prostate Brachytherapy to create one of the most successful programs that continues to this day. Aided by physicist Joseph Presser, PhD, and utilizing intra-operative treatment planning, radiation sources could be placed with more precision and accuracy within the gland, resulting in the most focused and tailored radiation treatment available for prostate cancer. Dr. Hsi also brought the Calypso localization system to Virginia Mason, adding greater capability for target localization in early stage prostate cancers. During that period, a temporary partnership with Evergreen Radiation Oncology brought Virginia Mason alumni, Drs. Eric Taylor and Michael Hunter back to the section for a few years.

The establishment of a partnership with St. Francis Hospital in Federal Way represented significant growth for the section, and a strong relationship developed with the Catholic Health Initiatives (CHI) system that continues to this day. This clinic, initially supported by Dr. Hsi and Christine Cha, MD, has continued to thrive in the South Sound community. Subsequently led by Huong Pham, MD (2001 – present) and Paul Mitsuyama, MD (2010 – present), along with staffing by Kas Badiozamani, MD (2004 – 2019), St. Francis recently upgraded its initial linear accelerator to a Varian Truebeam system, allowing state-of-the-art image-guided therapy and stereotactic therapy to become available to patients close to home in Federal Way and neighboring communities.

Additionally, the years shortly following 2000 saw the development of High-Dose Rate (HDR) brachytherapy at Virginia Mason. With the support of physicists Homayoon Parsai, PhD, and Paul Cho, PhD, the first HDR remote afterloading treatments at Virginia Mason were delivered by Dr. Badiozamani, which were the first HDR brachytherapy treatments in Seattle delivered with CT-based treatment planning. Guobin Song, MD, PhD, also arrived during this time (2005 – present).

The stereotactic radiosurgery program lead by Dr. Pham, Dr. Cho, (physicist) and Charlie Nussbaum, MD (neurosurgeon) was upgraded to the Brainlab system shortly after the installation downtown of the Varian Trilogy linear accelerator in 2010. With Brainlab software and the M3 collimator system, highly targeted therapy for brain tumors can be carried out with greater precision, resulting in better outcomes and fewer side-effects for patients.

Concurrently with the technological developments in the section, national research protocols and accreditation became core components of the program. Through the Radiation Therapy Oncology Group (RTOG, now the NRG), Virginia Mason was able to enroll patients in landmark studies through these cooperative group efforts, locally directed by Dr. Pham. In recent years, this work continues to be carried out in partnership with regional medical centers including CHI and Multi-Care, with support from the Benaroya Research Institute. The section also became the first private radiation oncology program in the city to receive accreditation from the American College of Radiology (ACR).

The years from 2010 to 2019 brought continued patient-centered innovation. Virginia Mason became the first hospital in the region to offer intra-operative radiation therapy (IORT) for early stage breast cancer. As a result of this popular treatment option, certain patients could receive adjuvant radiation therapy for breast cancer at the same time as their breast-conserving surgery, avoiding weeks of daily therapy. Michelle

Yao, MD (2007 – present) led these efforts, complementing her work in brachytherapy for breast and gynecologic malignancies. The use of the SAVI interstitial implant for breast cancer also became another highly desirable option for short-course partial breast treatment, reducing treatment time to a single week.

Over the past four years, the section has seen major developments in process, technology, and growth. The culture of safety was enhanced when Virginia Mason became an early adopter of the Radiation Oncology Incident Learning System (ROILS). This ASTRO-sponsored (American Society of Therapeutic Radiation Oncology) national program promotes reporting of "near-misses" and other safety concerns within a non-punitive environment that engages all team members to identify risks and improve processes. The transition to the state-of-the-art Raystation Treatment Planning System allows patients to receive better treatment plans more efficiently. Raystation also allowed greater networking capabilities across the section's CHI sites, ever more important as the partnership with CHI continued to expand.

In February 2018, Highline Medical Center in Burien became the second CHI site to partner with Virginia Mason to deliver top-quality radiation oncology care in the community setting. Utilizing the first Varian Truebeam linear accelerator within the section, patients in Burien gained access to cutting-edge care. Shortly thereafter, St. Francis in Federal Way also upgraded to the Truebeam platform, as the partnership with CHI and Virginia Mason extended each program's ability to improve technology and deliver better care to more patients.

A single radiation oncology program requires the dedication and coordinated teamwork of physicians, physicists, therapists, dosimetrists, nurses, and front desk personnel, in addition to a high level of administrative and technical support. Across three sites (including downtown Seattle, Highline Medical Center in Burien, and St. Francis Medical Center in Federal Way), the teamwork grows exponentially. It is impossible to adequately list and describe the remarkable contributions made by every member of our team during the past twenty years. Their great work, however, can be seen

274

and felt in the care delivered to our patients every day.

Physician Biographies

Maurice Dwyer, MD (1918 – 1943)

Dr. Dwyer's career is covered in the Radiology chapter in Volume 2 and will not be repeated here.

Thomas Carlile, MD (1942 – 1974)

See Radiology chapter in Volume 2.

John Hunt Walker, MD (1947 – 1979)

See Radiology chapter in Volume 2.

Kenneth D. Moores, MD (1956 – 1987)

See Radiology chapter in Volume 2.

Willis J. Taylor, MD (1957 – 1993)

See Radiology chapter in Volume 2.

Mark D. Hafermann, MD (1972 – 1999)

Mark Hafermann grew up in Minnesota, and attended the University of Minnesota School of Medicine, graduating in 1959. He did a one-year internship at Harborview Medical Center, and then spent two years in general practice at Group Health Cooperative in Seattle. This was followed by one year of residency in internal medicine at the University of Washington, and a radiology residency there, which included 2 years each of diagnostic radiology and radiation oncology training. This training was completed in 1967, when he moved to Bethesda, MD, to work as a clinical investigator at the National Institutes of Health for 2 years.

Dr. Hafermann then took a position as Assistant Professor of Radiology (Radiation Oncology) and Staff Radiation Oncologist at the University of Washington, where he worked for 3 years. He joined Virginia Mason in 1972, but remained associated with the UW, reaching the rank of Clinical

Professor of Radiation Oncology in 1994.

Dr. Hafermann served as Section Head of Radiation Oncology at Virginia Mason from 1983 – 1993, and Medical Director of the VM Cancer Center from 1993 – 1998. He retired on January 1, 2000, but did intermittent locum tenens work in the section both downtown and at Evergreen Hospital over the following year.

Dr. Hafermann was author or co-author of 46 peer-reviewed publications and 2 book chapters, including several in affiliation with the Northwest Medical Physics Center. He was coinvestigator on several national cancer projects, particularly on the topics of prostate and bladder cancer, serving as radiation oncology chairman and member of the executive committee for the National Bladder Cancer Collaborative Group A from 1980 - 1987. He was also a coinvestigator and protocol collaborator for the Lung Cancer Study Group from 1981 – 1989, and Vice-Chairman of the Committee on Public and Professional Communication for the American Society for Therapeutic Radiology and Oncology from 1986 – 1988. In addition, from 1983 – 1995, he assumed several positions with the Community Clinical Oncology Program at VMMC.

Dr. Hafermann and his wife, Vija, have 4 children and a home on Mercer Island.

Frank H. Allen, MD (1973 – 1981)
See Radiology chapter in Volume 2.

R. Garratt Richardson, MD (1975 – 1986)
"Garratt Richardson attended the University of British Columbia in Vancouver and received a B.S. in biochemistry in 1961. He then came to the States and the University of Wisconsin's graduate school, taking a M.S. in experimental oncology in 1953. He received his MD from McGill University in Montreal, Canada in 1968 and then moved to California for a series of post-graduate positions including: straight medical internship at University Hospital of San Diego County and therapeutic radiology residencies with Saroni Tumor Institute of Mount Zion Hospi-

tal and the West Coast Cancer Foundation in San Francisco. Before coming to The Mason Clinic, Dr. Richardson was Instructor at the University of Washington's Radiation Oncology Department." (from the *VM Pulse*, December 1975). He joined VM in 1975 and practiced there for 11 years.

Eric W. Taylor, MD (1983 – 1999; 2003 – 2007)

Eric Taylor grew up in the Seattle area, where his father, Willis Taylor, was one of the early members of the Radiation Oncology section. He attended the University of Washington for medical school, internship, and a residency in radiation oncology, which he completed in 1982. He joined Virginia Mason in 1983 and began practicing at Evergreen Radiation Oncology (an affiliated site) around 1986, where he has remained throughout his career. This affiliation was discontinued in 1999, but revived between 2003 – 2007, when Dr. Taylor again became part of VM. He continues to practice at Evergreen as of September 2019.

John J. Travaglini, II, MD (1986 – 2000)

John Travaglini attended the University of Massachusetts Medical School, graduating in 1981, and then did a residency in radiation oncology at the University of Washington, which he completed in 1985. He took a position at Virginia Mason in 1986, and has practiced at Valley Medical Center since then, first as a member of VM's radiation oncology section, and later remaining there after the affiliation was discontinued in 2000.

Sandra S. Vermeulen, MD (1987 – 1991)

Sandra Vermeulen attended Loma Linda University School of Medicine, graduating in 1983, where she also did an internship in internal medicine followed by a residency in radiation oncology. She joined Virginia Mason in 1987, where she practiced until 1991. She currently practices radiation oncology as part of the Swedish medical group in Seattle (as of September 2019).

John W. Rieke, MD (1988 – 2002)

John Rieke attended Oregon Health Sciences University for medical school, receiving his degree in 1982. He then did a residency in internal medicine at the University of Minnesota, followed by a residency in radiation oncology at Stanford Medical Center, which he completed in 1988. He worked at Virginia Mason for fourteen years. He currently practices radiation oncology at MultiCare Regional Cancer Center, based in Tacoma. He has been an active member of ASTRO for 27 years, serving on various committees.

Heath Foxlee, MD (1990 – 2002)

Heath Foxlee attended Michigan State University College of Human Medicine for his medical degree, which he received in 1982. He then did an internship in internal medicine at Beaumont Hospital, followed by a residency in radiation oncology at St. Mary's Medical Center in San Francisco, and a fellowship in medical informatics at UCSF. Dr. Foxlee joined the radiation oncology team at VM in 1990, and practiced primarily at the Sequim Radiation Oncology Center, which was affiliated with VM until 2002; he has continued to practice radiation oncology on the Peninsula to the present time (October 2019).

Michael A. Hunter, MD (1993 – 1997; 2003 - 2007)

Michael Hunter attended Yale University School of Medicine, graduating in 1989. He then did an internship at Abington Memorial Hospital in Abington PA, followed by a residency in radiation oncology at the University of Pennsylvania. He has been a member of the section for 2 intervals – one from 1993 – 1997, where he practiced at Valley Medical Center with Dr. Travaglini, and another from 2003 – 2007, where he practiced at Evergreen Medical Center with Dr. Eric Taylor, and where he continues to practice at the present time (October 2019). Dr. Hunter is very active in the Susan Komen Foundation, serving on the Board of Directors for Puget Sound and chairing the Grants' Committee.

Berit L. Madsen, MD (1993 – 2009)

Berit Madsen attended Stanford University School of Medicine, graduating in 1989. She then did a transitional year at California Pacific Medical Center, and a residency in radiation oncology at Stanford, which she completed in 1993. She joined the section at VM that same year, and led the effort to bring IMRT to Virginia Mason. She served as section head after the retirement of Dr. Hafermann. She left VM in 2009 to head up the Peninsula Cancer Center in Poulsbo, which is now part of Seattle Cancer Care Alliance.

Christine M. Cha, MD (1998 – 2003)
Christine Cha graduated from the University of Michigan Medical School in 1993 before completing a residency in radiation oncology at Memorial Sloan-Kettering Cancer Center in NY in 1997. She joined VM in 1998 and helped support the partnership with CHI Fransciscan in Federal Way. Dr. Cha left VM in 2003.

R. Alex Hsi, MD (1999 – 2009)
Alex Hsi graduated from the University of Michigan School of Medicine in 1991, and then did residencies in internal medicine there, followed by a residency in radiation oncology at the University of Pennsylvania. He joined Virginia Mason in 1999 where he practiced for 10 years, and served as section head for several years. He is a co-founder of the Peninsula Cancer Center in Poulsbo, WA and has served as Medical Director of the Prostate Cancer Center of Seattle.

Huong T. Pham, MD (2001 – present)
Huong Pham received her medical education at the University of Maryland, graduating in 1992. She then did a medical internship at St. Mary's Hospital in San Francisco, followed by a residency in radiation oncology at Cooper Hospital – University Medical Center, Robert Wood Johnson Medical School in Camden, NJ, which she completed in 1996, and a one-year fellowship in central nervous system tumors at UCSF.

Dr. Pham then joined the faculty at Case Western Reserve University in Cleveland from 1997 - 2000 where she was the co-director of the Gamma Knife Radiosurgery Program. In 2001, she joined VM and served as section head from 2009 – 2014; after Dr. Badiozamani left in the summer of 2019, she transitioned back to the section head role.

Kasra R. Badiozamani, MD (2004 – 2019)

Kasra (Kas) Badiozamani attended the University of Washington School of Medicine, graduating in 1995, followed by a residency in radiation oncology there. Dr. Badiozamani joined VM in 2004 and was section head from 2014 - 2019. He had a very busy prostate cancer practice and was instrumental in growing the prostate brachytherapy program at VM. He retired in the summer of 2019.

Guobin Song, MD, PhD (2005 – present)

Guobin Song received his medical degree from Shandong Medical University in Jinan, Shandong, PR China in 1988. This was followed by a rotating internship and a residency in cardiovascular surgery at Shandong Medical University Hospital, which he completed in 1991. Dr. Song then received his PhD, at Texas A&M University in College Station, TX, in 1997. This was followed by a general surgery internship at Greenville Hospital System, in Greenville, SC and a residency in radiation oncology at Indiana University School of Medicine Hospital in Indianapolis, which he completed in 2003.

Dr. Song joined VM in 2004 and is currently the medical director of the radiation oncology department at Highline Cancer Center.

Michelle Yao, MD (2007 – present)

Michelle Yao attended the University of Michigan at Anna Arbor, graduating with her medical degree in 1993. She then did an internship in internal medicine followed by a residency in radiation oncology at the University of Wisconsin, Madison, which she completed in 1999.

Dr. Yao then joined the faculty of the Department of Radiation Oncology at the University of Washington for several years before joining VM in 2007. She heads up the breast radiation program, which offers IORT and HDR brachytherapy accelerated partial breast irradiation at VM.

Paul Mitsuyama, MD (2010 – present)

Paul Mitsuyama graduated from the University of North Carolina School of Medicine at Chapel Hill in 2001. He did a transitional internship at the University of Pittsburgh Medical Center, followed by a residency in radiation oncology at the University of Washington, which he completed in 2006. He then was in private practice in Phoenix for several years. Dr. Mitsuyama joined VM in 2010. He practiced at both VM downtown and at St. Francis and is currently the medical director of the St. Francis radiation oncology department.

Physicists:

Doug Jones, PhD,
Joseph Presser, PhD
David Sterling, PhD
Paul Cho, PhD
Homayoon Parsai, PhD
Elizabeth Garver, PhD
Sreeram Narayanan, PhD
Ruth Velasco-Schmitz, PhD
Daniel Smith, PhD
Karen Claeys, PhD
Sangroh Kim, PhD

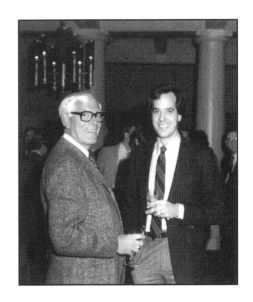

Will Taylor, MD, with
son Eric Taylor, MD
(PH 9132, VMHA)

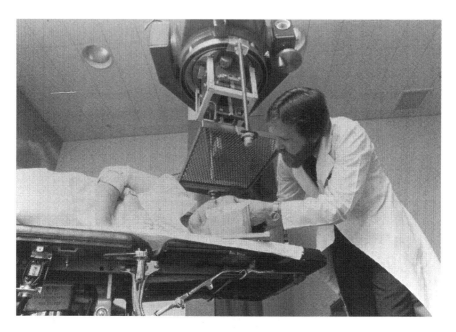

1982: Positioning a patient in Radiation Oncology
(PH 6715, VMHA)

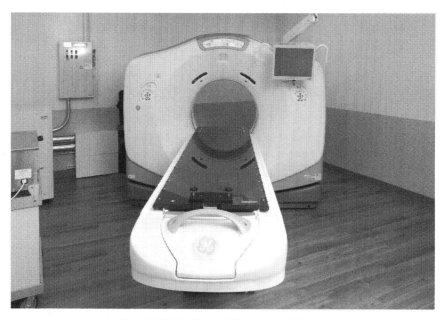

New CTS Radiation Simulator, 2015

17

Rheumatology

by Jeffrey Carlin, MD

The Virginia Mason Medical Center Section of Rheumatology was originally part of the section of Allergy and Immunology, established by **H. Rowland Pearsall, MD**, a Harvard-trained allergist who joined Virginia Mason in 1956. In 1964, recognizing that a rheumatologist was necessary to grow the section, he recruited **Kenneth Wilske, MD**, to join Virginia Mason.

Dr. Wilske grew up on a farm in Idaho and attended the University of Washington. Following a residency in internal medicine at Columbia Presbyterian Hospital in NYC he returned to Seattle for a 2-year fellowship in rheumatology at the University of Washington. He joined Virginia Mason in 1964 and spent 40 years at this institution. He was considered one of the giants of Rheumatology in his day, ultimately being selected to become a Master of Rheumatology by his peers at the American College of Rheumatology. He served as Section Head of Rheumatology for many years and was instrumental in establishing the Benaroya Research (BRI). He was a recipient of the **James Tate Mason Award** for his service to VMMC in 1999. For many years he sat on the board of the BRI and a research lectureship was established in his name. He also sat on the FDA Advisory Board for Rheumatology for many years. He published over 75 articles and chapters in various textbooks, but is especially renowned for the article he wrote with his partner, Louis Andrew Healey, MD, on "Remodeling the (Therapeutic) Pyramid" [1] in 1989, advocating more aggressive therapy for rheumatoid arthritis, and thereby establishing the therapeutic paradigm followed by rheumatologists today. Dr. Wilske unexpectedly passed away in 2013.

In 1968, **L. Andrew (Andy) Healey, MD,** was recruited to Virginia Mason from the faculty of the University of Washington, where he was on the faculty of the Rheumatology Division. Dr. Healey had grown up in NYC and went to Columbia Medical School, but came to Seattle for an internal medicine residency and a fellowship in rheumatology at the University of Washington. Dr. Healey published 51 papers and had a special interest in polymyalgia rheumatica and giant cell arteritis. He practiced at Virginia Mason for 25 years and was similarly named a Master of Rheumatology by the American College of Rheumatology. Dr. Healey passed away in 2015.

David Stage, MD, joined VMMC in 1975 to complete the triad of Virginia Mason rheumatologists who were so renowned throughout the nation. Dr. Stage had gone to medical school at Harvard and then did his residency and fellowship at the University of Washington. After spending a post-doctoral fellowship at the Pasteur Institute in Paris doing basic science research on the rheumatoid factor, he joined VMMC in 1975 where he practiced rheumatology until his retirement in 2005.

When VMMC and Group Health formed an alliance in 1997, **Jan Hillson, MD**, and **Wayne Jack Wallis, MD**, moved to VMMC from Group Health. Dr. Wallis left VMMC in 1999 to work for Immunex in drug development and was instrumental in bringing Enbrel® to market. Dr. Hillson also left VMMC in 2004 to move into the sphere of drug development.

With the retirement of Dr. Healey, **Daniel Furst, MD,** was recruited to join the Rheumatology Section after first being on faculty at the UCLA Medical School and then working for years in the pharmaceutical industry. Dr. Furst attended medical school and did his internal medicine residency at Johns Hopkins School of Medicine. He did his rheumatology fellowship at UCLA, thereafter joining the faculty there with a particular interest in scleroderma and rheumatoid arthritis research. While at VMMC he continued to publish and lecture world-wide. He left VMMC in 2000 to return to UCLA as a Professor of Medicine and is now Emeritus Professor with over 400 published publications.

Jerry Molitor, PhD, MD, was recruited from the University of Washington in 2000 to assist with Dr. Furst's scleroderma research studies. Dr. Molitor had gone to medical school at the University of Iowa after obtaining a PhD, in Immunology at Duke University. After completing his internal medicine residency and rheumatology fellowship at the University of Washington, he joined VMMC. Dr. Molitor worked part-time as a clinician and part-time as Director of the Arthritis Clinical Research Unit and Associate Director of Clinical Research. He left VMMC in 2007 for the University of Minnesota, where he is an Associate Professor of Medicine. He is the director of the Scleroderma Clinic there and has particular research interests in scleroderma and early rheumatoid arthritis.

Jeffrey Carlin, MD, joined Virginia Mason in 2002 when Dr. Wilske announced his impending retirement. He attended medical school at New York University and trained in internal medicine at the Medical College of Wisconsin. There, he fell under the tutelage of Daniel McCarty, MD, considered the leading rheumatologist of that time. After a rheumatology fellowship at the University of Washington, Dr. Carlin went into private practice at Northwest Hospital. After participating in multiple drug development trials, Dr. Carlin was recruited to work in the biotech industry, but was then recruited back to clinical practice by his mentors at VMMC. He served as Section Head of Rheumatology from 2007 - 2017 and is now the Director of the Arthritis Clinical Research Unit. Dr. Carlin is planning to retire in 2020 from clinical practice, but will continue to work with the BRI in his retirement.

Jane Buckner, MD, joined VMMC in 1999 as a post-doctoral fellow with **Gerald Nepom, MD, PhD**, at the Benaroya Research Institute. She attended medical school at Johns Hopkins and did her internal medicine residency at the University of Minnesota. A rheumatology fellowship followed at the University of Washington. She received the American College Rheumatology Senior Fellow Award during her training. She was named Director of Translational Research at the BRI in 2005 and Associate Director of the BRI in 2012. She was named President of the BRI in 2017. Dr. Buckner's laboratories have published extensively on the immunology of rheumatoid arthritis and type 1 diabetes. Despite her research and administrative commitments, she continues to see patients in clinic.

Florence Hsu, MD, joined VMMC in 2002 after a rheumatology fellowship at the University of Washington, but left in 2007 to join another Seattle-area clinic. **Jennifer Gordon, MD**, joined VMMC in 2004 after a rheumatology fellowship at UCSF, but left in 2008 to join Dr. Hsu. Dr. Gorman also left the section that year.

With the departures of Drs. Hsu, Gorman and Molitor, the Rheumatology Section was in tumult. Fortunately, **Elizabeth Jernberg, MD**, was recruited to join VMMC at that time. Dr. Jernberg had attended medical school at the University of Kansas and did her internal medical residency there as well. After working as an internist at Group Health, she went back and did a rheumatology fellowship at the University of Washington. Dr. Jernberg was in practice with Dr. Carlin in north Seattle until 2001. He was able to recruit her to join VMMC in 2007. In addition to working part-time at VMMC, she is an attending at Harborview Medical Center and is involved with the fellowship program, with a particular interest in musculoskeletal ultrasound. **Kori Dewing, ARNP,** was also recruited at that time to help out, but left in 2018.

Pedro Trujillo, MD, joined VMMC in 2009 after previously working at Group Health and the Cleveland Clinic. He had gone to medical school in his country of birth, Colombia, but did an internal medicine residency at Tulane Medical School and fellowship at the University of Washington. Dr. Trujillo left VM in 2015.

Stanford Peng, MD, PhD came to VMMC in 2009 from the biotech industry, but left in 2014 to return to biotech. He obtained an MD/PhD, at Yale, did his residency in internal medicine at Penn State and a rheumatol-

286

ogy fellowship at the Brigham and Women's Hospital. Prior to going into research, he was on the faculty of Washington University Medical School.

Vivian Stone, MD, joined VMMC in 2012 after being on the faculty of the University of Washington. She went to Rosalind Franklin University of Health Sciences/Chicago Medical School and did an internal medicine residency and rheumatology fellowship at Yale. Dr. Stone now serves as the Section Head of Rheumatology.

As the Rheumatology Section began to grow, additional rheumatologists were recruited from around the country. **Su Yin, MD**, joined VMMC in 2014 after 5 years of private practice in Plano, Texas. She attended medical school at the University of Texas Southwestern, followed by an internal medicine residency and rheumatology fellowship there. **Amish Dave, MD, MPH,** joined VMMC in 2016. He attended medical school at the University of Chicago and did his internal medicine residency at Stanford, followed by a rheumatology fellowship at the Brigham and Women's Hospital. He obtained an MPH at that time. In addition to practicing rheumatology, Dr. Dave sits on the board of the King County Medical Society and is interested in childhood lead poisoning.

Erin Bauer, MD, joined VMMC in 2106 after completing her rheumatology fellowship at UCLA. She attended George Washington Medical School and did her internal medicine residency at Kaiser Permanente in Los Angeles. Dr. Bauer has a particular interest and is board-certified in musculoskeletal ultrasound.

Meredith Morcos, MD, is the newest member of the team. She joined the section in 2018 after going to medical school at Emory University followed by an internal medicine residency and rheumatology fellowship at the University of Washington.

In addition to the physicians noted above, VMMC Rheumatology has inspired many of our VMMC residents to become rheumatologists. **Pam Sheets, MD**, practiced many years at the Polyclinic, but is now retired. **Christi Kenyon, MD,** is in solo practice in rheumatology in Seattle. **Amanda Nielson, MD**, is on the Rheumatology faculty at UNC Medical School, Chapel Hill. **Summer Engler, MD**, is currently practicing in

Anchorage, AK. **Heather Bukiri, MD**, is a fellow at UCLA and **Meriah Moore, MD**, is a fellow at the University of Michigan. Finally, **Stephen Slade, MD**, has been accepted to a 2020 fellowship at the University of Colorado.

References:

1. Wilske KR, Healey LA. "Remodeling the pyramid: a concept whose time has come." *J Rheumatol* 1989; 16: 565–7.

18

The Virginia Mason Sleep Disorders Center

by William DePaso, MD,
with contributions from Oneil Bains, MD

Kenneth Casey, MD, an early pioneer in clinical sleep medicine, arrived at Virginia Mason (VMMC) in 1987 and with **Neely Pardee, MD,** in the Pulmonary Medicine Section, created one of the first clinics in the Northwest to offer testing and treatment for patients with sleep disorders. Dr. Casey had developed *ProFox*, a computer program designed to analyze overnight oximetry patterns for signs of sleep apnea. This program was widely used across the country for decades.

Sleep disorders medicine is one of the newest medical specialties. Rapid eye movement (REM) sleep was discovered in 1955 at the University of Chicago and marked science's formal recognition of sleep as a distinct physiologic state. Previously, disturbances of sleep were thought to be psychiatric in nature, but then narcolepsy was determined to be a disturbance of REM sleep and in 1965 the syndrome of obstructive sleep apnea was first described. Stanford University opened the first sleep disorders clinic in 1971, but it soon closed due to a lack of patients with narcolepsy and absence of a tolerable alternative to tracheostomy, the only available treatment at the time for sleep apnea. In 1981, the first continuous positive airway pressure (CPAP) machine was developed in Australia by Colin Sullivan, PhD, BSc, MB and rapidly gained acceptance as a treatment for sleep apnea. Unfortunately, most patients remained undiagnosed and untreated due to a lack of trained physicians. The American Board of Sleep Medicine (ABSM) offered the first certifying exam in 1978. Physicians from the fields of pulmonology, psychiatry and neurology sat for the exam but their certification was not recognized by the American Board of Medical Specialties (ABMS) until 2007 when they assumed responsibility for board certification in sleep medicine. The American Academy of Sleep Medicine (AASM), formerly the American Sleep Disorders Association (ASDA), is responsible for accrediting sleep disorders centers and is the professional society for thousands of sleep providers.

In 1988, **William J. DePaso, MD,** became the first University of Washington (UW) pulmonary fellow based at Virginia Mason. He obtained additional training in sleep medicine during his fellowship and when he graduated, started the sleep medicine program at Valley Medical Center in Renton, WA, the fourth clinical sleep center in western Washington. Eventually under the tutelage of Carla Hellekson, MD, he became board-certified by the ABSM and the center was accredited by the ASDA. Interestingly, Dr. Hellekson was an intern at Virginia Mason and was not only the first person to take the certifying exam in 1978, but also the only person to obtain a perfect score!

Over the next decade, the sleep medicine program, under the Pulmonary Section leadership of Richard Winterbauer, MD, continued to grow. Drs. Pardee and Casey became board-certified by the ABSM; the sleep laboratory expanded and the sleep center became accredited by the ASDA. In 1989 there were two sleep beds in the laboratory and 29 studies were recorded that year. Pulmonary fellows **Steve Kirtland, MD** (1990), **David Corley, MD** (1993), **Vishesh Kapur, MD** (1999) and **Henry Su, MD** (2001) all obtained advanced training in sleep disorders at Virginia Mason and all four eventually became board-certified. Dr. Kirtland practiced part-time in the sleep center until 2010, and continues to practice pulmonology full time at Virginia Mason. Dr. Kapur has had a distinguished academic career at the University of Washington and is a national leader in the epidemiology of sleep disorders.

In 1993, **Nigel Ball, PhD** (in sleep physiology) became the director of the center and began the first clinical insomnia program in the region. In 1995, he recruited his colleague **Douglas Schmidt, PhD**, also a sleep physiologist as well as a certified sleep technologist, to run the technical aspects of the lab, which had now become larger (four beds and recorded approximately 1,000 sleep tests/year) and more computerized. He was also responsible for starting a novel home sleep apnea testing program. This program did not succeed due to technical and insurance reimbursement issues. Dr. Casey left VMMC in 1999 and has continued a prestigious academic career in sleep medicine as a prominent member of the Practice Parameters Committee.

That same year, **Daniel Loube, MD**, a pulmonary/critical care and sleep physician was recruited to serve as Medical Director of the Sleep Disorders Center. He was very productive clinically and academically. The lab expanded to five beds soon after his arrival and then to six beds in 2000. The growth within the sleep center mirrored the demand for clinical sleep services within the community. He started and coordinated multiple clinical research projects. He increased the visibility of the sleep center both within and outside the institution by speaking at professional meetings and to the media. In 2001, both Drs. Ball and Loube left Virginia Mason to join the Swedish Sleep Institute and Dr. DePaso was recruited back to VMMC by Bob Mecklenburg, MD (Chief of Medicine) and Neil Hampson, MD (Section Head, Pulmonary) to become medical director of the sleep center. Dr. Schmidt was promoted to Director.

In 2001, the sleep center, still a sub-section of the pulmonary medicine section, consisted of a six-bed laboratory with an adjoining clinic on level ten of the main hospital. Dr. DePaso was practicing 0.9 FTE in the sleep center and Dr. Kirtland was 0.1 FTE. Approximately 1,200 polysomnograms (PSG), or in-laboratory tests, were recorded that year. The demand for sleep consultation and testing grew rapidly and it could take as long as six months to be diagnosed and treated for sleep apnea. In 2002, **Oneil Bains, MD,** a general internist who completed a sleep medicine fellowship at Stanford University, joined Virginia Mason. His specialized training in the Stanford model to treat insomnia was utilized to create and maintain the premiere insomnia program in the Northwest. This approach, based on five, weekly group therapy workshops, is highly effective and satisfying to patients. Dr. Bains also started and continues to coordinate the pediatric sleep medicine program.

The sleep center continued to grow exponentially and with the administrative support of Drs. Mecklenburg and Hampson as well as **Patti Crome, MN, RN, CNA,** (VP Clinics), became a section independent of Pulmonary Medicine in 2003. Additionally, Dr. DePaso was appointed as Section Head and became a full time sleep medicine provider. A sleep medicine section, independent from the administrative control of pulmonary, neurology or psychiatry, was unique nationally. This increased visibility within the institution played an important role in the next phase of the sleep center's growth, which included the addition of another six beds to the laboratory, bringing the total to 12 in 2003.

Drs. DePaso and Schmidt had an early interest in the adoption of the quality management system developed by Toyota and adopted by VMMC. It soon became known as the Virginia Mason Production System. Under the excellent mentorship of **Liz Dunphy, RN,** they used these techniques to improve processes within the sleep center. The lead-time to diagnosis and treatment was reduced from six months to two weeks. The sleep lab was running with 99 percent occupancy, 362 days per year. Shadow charts were eliminated, the adoption of *Cerner Powerchart* was embraced, and computers were placed in the exam rooms using honorarium funds allowing dictation to be eliminated with real time documentation. Increased collaboration with **Ron Kuppersmith, MD,** a VMMC ENT sleep surgeon who understood the limited role of surgery in treating sleep apnea, created an even greater demand for consultation. In 2004, the section was fortunate to recruit **Matthias Lee, MD**, a psychiatrist and colleague of Dr. Bains from Stanford University. In addition to expanding the ability to treat insomnia, he subsequently coordinated multiple clinical research trials, several in collaboration with our Department of Anesthesia as well as with Edward Weaver, MD, MPH an ENT sleep surgeon from the University of Washington. Drs. Lee and DePaso are both clinical associate professors at UW and together have mentored numerous UW pulmonary and sleep medicine fellows.

In 2005, the lay press began to markedly increase community awareness of sleep disorders and their treatment. Locally, for the first time *Seattle Magazine* listed sleep medicine as a separate specialty in their annual "Top Doctors" issue and also featured a lead article about sleep disorders with a picture of Dr. DePaso on the cover. At this time, with 3.1 FTE sleep physicians and innovative administrative support for sharing revenue across the service line, the sleep center doctors used lap top computers to expand access to sleep consultations in the satellite clinics as well as on the main campus. Dr. Bains began seeing patients in Federal Way. The following year Dr. Lee started consulting in Issaquah, Lynnwood and Kirkland. Finally, Dr. DePaso started offering consultations in Bainbridge Island and Bellevue clinics.

When Dr. DePaso arrived in 2001, he brought an innovative approach to the dispensing of CPAP by durable medical equipment (DME) companies. He invited outside DME vendors into the sleep center during clinic hours so that CPAP could be dispensed immediately following a clinic visit with the provider. This often occurred in the morning following the completion of sleep testing the night before. This further shortened the time from diagnosis to initiation of treatment, and was greatly appreciated by patients and referring physicians alike. In 2004 Drs. DePaso and Schmidt were able to start VMMC's own CPAP/DME company and continue to serve as a high quality CPAP provider for approximately 1200 non-Medicare patients each year; as of January 2016, over 9,000 devices have been dispensed.

In 2007, **Sue Mystowski, MD,** a UW sleep fellow, practiced at the center for three months. She eventually practiced sleep medicine at the Evergreen Sleep Center in Kirkland WA, joining Dr. Henry Su. In 2008, **Nicole Philips, MD,** a neurologist who completed a sleep medicine fellowship at the University of Michigan, joined the sleep center and spent some time at the Sandpoint Clinic, where she practiced pediatric sleep medicine. She left Virginia Mason in 2010 and eventually practiced sleep medicine at Auburn General Hospital in Auburn, WA. Soon after her departure, **Christina Darby, MD,** another neurologist who completed a sleep medicine fellowship at Stanford University, joined our group and thanks to excellent collaboration with **Michael Elliott, MD,** was allowed to practice general neurology one day per week during her first two years. She left VMMC in March of 2016 to run a sleep center in her native Alaska.

Virginia Mason is a beta testing site for Cadwell EEG systems, giving them an opportunity to pilot their new home sleep apnea monitoring equipment. The sleep center used these systems as part of an expanding research collaboration with **Karen Roetman, MD**, and **Chris Bernards, MD**, of the Department of Anesthesia. The potential for these systems to reduce cost and increase patient satisfaction was immediately obvious, so clinical algorithms were developed to test these devices on patients during the summer of 2011. Fortunately this provided a significant lead over VMMC's competitors when the major insurance carriers decided to suddenly mandate Home Sleep Apnea Testing (HSAT) instead of in-lab tests in September of 2011, since everything was in place to immediately start a home sleep apnea testing program. Unfortunately, with the rapid growth in HSATs, there was a subsequent reduction in the need for in-lab sleep testing, and a commensurate drop in revenue. However, with innovation, Dr. Schmidt was able to scale down in-lab operations to eight beds in 2012 and six beds in 2014 at the same time that he cross-trained sleep technologists to increase the number of HSATs in most of the clinic locations. In 2015, 2101 HSATs and 1263 in-lab tests were performed. The overall financial performance of the operation peaked in 2010 when 3,538 in-lab tests were recorded.

In 2012, working with VMMC sleep surgeons **Tracy Eriksson, MD,** and **Geoffrey Deschenes, MD, Kasey Li, MD, DDS**, a world leader in sleep surgery practicing in Palo Alto, CA, was recruited to offer consultations to patients in the VM sleep center several times a year. With his highly specialized expertise in bi-maxillary advancement surgery, VMMC could now offer the full complement of surgical therapies for patients with sleep apnea. By seeing patients in Seattle, he obviated the need for patients to travel to his clinic in Palo Alto, CA for initial consultation and surgical follow up. When necessary, surgery was still performed in California during a week-long stay.

In 2013, Dr. Bains became Section Head of Sleep Medicine. In 2015, Dr. DePaso retired from clinical practice at VMMC. **Susan Rausch, MD, PhD**, a pulmonologist with a PhD in exercise physiology, started at Virginia Mason in August of 2015. The sleep center has undergone numerous reaccreditations by the AASM and all of its providers practice full time sleep medicine and are board-certified by the ABMS.

The overall success of the sleep center to date has been due to a highly functional collaboration between innovative physicians, excellent clinical/technical staff and a director with superb technical and administrative skills. The demand for sleep medicine consultations at Virginia Mason

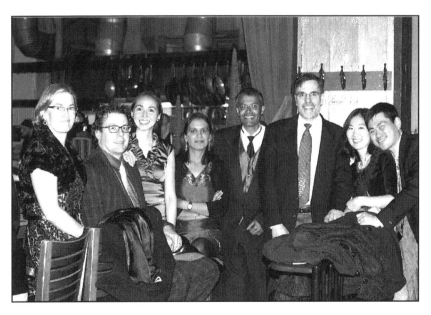

Sleep Physicians and their spouses at the Palace Kitchen en route to Virginia Mason Holiday Party, 2011
L to R: Barbara Ricker (spouse of Bill DePaso), Anthony Darby, Christina Darby, MD, Rattan Bains, DDS, Oneil Bains, MD, Bill DePaso, MD, Haejung Lee, Matthias Lee, MD

continues to increase. In addition to providing superb service, the regionally unique insomnia program is attracting large numbers of patients seeking help when other centers in the Northwest are downsizing due to lack of revenue from HSATs.

June 2019 addendum: Current physicians in the Sleep Disorder Center include Drs. Bain, Rausch and Lee, along with **Brandon R. Peters-Mathews, MD**, and **Amir H. Sabzpoushan, MD.** Dr. Peters-Mathews did a residency in neurology at the University of Minnesota followed by a fellowship in sleep medicine at Stanford University, which he completed in 2013. He has a special interest in utilizing cognitive behavioral treatment for insomnia (CBTI), and introduced a self-directed CBTI program at VM. This program is an online resource that allows patients to pursue CBTI through an online training course and has been well received by patients. Dr. Sabzpoushan did a sleep disorders fellowship at the University of Iowa Hospital and Clinics, which he completed in 2017. Sleep disorder services are offered downtown, and at 6 satellites, including Federal Way, Kirkland, Bellevue, Issaquah, Bainbridge, and Lynnwood.

19

The Department of Primary Care: An Overview

by John Kirkpatrick, MD, with contributions
from Catherine Potts, MD, and Ingrid Gerbino, MD

With the establishment of the Section of General and Screening Medicine in 1973 ("Screening" was dropped from the title in 1974), the first seed of the Department of Primary Care was sown. The department, created in 2010, includes the sections of General Internal Medicine at the Seattle campus, Pediatrics, the "Satellites" (now known as the Regional Medical Centers), and Concierge Medicine. These sections focus on the primary care needs of patients, and thus, when Catherine Potts, MD, was appointed as the first Chief, she focused on integrating and aligning these sections and the family practice physicians, internists, pediatricians, and advanced care practitioners who worked in primary care throughout the medical center. Under her tenure, and that of Ingrid Gerbino, MD, who assumed the role of Chief in 2010, the Department of Primary Care has continued to grow and is now the largest department in the Medical Center.

In the following 4 chapters, the stories of the development and growth of these sections are told. Jim Simmons elucidates the remarkable story of the fledgling section of General Internal Medicine, which has grown to be the largest on the downtown Seattle campus. Richard Dion, MD, the founding member of the section of Pediatrics in 1962, relates the history of the growth and subspecialization of this section, which eventually moved to a more primary care focus both downtown and in the satellites. A third chapter represents an overview of the birth, growth, and present day status of Virginia Mason's regional centers (originally known as the Satellites), which have had a tremendous impact on the course of the medical center. The story tells of the events leading up to the opening of the first satellite clinic, Mason Clinic East in 1982. A few years later, Gary Kaplan, MD, was asked to oversee the opening of a satellite in Federal Way and was eventually named Chief of the Satellites. Over the next fifteen years, the satellite network grew to 14 sites. Existing community clinics were purchased and many Virginia Mason Residency graduates joined these sites as providers. Expansion occurred quite rapidly, but ultimately had to be scaled back as several of the sites did not prove to be profitable. Several excellent locations remain, however, and provide both primary and specialty care, as many of the downtown VM specialists spend some of their workdays in the outlying communities.

Finally, you'll read the history of Virginia Mason's Concierge Medicine section, an innovative program that was initially called the "Lewis and John Dare Center", and provides "concierge medicine" to its patients. It was named after The Mason Clinic's first administrator Lewis Dare and his son John, also an administrator at The Mason Clinic, both of whom stood for quality and service and provided excellent administrative oversight for over 50 years.

From these early beginnings, the department has evolved into a robust force within the medical center, and, under the leadership of Dr. Ingrid Garbing, one imagines a bright future ahead.

20

General Internal Medicine - Seattle Campus

by James Simmons, MD

The Section of General Internal Medicine (SGIM), established in October 1973, was the first Virginia Mason Medical Center (VMMC) section dedicated specifically to providing primary non-obstetric care to adults. The initial name was "Section of General and Screening Medicine" but this was changed to General Internal Medicine after Jim Simmons, MD, and Dave Gortner, MD, were recruited and requested the change. Approaching The Mason Clinic's 100th anniversary in 2020, the SGIM looks back on what will then be its forty-sixth full year of participation in the clinic's history. During that time they have been early adopters of many of the medical zeitgeist's incubating movements, introducing new ideas into practices, using new technologies, and trying new ways of doing work. In chronological order these include:

• **Keeping Problem Lists, Drug Lists, and Screening Test completion dates on patients.** Jim Simmons and Dave Gortner used pen and paper for this in the 1970s and 80s. When desktop computers became available in offices in the 1990s, Dr. David Gortner was the first VM MD, to have problem lists on a computer, which could be accessed and printed should the paper chart be unavailable.

299

- **Working at improving patient access to the Clinic and Section.** The section provided same day access for patients who needed to be seen but whose provider could not accommodate them, by having an "Emergency Call" physician who started their day with multiple open slots. Later, experimentation with "double booking" into full schedules was tried, but proved unpopular with patients and staff and was discontinued.

- **Increasing our medical resident and other teaching commitments.** Beginning as rotating attendings for hospital and outpatient internal medicine housestaff in the 1970s and 80s, section members progressed in the 1990s to leadership roles in the VMMC's Internal Medicine Residency program with more focus on outpatient teaching. By the second decade of the 2000s SGIM physicians were partnering with residents in 3-year "collaborative practice" mentoring roles while also welcoming more residents to rotations in the section. VMMC Continuing Medical Education (CME) courses, previously occasionally organized by SGIM, have become an annual event with the "10th Annual Topics in Primary Care" course occurring in 2018, and an 11th scheduled for 2019.

- **Hiring women physicians and making women's health a focus.**

- **Hiring MDs trained in geriatrics.** Although practice dedicated solely to frail elderly patients was never the goal, knowledge gained from those section members trained in geriatrics benefited SGIM and the Clinic as a whole.

- **Learning, practicing, and teaching Evidence-Based Medicine.**

- **Forming or helping form and staff new VMMC services,** some surviving, others not. These included:

  A) **The Center for Women's Health** – staffed by female providers for women patients. Section members Karen Rosene, MD, and Judy Bowen, MD, were cofounders.

  B) **The Specialty Clinic** – a subsection of the Medical Residents'

Continuity Clinic, housed in the section, including SGIM attendings with a special interest and expertise in HIV/AIDS. Early in the epidemic this served as an entry point into the VMMC system for these patients to get continuing care and to provide residents experience and training managing their problems.

C) **Asian American Clinical Program** – a subsection of SGIM organized and led by John Kirkpatrick, MD, to provide continuing care for patients of Asian heritage who felt more comfortable with staff and providers fluent in their native language and knowledgeable about their culture.

D) **Experimentation with a section-based hospitalist system** – though we soon abandoned this effort, section member Roger Bush, MD, was later instrumental in the formation of the permanent Hospitalist department.

E) **Concierge Medicine Department** - co-founded by John Kirkpatrick, MD, and Bruce Nitsche, MD.

F) **Integrative Medicine Department** - Astrid Pujari, MD, trained in both western medicine and phytotherapy, joined SGIM in 2001. She left GIM in 2005, though she continued to consult in the VM Cancer Institute until 2018. She became a founding member of the new Department of Integrative Medicine in October 2018 and is certified in that specialty by the American Board of Physician Specialties. [1]

• **Using computers and an electronic medical record in exam rooms.**

• **Using speech to text technology to generate medical record documentation.**

General Internists at Virginia Mason
Preceding the Section of GIM

General internists were vital contributors to The Mason Clinic (MC) for the 53 years preceding the establishment of the Section of General Internal Medicine in the fall of 1973. James Tate Mason, MD, began his solo practice in Seattle in 1909, practicing both general internal medicine and surgery. [2] In 1917, while attending a meeting at the Mayo Clinic, he befriended John M. Blackford, MD, and invited him to leave his internal medicine practice there and join him in Seattle. [3] Dr. Blackford is credited with being "the group practice guy" [4] among the founders (he is the one with a cigarette in his hand in the portrait previously in the lobby of the Buck pavilion). They were joined in 1918 by Maurice Dwyer, MD, a radiologist. This trio of physicians, the nucleus of the future Virginia Mason Clinic, was practicing together by 1919 [5], located in the Joshua Green Building [2] on 4th and Pike. Brothers George Dowling, MD, and J.T. Dowling, MD, an internist and otolaryngologist respectively, joined their partnership in 1920, as did Lester Palmer, MD, a diabetologist. [5]

Thus two of The Mason Clinic's six founders were identified solely as general internists and Dr. Mason, the ultimate founder, included general internal medicine in his practice. [5] Dr. Lester Palmer, in 1923, was the first physician in the Pacific Northwest to administer insulin to a diabetic patient. [6] He and J. T. Dowling, an otolaryngologist, presaged VM's long and continuing excellent reputation for subspecialty medicine and surgery. Dr. Mason was the first Chairman of VMC. After his death in 1936, Dr. Blackford followed him in that role and is credited with "rounding out the clinic in various specialties". [4]

The American College of Physicians was founded in 1915 "to promote the science and practice of medicine". [7] There were no specialty-certifying boards of American medicine until 1933. [8] The American Board of Internal Medicine (ABIM) was founded in 1936, and that of Surgery in 1937. [9] Earlier members of VM were grandfathered into the specialty they had been practicing. Dr. Mason died in 1936, before having the chance to decide whether to be certified as an internist or a surgeon. [10] He was listed as both in the earliest roster of future VM physicians in 1918. [5] Evidence suggests he would have chosen to join the surgeons. He had published papers on surgical topics [11]; was elected to the American Surgical Association in 1930 [12]; and trained Dr. Joel Baker, VM's third Chairman, as a surgeon [13].

Since the 1940s board certification has been a requirement to be a partner of The Mason Clinic, which dissolved in 1986, or a member of the nonprofit corporation succeeding it. Before SGIM's establishment all partners in medical subspecialty sections were board-certified general internists and saw patients for general medical care as well as care in their subspecialty. The ACP Council on Subspecialty Societies was founded in 1977. [14] The first organization solely for general internists, The Society for Research and Education in Primary Care Internal Medicine (SREP-CIM), was founded with funding through the ACP from the Robert Wood Johnson Foundation and had its first meeting in 1978. It was renamed SGIM (Society of General Internal Medicine) in 1988 [15], and is currently more focused on the needs and interests of academic teachers and researchers than those of clinicians.

Preceding SGIM, VM's Department of Medicine (DOM) had grown to include the medical subspecialty sections listed below. [16] The parentheses contain two dates – the first and boldfaced, is the year that ABIM recognized the subspecialty [14]; the second is the year of arrival of the first VMC physician in the section [5]. The listed names are the medical subspecialty section founders who were still practicing during the early years of SGIM.

- Diabetes/Endocrine (**1972;** 1920)
- Cardiology (**1921**; 1941)
- Hematology/Oncology (**1972/1973**): Randy Pillow (Hematology, 1954); Robert Rudolph (Oncology, 1972)
- Pulmonary (**1941**; 1950): Ed Morgan
- Dermatology (**1933**; 1936)
- Immunology & Rheumatology (**1972**): Roland Piersall (Immunology, 1966); Ken Wilske (Rheumatology, 1968)
- Nephrology (**1972**/1964): Dick Paton (1964)
- Neurology (**1935**/1968): Richard Birchfield (1968)

In his 1952 Chairman's report Dr. Joel Baker, a venerated, VM-trained surgeon and the third clinic chairman, thoughtfully noted his concerns about the clinic becoming "too specialized":

"Although the past few years has forced us more and more into handling a higher proportion of referred work, it may be possible that we are becoming too specialized – or rather in so doing we may sacrifice a large future source of local practice requiring specialists. For instance, we find it difficult to handle general practice cases that show up daily at the Clinic, and we are not well organized to handle local family practice in the manner that the family physician used to do. Our teaching programs are aimed only at the specialty fields, and we offer very little home call service. Our position is different from the Mayo Clinic. We are in a metropolitan area, now well supplied by a number of young well-trained competing specialists, several hospital groups, and a University Medical School. Do you think that we dare put all our eggs in one basket, i.e. referrals from several hundred friendly doctors, or would our future in a big city be better protected by taking care of our proportion of the general populace so that our basic source of specialty tools is much broader, and less destructible? The problem needs thought." [17]

In the late 1960s and early 1970s clinic partners had two major concerns. First, that continued growth would erode the perceived cultural benefits of a smaller group. Second, that adding medical generalists could threaten their identity as a specialty clinic and reduce quality of care. "You need to be narrow to be sharp" was rumored to have been quoted in discussions about establishing SGIM. The fourth clinic chairman, John Walker, MD, championed both growth and adding SGIM, as did then DOM Chief, John Allen, MD. In 1969, after reviewing the last 17 years of Chairman's reports, Dr. Walker observed "difficulties faced in the future over the years have been about the same. We have always been concerned about clinic growth and ultimate size. There was as much concern of doubling the Clinic from 25-50 as there is from 50-100." [18] He echoed Dr. Baker's assessment of a role for generalists, stating "because we are reluctant to turn away people who seek our services, we thread them through our system, which is not well designed to satisfy their requirements". [19] "Going through the clinic" was the phrase patients used for seeing multiple doctors for different complaints or findings. Indeed, a single patient might be sent to a nephrologist for a mildly elevated screening blood pressure reading, a neurologist for a complaint of headache, a pulmonary doctor for a complaint of dyspnea, a cardiologist for chest pain, and a hematologist for a complaint of fatigue.

The Earliest Years of SGIM

The first physician hired for the new section in the fall of 1973 was Nicholas Sinally, MD, who previously served 20 years in the US Public Health Service (USPHS). He headed the outpatient medicine clinic in the USPHS Hospital, a Beacon Hill landmark sitting high above interstate 5 and later the home of Pacific Medical Center and Amazon. Second was James Simmons, MD, coming in July 1974 having worked two years' in that clinic, fulfilling an obligation for national service after finishing his residency at Grady Memorial Hospital in Atlanta. Third was David Gortner, MD, who came in March 1975. He had been chief resident at the University of Minnesota and the medical officer on an atomic submarine, and moved to Seattle for family reasons. Next came John Kirkpatrick, a native Washingtonian and UW Medicine graduate, who arrived in 1976 following his residency at the Mayo Clinic. James Bender, MD, joined us at the completion of his residency at VM in the summer of 1977. He was the first member recruited by SGIM physicians, earlier ones having been recruited by Dr. John Allen. Dr. Sinally resigned in the fall of 1974. The remaining quartet all retired from VM. Three of them, Drs. Simmons, Gortner, and Bender were Section Heads. Dr. Kirkpatrick co-founded the Department of Concierge Medicine with Bruce Nitsche, MD.

When SGIM began, physicians were expected to participate in patient care, education, and "PAGE" (Professional Activity and Group Effort). Examples of the latter included activities such as serving on or chairing clinic, local, and national committees, presenting to medical groups, and publishing in medical journals. SGIM's activities in these categories are reviewed by decade in the following sections.

PATIENT CARE

In 1920 the founders insisted, as did the Mayo Clinic, that all decisions be made with the patients' best interests in mind. [20] The group recommitted to this ideal in the early 2000s. The year before the "Virginia Mason Production System" (VMPS) was implemented, CEO Gary Kaplan, MD, had the following "ah-ha moment". The Virginia Mason Board of Directors asked him, "Who's the customer?" Of course, his answer was, "It's the patient". The board suggested taking a closer look, which clinic leadership did. "We did a deep dive on our processes, and (ah-ha!) found out most of them were designed around us – the physicians, nurses and other team members – not the patient." [21] The VMPS Strategic Pyramid has the patient at the apex, with the "vision to be the quality leader" just below. [22] One of the reasons John Blackford wanted to build a hospital in 1920 was his desire to assure quality control in the clinical laboratory. [23] Belonging to a group striving to provide the highest quality medical care and in which world-class consultation was available for almost any medical or surgical problem has always been relished by SGIM members.

The 1970s

SGIM was expected to attract and retain new patients for VM. This occurred; the section became the leader in New Appointment Desk (NAD)-filled appointments. In addition to local patients, there were a lot of people from the rest of Washington as well as Alaska, fewer from Oregon, Montana and Idaho. They came for primary and secondary care. They came for "routine physicals". VM offered a service of shorter appointments for patients requesting a physical exam. Those appointments were for 30 minutes, while a new patient appointment to establish care was typically for an hour at that time. SGIM physicians each had an afternoon a week when six of these visits were scheduled. A prehistory questionnaire was fed into a mainframe computer, resulting in an accordion-folding printout. Some were so long they could have reached from the exam room floor to the ceiling or further. Many of these patients had not been able to get a timely appointment any other way. SGIM also participated in VM's "Executive Physical" program in which company's sent higher-level employees for examinations, typically with a battery of tests agreed on by VM and the sponsoring company done in advance of the appointment. Many of those executives and their family members became long-term section patients.

In the early years, travelling in Washington meant recalling patients who had come from towns we passed through. Alaska also was a common source of patients. Seattle was then described as "the only American city with a state as a suburb". The Alaskans might be "Triangle-ing" in the winter, meaning going to Hawaii for sun, then coming to be seen at VM before returning home. Part of the trip was tax-deductible because of the medical visit. Some, having previously been seen initially by VM medical subspecialists for these visits, were expecting to "go through the clinic". Some were delighted to find that unnecessary; others felt they were not getting what they expected when consultation was not thought to be need-ed. When the Alaska Pipeline was under construction between 1974 and 1977, it seemed that half the workers (many from Texas) and residents from the North Slope and Fairbanks came for symptoms exacerbated by the stresses associated with that project in that setting. Alaska was truly the "last frontier" - both geographically and medically. A memorable Alaskan patient sent for a medical exam before surgery for laryngeal cancer could barely be heard, but did not know exactly when his voice started to change. He lived alone working as a fur trapper and had scarce opportunity to talk to people. One day he could not shout at his dog "chasing a varmint." When he went to town to resupply, his voice was barely above a whisper. Another, a dedicated teacher in a small native village, was found to have cervical cancer on a Pap smear done during a check up on her way back from California. At that time Pap results took several days to return and were not available until she had reached home. Travel out would be dif-ficult and she did not want to leave her students without a teacher, so she came back in the summer, when she observed, "Well, Doc, I earned it. I slept with every white man who came to that village!"

The section followed their patients in the hospital. They consulted on patients referred from within and outside VM. The VM referrals came mostly from surgeons for preoperative medical evaluations, neurologists (example, "This man has a paraneoplastic neurologic syndrome. I want you to find the cancer"), occasionally from medical subspecialists for diagnostic help should no subspecialty diagnosis be apparent. Retiring medical subspecialists sent their general medical patients to SGIM for continuing care. Outside physicians sent patients to evaluate and decide which, if any, subspecialists they should see. Outside clinical psychologists asked for evaluation of patients for medication management, if that seemed indicated and safe. Their diagnoses included major depression, panic disorder and anxiety disorder. One busy, frequently referring psychologist eschewed psychiatry involvement fearing they would "steal" her patient.

In the four months that Dr. Simmons was the only member of SGIM, he shared weekend call with the Section of Immunology and Rheumatology. He was told to call should a patient of theirs present problems he felt uncomfortable managing. To his relief no such calls were needed. The patients presented with common medical problems like pneumonia, congestive heart failure or heart attacks (which did require consultation with on-call cardiologists to be admitted to the coronary care unit). He did receive one memorable call from a patient of Dr. Ken Wilske, a renowned rheumatologist who also had a large general medicine practice. His patients included a host of Seattle's dignitaries and civic leaders. Dr. Simmons and his wife were having dinner with an elderly neighbor couple. The husband had been laid off from a local company during a business downturn, shortly before reaching his retirement age. The VM operator called with a patient of Dr. Wilske's and the following exchange ensued: "Hello, John Doe of Company XYZ". "Hello, Jim Simmons of Virginia Mason," was the reply, knowing the company but not the person nor his position. His question was about a grandchild and he was transferred to the pediatrician on-call to be sure he got VM's best advice on the subject. Dr. Simmons did not know that the caller was his company's Chairman of the Board at the time, but his neighbor did and was delighted with the conversation.

When Dr. Gortner arrived in March 1975, he and Dr. Simmons did

308

every other week call till Dr. Kirkpatrick joined them. The GIM weekend on-call physicians had Saturday morning office visits scheduled before afternoon hospital rounds. As the section grew, the weekend on-call hospital list and the number of telephone calls from or about patients did also.

In 1978 SGIM recruited and hired Lisa Taylor, MD, the first woman clinician to be on a partnership track at VM. She resigned in 1980 to move with her physician husband to a new location where he had obtained a job. She would have become eligible for partnership in 1981. Instead, Susan Detweiler, MD, a pathologist, was hired in 1980, and became the first woman partner at VM in 1983. [5]

The DOM had a rotating "Emergency Call Service" designed for patients with general medical problems and not established with a DOM member. SGIM took over the service in 1978. Any patient seen for the first time became the patient of the physician who saw them then.

In addition to fostering decades-long patient relationships, the section saw and diagnosed many "interesting cases" including:

- pituitary apoplexy
- panhypopituitarism (with previously masked diabetes insipidus revealed clinically when cortisol was replaced, in one case)
- two insulinomas ("hypoglycemia" was the culture's faddish explanation for multiple nonspecific symptoms at the time and a frequent complaint)
- all subcategories of hypothyroidism, from primary (alone and with primary adrenal insufficiency – "You look very tan for an Alaskan") to tertiary.
- Pheochromocytoma, including recurrent ("You don't think I could have another pheochromocytoma, do you, Doc?")
- acute intermittent porphyria (the patient, whose diagnosis had not been established, was transferred from the hospital in Forks with an acute attack, and the ambulance stopped at every ER on the trip for pain meds)
- multiple cases of subacute endocarditis
- several cases of bacterial vertebral osteomyelitis

- chronic carbon monoxide poisoning (an interest of Dr. Kirkpatrick's)
- ergot toxicity
- periarteritis nodosa
- sclerosing mesenteritis
- secondary syphilis with and without Herxheimer reactions with treatment

Drs. Simmons and Gortner maintained problem lists on their patients – uncommon at the time.

The section shared a small space with Dermatology on the 8th floor, which later became the north side of the Buck Pavilion.

The 1980s

The section continued to grow.

Laurie Witcher (then Laurie Fields), a Certified Physician's Assistant (PA-C), became the section's first non-physician practitioner, transferring from VM's Ob-Gyn Section in 1980, soon after Lisa Taylor resigned. She brought not only an excellent knowledge of general medicine but was the first long-term section provider particularly knowledgeable and accomplished in women's health. She quickly became a fount of knowledge to the male providers for outpatient women's health issues.

Bob Aduan, MD, joined the section in 1981. He had been a "Teacher of the Year" where he practiced before and tried to educate us about cholesterol particles before any of us had ever heard of them. He was diagnosed with Chronic Myelogenous Leukemia in 1985 and died from pulmonary aspergillosis following a bone marrow transplant at VM. He left a wife and children behind.

Karen Rosene, MD, joined the section in 1982, giving us seven medical providers. She was the only internist in North America to complete a two-year fellowship in Maternal-Fetal Medicine and came with the understanding that she would have one day per week to attend and teach at the University of Washington, where she had done her medical residency. She was thus the first "part-time" clinician in the section. She later co-founded the Center for Women's Health (CWH) at VM in 1988. She resigned to go to Brown University in 1989.

Paul Smith, MD, and Roger Bush, MD, joined SGIM in 1984, beginning long and impactful careers in the section, medical center, and regionally. Paul had been chief medical resident at the University of Rochester after graduating from the UW Medical School. Roger graduated from UCSF and was an outstanding medical resident for VM.

The HIV/AIDs epidemic reached a tipping point in this decade. For a period of time, HIV/AIDs was deemed a "primary care disease" and section members followed a number of these patients. In 1979 while a medical student at UCSF, Roger Bush admitted a young man, whose name he still recalls, straight off a plane returning from a year's stay in Zaire. The patient's chest x ray had diffuse patchy infiltrates and large blebs and he had bluish spots all over his body. Dr. Bush dictated the patient's death summary, but the cause of death was a mystery. He states that his "interest and involvement in AIDs went from trickle to a torrent about 1985-1987." Soon after hearing a talk about the "new syndrome" at a local SREPCIM meeting in February 1985, he saw a hemophiliac with a persistent cough and diffuse infiltrates on his chest film and realized that the patient had this new syndrome. The first commercial blood test for HIV was licensed in March 1985. Dr. Bush estimates that within the next one to two years he was following 50 to 100 infected hemophiliacs and a large number of infected gay men. He estimates signing about 200 death certificates, and feels that he was a palliative care specialist before that became a recognized field. He learned to do skin biopsies because of the difficulty getting them done by dermatologists. [24] Other SGIM physicians also followed HIV/AIDS patients but not in such numbers.

Lesley Althouse, MD, the first section member with a special interest and training in Geriatrics, joined the section in January 1985. She did her undergraduate, medical and internal medicine residency at Oxford University in England and a fellowship at Johns Hopkins in 1984. Section members shared covering for her when she was on maternity leave. Making rounds on nursing home patients was an eye-opening experience for most of the section's physicians. Kathy Kundert, PA-C came in 1986, having received specialty training in geriatrics at Stanford the year before. In 1989, they were joined in their work with geriatric patients by nurse Nancy Becker Lencioni, who transferred from the Endocrinology Section. A second geriatrician remained only a year from 1987 to 1988.

Judy Bowen, MD, in 1985, became the third former VM medical resident to join the section, transferring from her practice in an early VM satellite clinic in Mountlake Terrace. She was a co-founder of The Women's Center and a Program Director of the Medicine Residency Program before moving on to a position at the University of Oregon Health Sciences in 1996; by 2019 she had risen to the position of Head of the Division of General Internal Medicine and Geriatrics. [25]

In 1988 Karen Rosene and Judy Bowen left SGIM to found the separate Center for Women's Health. This was the first of several offerings of clinical services to subsets of the general medical patient population in which section members were founders or early participants.

The 1980s was the decade when prepaid medical care became more common in American medicine and Virginia Mason participated, even owning an HMO. This was not VM's first experience with prepaid care. Towards the end of the clinic's first decade in the 1920s, the Great Depression struck and many patients could no longer afford to pay their medical bills. VM survived then by selling prepaid medical contracts to private companies and government institutions with large groups of employees, such as Boeing, the U.S. Post Office, and the Police Department. [26] The 1980s and 90s HMO phenomenon was propelled by the rising cost of medical services, some of which was believed to be due to unnecessary testing and care. SGIM members served as primary care providers (PCPs) but did not have a large number of HMO patients – in 1984 a study of the first quarter of the year showed that 17% of new patient visits were HMO enrollees. [27] Other physicians serving as HMO PCPs in the downtown clinic were in the Section of Endocrinology and Diabetes, some of whom later admitted to a heightened appreciation of the medical knowledge base needed by, and administrative burden assigned to, primary care providers. The PCP role in an HMO could indeed be burdensome. There were calls in the middle of the night from emergency rooms because a patient was there and permission or denial from a PCP was believed necessary to evaluate them. There were forms to sign if specialist's orders were to be followed. There were forms to sign to consult a specialist. There were patient requests for medically unnecessary consultations, tests, or prescriptions. A patient whom Jim Simmons had agreed to refer to his chiropractor for chronic back pain filed a complaint with the King County Medical Society when refused such consultation for hay fever. VMC had a financial loss in 1988 due to decreased reimbursement for care by all payers including VM's HMO. [28]

The 1990s

The 1990s was the decade when the "Evidence-Based Medicine" movement coalesced; GIM was an early adopter of that approach and continues to supply expertise in its concepts and methods to the group and community.

The 1990s was also a decade that saw the section experimenting with different ways to provide care to two subsets of patients:

• **Patients of Asian Heritage:** Dr. John Kirkpatrick founded The Asian American Clinical Program (AACP), a subsection of SGIM, in the late 90s. Though it did not survive, SGIM gained valuable members when it disbanded. Several of them were Asian American graduates of VM's medical residency who did not stay with VM for their entire careers. The physician originally recruited for the AACP who stayed the longest and had the greatest impact on VM patient care was Keith Dipboye, MD. He qualified for the AACP by finishing an undergraduate Japan Studies program, then attending Osaka University in Japan as a Fulbright Research Fellow. He also brought considerable information systems skills that were tapped when VMMC was choosing and implementing an electronic medical record (EMR) the following decade.

• **SGIM patients hospitalized in Virginia Mason Hospital**: From its inception GIM physicians saw their patients in the hospital as well as patients scheduled in clinic Monday through Friday. On weekends and clinic holidays a lone section physician rounded on all the section's inpatients. On Saturday mornings a half-day was spent seeing patients in the clinic as well. As the number of providers grew, the weekend doctor might be rounding on 30 or more inpatients. In hopes of easing this increasingly oppressive duty, SGIM began an experiment by having two section physicians cover hospitalized patients on weekdays for two weeks, while having no routinely scheduled clinic visits. This trial began in 1995. However, the arrangement proved unpopular with physicians, patients, and staff and was discontinued in early 1996. Nonetheless, GIM played a major role in the creation and staffing of the Section of Hospital Medicine. In the late 1990s, VM's medical house staff grew restive about their heavy workload. Roger Bush, MD, then the Internal Medicine Residency Program Director, attended one of the earliest meetings of the Society of Hospital Medicine, founded in January 1997. During a break, he met Barry Aaronson, MD, in the men's room. Barry was not content in his hospitalist job in Tacoma. On his return to Seattle, Roger worked to convince VM to start a hospitalist service with Barry as the first member. Initially he worked daytimes Monday through Friday. Night coverage was provided by a Non-Housestaff Admitting Service (NHAS), staffed by UW fellows and headed by Dave Gortner, which managed hospital admissions at night as well as Barry's patients. SGIM physicians continued to cover their patients admitted on the house staff service. [29,30].

The late 1990's were again economically challenging times for American medicine. VMMC lost money in 1998 and 1999, a fate shared by many medical centers. The experiments with managed care in the 1980s and 90s were at least partially to blame. [31]

Notable additions to the section's providers in the 1990s included:

• Julie Pattison, MD, came to VM in 1992, working half-time in CWH and half in GIM. She became full-time in SGIM when CWH disbanded and remains, having been a section and clinic wide promoter of VMPS (Virginia Mason Production System) as well as Section

314

Head in GIM.

• Gail Gregerich, MN, ARNP. She was the section's first long term nurse practitioner, joining us in 1995.

• Dan Hanson, MD, joined us in 1995 after his chief medical resident year at VM. He served as an associate program director of VMMC's Medical Residency Program; after moving into the Hospitalist Department he served as Section Head and has become a Fellow in The Society of Hospital Medicine.

• Steve Hayashi, MD, came to VM in 1997. He had been a "Teacher of the Year" before joining SGIM and has been a perennial favorite on various "Seattle's Best Doctors" lists since.

• Carrie Horwitch, MD, MPH came in 1999 to fill a vacated Assistant Program Director (APD) position, bringing expertise in HIV/AIDS. She has been a stalwart teacher for her physician and resident colleagues. None who saw it can forget her mirthful GIM Journal Club presentation, introducing us to the multiple health benefits of laughter and leading us in a mindful laughing exercise. She has become a certified leader and teacher of laughter therapy. [32] She was also certified as an "HIV Specialist" by the American Academy of HIV Medicine in 2000. [33].

• Keith Dipboye, MD, came in 1999 and contributed to the functionality of VM's EMR by creating two very useful "apps" for it.

The 2000s

The first two decades of the new century were transformative for VMMC and SGIM. Gary Kaplan, MD, became the seventh Clinic Chairman in 2000. He was a superlative VMMC chief medical resident in 1980-81, after which he was instrumental in developing and leading the medical center's satellite system. He is the second general internist and VM-trained MD, to be Chairman. The first general internist and second Clinic Chairman was John Blackford, MD. Joel Baker, MD, the third Chairman, was a VM trained surgeon. When Dr. Kaplan became Chairman, VMMC, along with many other U.S. medical centers, had lost money for two consecutive years. Soon after taking over, he told leaders, "We change, or we die". [34] This dire warning followed not only the financial losses in 1998 and 1999, but also concerns fueled by two reports from The Institute of Medicine addressing medical errors as defects in quality of care creating wasteful high costs. [35] The actions taken in response to these challenges led to the development and deployment of the Virginia Mason Production System (VMPS) which has since garnered interest and attention nationally and internationally.

By 2001 the section had grown to 25 providers (21 MDs, 2 PAs, & 2 NPs) and occupied the entirety of the 8th floor of the Buck Pavilion. [36] This was the decade when:

- We ceased managing our patients in the hospital.
- We became a section in a new Department of Primary Care rather than the Department of Medicine, a potentially advantageous political and administrative change.
- Dr. John Kirkpatrick, among the founding trio of SGIM, left the section to cofound the Dare Center, now called Concierge Medicine.
- The Virginia Mason Production System (VMPS) and the Electronic Medical Record (EMR) were introduced and refined, revolutionizing our daily patient care. SGIM was the downtown campus test group for both of these innovations.
- Section nurses began case-managing patients with chronic medical problems, diabetes being the first.
- Clinical Pharmacists, Psychotherapists and Social Workers began seeing patients on site on Buck 8.
- The increasing complexity of the section led to reorganization of providers and staff into 6 pods with initially 4, then 3 deputy heads. The section held weekly business meetings three times per month; the pods every other month. [37]
- Physician Assistants and Nurse Practitioners (PAs and NPs) were now referred to jointly as Advanced Practice Clinicians (ACPs) at VM. Their numbers increased and roles expanded within the section.
- The section continued to grow.

316

Sometime in 2000 the hospitalists "slowly started covering some SGIM inpatients." [30] By the Spring of 2006 the Section of Hospital Medicine had grown large enough to accept all of SGIM's hospitalized patients. [38] This was better for patient care for a variety of reasons, high among them being the enlarging knowledge bases for both outpatient and hospital medicine, which continued to grow rapidly. Many of the hospitalists transferred from SGIM, including Dan Hanson, Tom Gunby, Michael Ingraham, and Roger Bush. For some, the change to being solely outpatient doctors was bittersweet. The hospitalists' timely and factual hospital discharges could not totally replace existential and emotional memories gained at the patient's bedside.

John Kirkpatrick cofounded the Dare Center in 2000. It was named for John and Lewis Dare, father and son and VMCs first and second clinic administrators. Physicians' panels were limited to about 300 patients who paid an annual fee to enroll and whose insurances were also billed for services delivered. Patients had 24/7 access to their physician by cell phone or pager, same day appointments, longer routine appointments, and nursing or patient's home visits if indicated. Coordination of complex care might include the Dare Center physician attending a patient's appointments with consultants. SGIM members who migrated to Concierge Medicine practices have included Lesley Althouse, MD, nurse Nancy Lencioni, Tammira Price, MD, Paul Kassab, MD, and Eileen Bailey, MD.

Jim Bender, Keith Dipboye, and Dave Gortner were among the group of providers who helped VM decide on which EMR to use. Section members were queried about desired functionality. GIM was the first section to have computers in all exam rooms and the first to use Cerner in the downtown clinic. Keith Dipboye wrote two very useful applications enhancing the program. The first was a computerized version of a Primary Care and Prevention tool. A patient and medical assistant (MA) flow manager could jointly review the PCP report. The MA could administer any routine vaccines when due, determine what testing was due, and schedule some for the patient. The screen would be left open for the provider to see what had been done. Keith's second "app" was a semi-automated letter reporting patients' test results. A provider could add a greeting and perhaps a personal message, along with any needed explanation or follow up needed. Patients appreciated this as it decreased the time it took to receive test results. The staff liked it because it decreased patient calls about results.

The Virginia Mason Production System (VMPS), adopted in 2002, grew out of VMMC's leaders search for a management framework that could achieve and maintain the group's goals of putting the patient first and being "the quality leader". They believed that realizing those goals would promote financial viability by improving the quality and safety of outcomes while decreasing costs. [39,40] After studying TPS principles in depth for a year, and following in Boeing's footsteps, clinic, physician and administrative leadership visited Japan in June 2002 to see TPS in action. [41] During an immersive two-week experience, the group realized that the TPS framework could be adapted to health care and become VMPS. [42]

Kim Pittenger, MD, a family practice physician in the Kirkland satellite clinic and Ken Gross, MD, an endocrinologist, designed the PCP (Primary Care and Prevention) report. When this was developed and implemented in 2002, the clinic was still mostly using paper medical charts, though billing and lab data were computerized. A program was written that enabled mining of these databases to produce a printout made available when a patient was seen for a scheduled appointment. The provider could see at a glance which screening or disease management tests had been done, and some results. [43] This saved the time and effort of providers trying to keep track of such information by a method of their own. Later a system to call back diabetics who had not been seen for appropriate follow-up was also introduced.

The second major VMPS innovation in primary care delivery, conceived and first implemented in Kirkland, was the "flow station." Morale was at a low nationwide among primary care providers, largely due to the increasing burden of "indirect care" – work done for absent patients requesting medication refills, lab results and interpretation, forms filled out and signed, questions answered, and the like. The concept was to come

318

up with a way to get the indirect work done in "flow" rather than being "batched" and done at the end of the time spent seeing a day's patients. "Batching" is known to reduce quality and increase time to complete tasks compared to doing things in "flow." [44] After planning, trialing, and implementing flow stations, Kirkland primary care doctors were able to see more patients in the same number of work hours; patient satisfaction improved; and negative profit margins became positive. [45]

When SGIM was urged to get up to speed in VMPS, we were operating in a disorderly environment with considerable waste and lack of teamwork. Despite VMMC's sobriquet of "Team Medicine," SGIM's five teams failed to make a whole functioning section. Generally physicians, not patients, remained atop the pyramid, contradicting our professed goal. Cindy Rockfeld became administrative director of SGIM in 2003 and soon realized that "breaking down silos" and "fixing our foundations" had to be done first. [46] To assist us along the VMPS path, Joyce Lammert, MD, then Section Head of Allergy and Immunology, a medical center leader and trained in VMPS, was appointed by CEO Gary Kaplan as interim SGIM Section Head. The change was announced at an assembly of all SGIM members. When Gary delivered this message, many in the group were stunned and dismayed. Jim Simmons spoke up saying that in the past SGIM had had difficulties having assets allocated to it; Dr. Lammert was a valuable VMMC asset and leader and we should be grateful to Gary for loaning her to the section and welcome her.

The first project was to standardize the exam rooms that were not being utilized efficiently. Each provider was assigned certain exam rooms, stocked to match their preferences, including idiosyncratic and sometimes out-of-date patient education materials. Interrupting a patient visit to look for and retrieve something needed but missing in the room was agreed upon as the most disruptive activity in a provider's day. After getting buy-in and input from providers and staff, one busy weekend was spent stocking all exam rooms identically, with the same items located in the same places. Exam rooms were thereafter checked daily to replace anything missing. The improvement was promptly noted and appreciated by section providers. The next step was to add stand-up flow stations in the halls so that the provider and medical assistant (MA) "Flow Manager" could try to keep up with the day's work during regular working hours. A few minutes between patient visits were to be devoted to doing a few medication refills or patient's messages, rather than waiting till the end of the day to get to any but the truly urgent ones. Drs. Julie Pattison, Keith Dipboye and their MAs were the first in the section to trial this, again successfully. [47] After these two VMPS methods were introduced, any provider could work with any MA, using any section exam room.

Section nurses' case management services began with SGIM's diabetic patients. A clinic visit would begin with the nurse meeting with the patient, getting an interim history of problems or questions. The provider was paged and might obtain additional history or exam, then devised a plan with the patient and nurse. The nurse then reviewed the visit and plans with the patient. Between visits, nurses checked in with the patient by phone to see how things were going. Patients, nurses, and providers all liked this system. Many patients were delighted to see improvement in their numbers related to diabetic and cardiovascular risk factor control. Patient satisfaction with their care also improved. Later section nurses began doing managed care with a variety of chronic medical diseases for patients not doing well or needing more education. [48,49]

Some time after 2011, clinical pharmacists, clinical social workers, and psychotherapists joined Certified Physician Assistants and Certified Nurse Practitioners on Buck 8 providing direct and indirect care for SGIM patients. [50,51] The two Clinical Pharmacists help patients primarily for blood pressure management, and also with lipid control and poly-pharmacy. While available appointments with psychiatrists were still limited, short and medium-term psychotherapy were easier to access with a clinical social worker and 2 clinical psychologists. [49]

Nurse Practitioner Terry Cunningham continued to provide excellent care to his panel of patients. He was the only Advanced Care Practitioner (ACP = PAs & NPs) to have his own panel of patients. [51] The rest of the on- site ACPs were doing mostly indirect care and direct care for their pod, seeing occasional new patients [50,51] rather than having their own panel of patients. Laurie Witcher, PA-C, the section's first ACP in 1980, was the first to focus on indirect care in the earlier 2000s. By 2019 she had transitioned to doing an estimated 90% of her work from home, using the EMR, My VM's patient portal, her work cellphone and also using Skype for team communication, She estimates that the bulk of her work involves "Provider Out Indirect Care". Time permitting, she also does "enhanced coverage" for providers in the clinic who "are struggling to keep up", which she identifies by viewing their "Cerner Box", a folder in the EMR to which she has proxy. She then does what she can to help them and notes those needing more support. [50]

Providers joining the section included [52]:

VMMC Internal Medicine Residency Graduates:

- Alisse Ryan, MD, in 2002 after her year as VMMC's Chief Medical Resident
- Jason Eintracht, MD, in 2005
- Eileen Bailey, MD, in 2006
- Minori Yoshioka, MD, in 2007
- Ellen Frechette, MD, in 2007
- Nkeiruka Duze, MD, in 2009
- Sandra Lord, MD, in 2015
- Monica Waldie, MD, in 2015
- Leah Geyer, MD, in 2015 after her year as VMMC's Chief Medical Resident
- Camille Johnson, MD, in 2016 after her year as VMMC's chief medical resident
- Travis Gerrard, MD, in 2019 after his year as VMMC's chief medical resident

And Graduates of Other Medical Residencies:

- Astrid Pujari, MD, in 2001 with training in traditional medicine and Phytotherapy.
- Lee Ferguson, MD, in 2006
- Michael Soung, MD, in 2007 after his Medical Chief

Residency year at The University of Washington
- Joy Bucher, MD, in 2010 after her year as Chief Medical Resident at The University of Washington
- Lauren Crowley, MD, in 2011
- Nicholas Moy, MD, in 2012
- Soheila Hedayati, MD, in 2015
- Brandon Auerbach, MD, in 2017
- Kevin Means, MD, in 2018
- Michelle Lam, MD, in 2019

At Dr. Bender's "retirement from clinical medicine" party, he told Dr. Simmons, "The section has been recruiting such good people lately that we would have never gotten a job."

TEACHING

The English word "doctor" came directly from a Latin word meaning "teacher" [53], a fact oft cited by J. Willis Hurst, MD, Department of Medicine Head at Emory University, to his residents during morning report at Grady Memorial Hospital in Atlanta, where Jim Simmons trained. Teaching has been an important part of VM's mission from its early history to the present. Internships were begun in 1925. Medical and Surgical residencies, the first in the region, were added in 1939. [6] "Education" is among the foundational elements in the VM Quality Pyramid, resting just above "Virginia Mason Production" at the base with "The Patient" at the apex. The chance to teach and learn from residents has long been an important factor in many providers' and staff's desire to work at VMMC. SGIM has carried on this tradition from the section's beginning.

The 1970s and 1980s

Like other members of the DOM, SGIM members taught medical residents mostly on the hospital wards. A member would be assigned to a resident team for a period of time, typically a month with 2-3 meetings a week. The format was usually that an intern, with the patient's consent, would present the history in a conference room, the team would go to the patient's bedside, review the history and any "teachable" physical findings, and then retreat back to the conference room to discuss things.

There was also an outpatient resident's clinic that the attendings would supervise in rotation with other members of the DOM with a similar format. Paul Smith, since joining SGIM in 1985 to the present, has exemplified dedication to teaching outpatient medicine to VM's medical residents.

When Dr. Bender joined the section as the fourth member, he suggested that a journal club be started, having attended those of other DOM sections he had rotated though as a VM house officer. In 1977 section members began reviewing recent journal articles for the group on a weekly schedule.

Dr. Simmons was the first SGIM member to present at VM's Grand Rounds. Much to Dr. Bender's dismay, the topic was "Hysteria", at the time a diagnostic term for a syndrome, which would now be classified by the Diagnostic and Statistical Manual-5 (DSM-5) under the rubric "Somatic Symptom Disorder: Severe". The word was derived from a Greek word, hystera, meaning womb, and was applied to emotional and physical symptoms thought by the ancient Greeks to be "peculiar to women". [54] These patients had a history of seeing multiple physicians for multiple recurring symptoms and having surgeries for which no physical cause had been found. Dr. Bender feared the presentation might seem a solicitation to colleagues to send patents suspected of it to SGIM. Every physician was seeing these patients. Indeed, most of the physical morbidity of the syndrome was iatrogenic – unnecessary surgery, too many medications, too many consultations. It was among the earliest psychiatric disorders for which there were diagnostic criteria and one of only a few psychiatric diagnoses that could reliably be made in the 1970s. The diagnostic criteria came from research done by the Department of Psychiatry at Washington University in St. Louis. Dr. Simmons first learned about it from a psychiatrist just out of a residency in that department also working in the USPH outpatient clinic in Seattle. Psychiatric co-morbidity was typically present. Most physicians found them frustrating patients. In addition to a diagnostic protocol, there was a known prognosis (chronic) and morbidities (mostly iatrogenic). There was also a management strategy emphasizing establishing a relationship with the patient, being attentive for any clues to a physical disease coming from new symptoms or signs, and trying to shield them from unneeded surgery, medication, or invasive testing. Dr. Simmons appreciated having Dr. Richard Winterbauer, MD ("Buddha", to the medical residents), say to him afterward that the presentation was "very scholarly". Over time, as the culture got more medically sophisticated, it seemed there were fewer such patients.

SGIM's first Continuing Medical Education (CME) course featured general Internists from both the downtown SGIM and satellite clinics addressing topics such as screening, lipids, and venous thromboembolism. A guest speaker, Richard Deyo, MD, then on the UW Medical School faculty, was and remains an expert on low back pain in primary care. His talk centered on when to order plain lower spine X-rays on patients with this complaint and which few findings on them correlated highly with clinical symptoms. This selective testing strategy was contrary to the widely taught and implemented practice at the time for plain X-rays to be ordered in all patients with low back pain.

The 1990s

This was the decade when "Evidence Based Medicine" as an approach to medical practice was introduced and GIM providers were early adopters. It was also the decade when GIM's involvement in medical resident teaching burgeoned.

In 1993, non-academic centers faced new rules to remain certified to offer an internal medicine residency program. These consisted of requiring physician staff to include a Program Director (PD) as well as 4 Assistant Program Directors (APDs) spending at least 20 hours per week working on Program needs and away from their clinical practice. At the time, Judy Bowen, MD, was the PD. She invited four section members to serve as APDs: Roger Bush, Paul Smith, Lucy Sutphen, and Jim Simmons. The major teaching activities overseen were the Medical Resident's Continuity

Clinics including The Specialty Clinic (HIV/AIDs). The GIM conference room, some exam rooms as well as space in several VMMC affiliated clinics in the community housed these activities. There was also a GIM Noon Conference once per month, joining the other medical sections that had long had such lecture-based teaching sessions in an auditorium on the 4th floor of the hospital. The APDs were assigned responsibility for heading up the following aspects of the program:

Lucy Sutphen - Administrative details of the Medical Residents' Continuity Clinics. These included the "IMA" (Internal Medicine Associates) housed in SGIM, as well as Community Clinics, including Pike Place Market, Country Doctor, Carolyn Downs, and for a while, Rainier Valley. Dr. Sutphen also ran career-planning workshops for the residents. [55]

Roger Bush – The Specialty Clinic (HIV/AIDs). Beyond the educational objective, this was important in providing patients access to up-to-date HIV care at VM. As more treatments for the infection and its complications and better ways to monitor that treatment came along, it became difficult for GIM providers to keep up with them. There was no Infectious Disease Section at VM at the time.

Jim Simmons - curriculum for the Medical Residents' downtown and community clinics didactic sessions as well as for the GIM noon conference. A didactic session preceded the first scheduled patient visits of the day. The week's topic was announced in "The Weekly Reader" delivered before the week in which they were used, with one of the residents acting as the presenter. The curriculum came from Dr. Simmons experience as well as data from national surveys tallying the most common reasons patients visited general internists. The "Weekly Reader" included the topic and why it was important for generalists to be knowledgeable about it, along with learning goals for the reading and didactic session. It was distributed along with a copy of a faculty-chosen review article from the medical literature for the first several years. Later all residents were given a copy of Goroll's *Primary Care Internal Medicine* textbook with a suggested chapter or chapters to read. Topics began with the theory and practice of screening, followed by a segment on cardiovascular risk factors. Disorders with seasonal patterns were done in season; subspecialty problems a general internist should be able to manage were also done in blocks. The noon conference was used to cover primary care topics not covered in the didactic sessions. Speakers were invited by Dr. Simmons and not always members of SGIM.

Paul Smith – evaluations of medical residents by their attending physicians. These were requested from attendings on all clinic and hospital rotations to be sure each resident was on track in acquiring the medical and professional knowledge required to become eligible for board certification.

The residents seemed to value their continuity clinic experience, voting the annual "Internal Medicine Teacher of the Year" award to Lucy Sutphen for 1993-94 and Jim Simmons for 1994-95. When one of the residents asked Dr. Simmons what he wanted from the residents, the reply was, "To be proud of you". When Dr. Simmons resigned his APD position to return to full-time clinical practice, he was presented, with a nod to his love of classic rock music, a Lava Lamp with the base inscribed: "Dr. Simmons, Thanks for Lighting the Way!".

GIM Journal Club continued, with a procedural change – Jim Simmons and Paul Smith chose the articles and sent copies out with a cover sheet detailing why they were chosen. In early November 1993, Jim Simmons chose "How to Get Started" the first article of a new *JAMA* series, "Users' Guides to the Medical Literature" and delivered a copy to section providers with the message that it was for the coming week's GIMJC "and for posterity." Subsequent articles in the series were reviewed as they appeared.

Roger Bush was the first person to give a VMMC Grand Rounds using EBM concepts. The program featured a vascular surgeon reviewing the results of a randomized trial of surgery for asymptomatic carotid stenosis. The results appeared favorable for the procedure and a general internist was requested to talk about screening for this condition. Instead, Roger focused on the EBM concepts of ARRs (Absolute Risk Reduction) and the NNT (Number of procedures needing to be performed to help one person). He recalls using a grease pen on a transparency projected overhead to demonstrate the calculations. At the time, the typical way to present results of treatment trials was to cite a "Relative Risk Reduction (RRR)", the percentage of patients benefiting from the treatment. At first blush, RRR outcomes could seem quite impressive. Those same results viewed as NNT & ARR could be much less affecting. Roger vividly recalls Fritz Fenster (a highly respected hepatologist, and teacher), "approaching me afterwards to offer a huge 'attaboy', which meant a lot to me ...." [24]

Primary Care of Women, the first textbook on the subject, was published in 1995. [56] Two of the three editors were Dawn Lemcke, MD, and Julie Pattison, MD, who were then in the Center for Women's Health. Both were welcomed into SGIM when the CWH was dissolved. They also authored the chapter on "Menopause and Estrogen Replacement Therapy" and Dawn Lemke added a chapter on "Osteoporosis". Other chapter authors who were SGIM members included [57]:

- "Adolescent Medicine" by Jane Becker, MD
- "Geriatric Medicine" by Deborah Fetherston, MD, and
  Lesley Althouse, MD
- "HIV Infection" by Roger Bush, MD
- "Preventive Services" by Paul Smith, MD,
- "Venous Thromboembolism: DVT and PE" by Jim Simmons, MD

The book received a good review in *The New England Journal of Medicine*. [58]

The 2000s

SGIM's contributions to teaching within and outside of VMMC grew during this period more than any other period in the history of the section.

VMMC's medical residents' involvement with SGIM mushroomed. The Continuity Clinic was replaced with "Collaborative Practice", a 3-year mentor/preceptor relationship with a general internist. Most SGIM physicians participate and about a half of the medical residents have this experience in SGIM. A rotation in SGIM is required of all IM residents. Residents in the Primary Care Track also have rotations in GIM in their second and third years, but most are taken in satellite clinics. [49]

The only SGIM member who remains an Associate Program Director in Medicine is Joy Bucher, MD, who continues to devote half her time to the program. Paul Smith, MD, and Michael Soung, MD, are "Core Faculty" [59], with special program duties but are not bound to spend 20 hours per week devoted to them. Michael Soung received the 2015 "Teacher of the Year" award from the internal medicine medical residents. [60]

GIM Journal Club continues and is held once monthly. Ellen Frechette, MD, and Minori Yoshioka, MD, schedule the providers who lead the meetings. Typically the program includes presentation of an article chosen by the speaker and passed out before the meeting, followed by a case. Periodically, a Morbidity and Mortality conference is on the program. Both formats include questions and comments from attendees. [61]

VM Grand Round presentations by SGIM member have accelerated. After reviewing the total list of GR presenters since 2015, Michael Soung found five section members listed. Carrie Horwitch has also organized sessions with VM IM residents presenting case studies of patients they have seen, or details of their research activities and findings. [49]

SGIM has organized an annual daylong "VM Primary Care" course for the last 10 years. Paul Smith has been a co-chair for each of these. Michael Soung and Joy Boucher have been among the other co-chairs. [49]

Michael Soung and Carrie Horwitch are frequent presenters at Washington American College of Physicians (ACP) meetings and Carrie and Paul Smith have presented at the national ACP meeting. [49]

"PAGE"

"PAGE" was used as part of the formula to determine providers' incomes and was categorized as activities within VMMC, Regionally, Nationally, or Internationally.

VMMC

SGIM Section Heads and Their Tenures:

1. **Jim Simmons (1974 – 1989):** Dr. Simmons was the first SGIM member to retire from a career spent only at VMMC. In his position acceptance letter to then Clinic Chairman, John Walker, he "looked

forward to a long career at VM and hoped to maintain the group's tradition of dedication to excellent patient care." As Section Head his major goals were growing the section and maintaining our learning about the ever-expanding knowledge base useful to SGIM practitioners. Clinic leaders always anticipated SGIM becoming the largest downtown section but had trouble finding space to accommodate that goal until the Buck Pavilion was opened. Recruiting providers and advocating for additional allocation of space were major Section Head activities, with much help from other section members. SGIM members were willing learners and teachers. There was the luxury of having journal clubs weekly at first, then three times per month with one "business meeting". Dr. Simmons resigned when the job had grown complex enough to require skills he lacked and was unlikely to acquire. Dr. Jim Bender was the one with a lot of ideas for the section and how to accomplish them.

2. **Jim Bender (1989 - 1994)**: Dr. Bender brought not only a seemingly easy excellence as a clinician, but also an engineer's skill at analyzing a problem, along with a desire to make things work better. He was destined to be the section member to use his talents the most in VMMC-wide positions.

3. **Dave Gortner (1994 - 2005)**: Dr. Gortner was the third member of the section's founding quartet who became a section head. He presided over a period of growth in the number of providers, including more part-time providers, and a period of increasing use of computers in patient care. He served in leadership or member positions on a number of VM's committees and in the DOM. He retired from VMMC to move to sunny Arizona, where he continued to be active clinically and in teaching till his retirement in 2017.

4. **Joyce Lammert (2005 - 2006)**: Dr. Lammert was Section Head of Asthma and Allergy when she was appointed by Gary Kaplan to serve as a temporary section leader in 2005 to help the transition to a VMPS-based work flow. She had been among the first clinicians to become expert in VMPS and greatly facilitated SGIM's adopting its

methods.

5. **Julie Pattison (2007 - 2009)**: Dr. Pattison worked tirelessly in 2005 and 2006 helping the section implement VMPS. She became the Section Head when enough progress had been made for Joyce to leave. She has continued to support VMPS in the section and clinic wide. Dr. Pattison retired in late 2019.

6. **Jason Eintract (2009 – present)**: Section provider growth has continued apace, including physicians and Advanced Practice Clinicians (APCs - which include Physician Assistants and Nurse Practitioners). Innovations in patient care have included having clinical pharmacists, social workers, and psychotherapists see SGIM patients on the 8th floor where SGIM is housed. Subsection Heads have been added to the group's administrative leadership.

Other VMMC Positions Held and Other "PAGE" Activities by SGIM Members [62]:

Jim Bender served on VM's Partnership's Executive Committee for two terms in the 1990s and was an ex officio member of VMMC's Managing Committee in 2002, while serving as the Chief of Hospital Medicine. He became the medical director of managed care in 1994 and the acting medical director of VM's short-lived managed care insurance plan (VMHP) during its transition to Aetna in 1997. He, Dave Gortner, and & Keith Dipboye were influential in the decision about which electronic medical record to deploy for the Medical Center. He later served as the Medical Director of Information Systems.

Judy Bowen was the Internal Medicine Residency (IMRP) Program Director from 1993 – 1996 and was on the Executive Committee in 1995.

Roger Bush was the Director of VM's Home Health Service from 1989 – 1994. [24] He was among the 4 SGIM APDs in the IMRP from 1993-1996, at which time he became its Program Director, serving in that role until 2007. He founded and was the director of the HIV Clinic within the VM Medical Residency. He was instrumental in the formation of VMMC's Hospitalist Department and piqued Barry Aaronson's interest in becoming its first member. He, David Gortner and Barry Aaronson were on the committee that successfully argued for establishing a Hospitalist program.

Keith Dipboye was the Program Director of the Transitional Medicine Residency Program in the 2000s. He served as Associate Director of Medical Informatics from 1999 to 2015.

David Gortner was elected to the partnership's Executive Committee as well as to its Compensation Committee. He was influential in developing the group's processes for accessing patient information -both analog (paper charts) and digital (Cerner EMR) - serving as a long time member and Chairman of the Medical Records Committee, and as participant in the choice and implementation of Cerner. He was Section Head when SGIM pioneered Cerner in the outpatient setting, putting computers in every exam room.

Carrie Horwitch joined the section in 1999 to fill a vacancy in the Associate Program Director position of VMMC's Internal Medicine Residency and took over as leader in the Medical Residency's HIV clinic. She has gotten advanced training and a certificate in HIV care. She made Laughter Therapy available to VMMC patients.

John Kirkpatrick was the Associate Program Director of VM's Wellness Program (SENSE) from 1983 to 1990. He served as Director of Home Health Care from 1984 to 1989, as well as Medical Director of the Executive Health Program from 1988 to 1999.

Jim Simmons got his second home computer in the early 90s as an inducement not to resign as chairman of the VMH Utilization Review Committee. It was very difficult to get physicians to accept an appointment to membership on the committee. He accepted the computer and another term on the job if allowed to address the VMMC Board of Directors. The message delivered was that the specially trained nurses were the experts on the Medicare and private insurance rules and could reliably determine when an admission put the hospital at risk for penalty. A physician's review was not needed for every such determination, but should be available when the nurses had questions about medical issues that might justify guideline deviation or to deal with attending physician pushback. This was the process soon adopted.

Michael Soung is used as a consultant on evidence-based medicine issues by Dr. Bob Mecklenburg, Director of the Center for Healthcare Solutions at VMMC. The Center's goal is to get the message out to insurance and large companies about VMMC using the best available evidence to produce our recognized stellar clinical outcomes. [63]

Norris Kamo, MD, is the Section Head at University Village regional medical center, after starting in SGIM.

Nicholas Moy, MD, is an Associate Medical Informatics Officer, serving as a liaison between providers and the IT department. He has also developed Chronic Disease Dashboards for the Department of Primary Care providers to use tracking how they are doing in meeting goals for management of care recommended for diabetes, hypertension, colorectal cancer screening, and statin therapy. [64]

Seattle and Washington State "PAGE" Activities
American College of Physicians (ACP) Involvement:
SGIM members have played major roles in the Washington Chapter of the ACP, especially in the 21st century, serving in leadership roles, garnering many chapter honors and organizing and presenting at CME programs at chapter meetings.

Carrie Horwitch served as governor of the chapter from 2010 - 14.
Roger Bush was on the Governor's Council of the chapter from 1996 - 2004.

Current or former SGIM members who have been awarded the FACP (Fellow) designation include [52]:
- **Lesley Althouse**
- **Joy Bucher**
- **Nkeiruka Duze** [65]
- **Ellen Frechette**
- **Paul Kassab**
- **John Kirkpatrick**

- **Julie Pattison**
- **Elaine Sachter**
- **Jason Eintracht**

Roger Bush in 2011, **Carrie Horwitch** in 2014, and **Paul Smith** in 2016, became Laureates of the Washington ACP chapter, the ultimate rung in the state ACP's hierarchy of awards. It is given in recognition of having "demonstrated by their example and conduct an abiding commitment to excellence in medical care, education, or research and in service to their community, their Chapter, and the American College of Physicians". [66]

Paul Smith was named "Internist of the Year" in 2015. [67]

Carrie Horwitch and **Michael Soung** have been frequent presenters at Washington ACP CME courses. [49]

Jim Simmons (2001) and **Margaret Adam** (2017) received the "Golden Apple" award for community-based excellence in teaching. Maggie Adam was no longer a SGIM member in 2017; instead she was working as Medical Director of the Pike Place Market where she served as attending to VMMC internal medical residents seeing patients there. [67]

Recognition On Seattle Best Doctors' Listings:

Since at least the 1990s various local magazines have published lists of doctors receiving the most votes from their peers as being among the best doctor in their specialty. Not surprisingly, VMMC physicians have done well. Unfortunately a complete historical listing of the many SGIM doctors on these listings is not available, but a convenience sample of their performance on them can be gleaned from reviewing online lists available on the websites of *Seattle Magazine* from 2013 to 2019 [68], and that of *Seattle Metropolitan Magazine* from 2008 to 2019. [69] Each year's listing must be looked up separately. John Kirkpatrick found the lists from *Metropolitan Magazine* for the years 1996, 2000, and 2002 as he was going through memorabilia saved from his VM career. [70] *Seattle Magazine*'s available lists online include the following information [68]:

- **Steve Hayashi** is distinguished by the milestone of his tenth listing as of 2018.
- **Carrie Horwitch** has been named four times since 2015, and was featured in a profile and Q & A section in a 2018 article.
- **Michael Soung** has also been named three times since 2015.
- **Astrid Pujari** was named twice, in 2006 and 2013 [71]
- **Joy Bucher, Keith Dipboye, Ellen Frechette, John Kirkpatrick,** and **Julie Pattison** were named once each.

Seattle Metropolitan Magazine's "Top Doctor" lists from 1996, 2000, and 2002 include [70]:
- **Jim Bender, Dave Gortner, John Kirkpatrick** and **Jim Simmons** three times
- **Roger Bush** and **Lael Paul** twice
- **Judy Bowen, Tom Gunby, Steve Hayashi, Dan Hanson, Julie Pattison, Rebecca Ruud, Paul Smith,** and **Lucy Sutphen** once each.

Seattle Metropolitan Magazine's "Top Doctor" lists available on line include [69]:
- **Paul Smith** from 2013 – 2017 [52,69]
- **Astrid Pujari** from 2008 - 2010 [71]
- **Micheal Soung** twice
- **Steve Hayashi** and **Carrie Horwitch** once each

Recognition by "America's Best Doctors" Awards:

Despite the title, the award is voted on by a state's physicians who have been previously given this award. Jim Simmons remembers getting a call from Dr. Ken Wilske in 1994 or 95, saying he was planning to vote for him and asking "who else should I vote for in your section?" Several SGIM doctors were mentioned. John Kirkpatrick remembers a similar call from Dr Wilske as well and getting follow-up mailings from the organization offering wall plaques for sale. [70] There is no public historical or current list available of those named on this listing. SGIM members known to have been on the list from memory, a saved letter to Jim Simmons from the organization, a congratulatory letter from Gary Kaplan in 2007, and a CV [24] are:

- **Jim Simmons** in the middle 1990s and in 2007
- **John Kirkpatrick,** probably also in the mid-1900s
- **Roger Bush** in 1996 [24]
- **Astrid Pujari** from 2004 -2010 [71]

Recognition by Center for Study of Services [72]:

This organization provides information based on patient experience ser-veys. Dr Kirkpatrick has a letter from 1999 including a state by state listing of the top vote getters in each state. SGIM physicians listed for Washington state were **Lesley Althouse, Roger Bush**, and **John Kirkpatrick**. [70]

Regional PAGE Activities

Roger Bush was the president of The Society of General Internal Medi-cine Northwest Region in 1998. [24]

National PAGE Activities

Carrie Horwitch has been active in a leadership role in the ACP nation-ally. She was an ex-officio member of the ACP's Board of Governors from 2010 to 2014. In 2014, she began a term on the Board of Regents, the main policy-making body of the College. She has served on "several na-tional ACP committees, including the Ethics, Professionalism and Human Rights Committees, the Clinical Skills Subcommittee and ACP's High Value Care Committee". [73]

Roger Bush has been active on a national level in the ACP. He was chairman of the National Clinical Skills Subcommittee from 2008 - 2012 and on the National Education Committee from 2008 - 2010. He was on the National Nominating Committee of the Association of Program Di-rectors in Internal Medicine in 2001. [24]

Roger Bush, Paul Smith, and **Carrie Horwitch** have received the

Master award (MACP). [74]

International PAGE Activities

John Kirkpatrick was the Medical Director of VM's International Medical Services. He led VM's team supporting the November 1993, Asia-Pacific Economic Cooperation (APEC) conference in Seattle. [75] He also visited China with then Washington Governor Gary Locke in 1997 and 2003. [76]

The Section of General Internal Medicine as VMMC Approaches its One Hundredth Anniversary

The establishment of SGIM in late 1973 can be traced to the realization of the importance of having a group of physicians committed to providing primary care by VMMC's third and fourth Chairmen, Joel Baker and John Walker, combined with the efforts of the long-serving Chief of the Department of Medicine, John Allen. In its nearly forty-six years of existence it has grown to be the largest section on the downtown campus and in the Department of Primary Care. [51]

Throughout those years our members have been dedicated to patient care, teaching, and continued learning. Many have been recognized for excellence in these endeavors by other medical care providers, as well as patients. Current providers get uniformly excellent scores on patient satisfaction questionnaires.

VMMC and SGIM's past and current members can be proud of their accomplishments and of being contributors to the excellence of a demonstrably world class medical center, whose goal is to put patients first.

Optimism and expectations for continued achievement and success in leading the way in patient care, education, and innovation are appropriate.

Acknowledgements and Thanks

Especially to:

Jeni Spamer, VMMC archivist, for her invaluable aid in finding physical documents in the archives; huge help in retrieving some correct citations when I could not read all the details in my "doctor's

336

handwriting" notes I made for them; and with amazement for the Joel Baker quote on sixth page of this chapter, which she copied and forwarded to me after coming across it in her work, recalling I was looking for information on how and why the decision to form a Section of General Internal Medicine had been made in the first place.

John Kirkpatrick for his patience with my desultory activity in finishing the project.

Katherine Galagan for her invaluable editorial help.

Dave Gortner for his "GIM HISTORY: 1973 to Present", four-and-one-quarter pages of information from 1973 to 2003, which he kept contemporaneously by year. It was the main source I had for much of the information on PAGE activities at VMMC for section members.

Roger Bush for his memories of the early HIV/AIDS epidemic and SGIM's first Grand Rounds presentation.

Michael Soung, Jason Eintracht, and **Laurie Witcher** for their detailed information on section activities after 2011.

To all the other section members listed in the references for answering questions posed to them about their activities and memories of SGIM.

And Most Especially to:

My wife and life's love, **Jytte Simmons,** for her gentle kindnesses and encouragement during this project and our life together.

References:

1. Pujari A. E-mail to Dr. James Simmons responding to questions on 10/18/2019.
2. Ross A. *Visions and Vigilance. The First 75 Years Virginia Mason Medical Center 1920 –1995.* At: https://vnet.vmmc.org/orgs/99580/documents/Vision_and_Vigilance.pdf; page 2; accessed 9/27/18.
3. Ibid, page 12.
4. Steenrod WM. "Interview of John Dare 10/11/85", page 22, Virginia Mason Archives.
5. VMMC Historical Physician Partner and Member Roster: 1918 – 2009, Virginia Mason Archives.
6. Ross A. *Visions and Vigilance. The First 75 Years Virginia Mason Medical Center 1920 – 1995.* At: https://vnet.vmmc.org/orgs/99580/documents/Vision_and_Vigilance.pdf; page ii; accessed 9/27/18.

7. American College of Physicians timeline. At: https://www.acponline.org/about_acp/history/timeline/index.html; accessed 9/27/18.

8. "ABMS History of Improving Quality Care." At: https://www.abms.org/about-abms/history/; accessed 9/27/18.

9. "ABMS Member Boards." At: https://www.abms.org/about-abms/member-boards/; accessed 9/27/18.

10. Walker J. "History of Specialization of Medicine @ Virginia Mason Medical Center", an abbreviated synopsis delivered at grand rounds 11/9/1990; Virginia Mason Historical Archives.

11. Mason JT. "Mistakes in 100 Thyroidectomies." At: https://vnet.vmmc.org.orgs/99580/documents/The _ Mason _ Family _ virtual _version_pdf, page 8; accessed 8/27/18.

12. Mayo WJ. Letter to Dr. James Tate Mason, 5/20/1930. At: https://vnet.vmmc.org/orgs/99580/documents/The_Mason_Family_virtual_version.pdf, page 11, 21; accessed 8/27/18.

13. Traverso LW, Jolly CP. "Joel Wilson Baker MD." *Arch Surg.* 1999,134(9);970. doi:10.1001/archsurg.134.9.970.At: https://jamanetwork.com/journals/jama-surgery/article-abstract/390369; accessed 8/27/28.

14. American Board of Internal Medicine. "Exam Administration History." At: https://www.abim.org/about/exam-information/exam-administration-history.aspx; accessed 8/27/18.

15. "SGIM History." At: https://www.sgim.org/about-us/about/history-and-by-laws; accessed 10/3/18.

16. Department of Medicine Roster, 1975. VM Historical Archives.

17. Baker J. Virginia Mason Chairman Report 1952, page 5. Virginia Mason Archives.

18. Walker J. Chairman's Report, 1969, page 38. Virginia Mason Archives.

19. Walker J. "Remarks for Port Ludlow Conference-April 8-9,1972". Dr. John Walker's Papers 1964-1976." page 8. Virginia Mason Historical Archives.

20. Ross A. *Visions and Vigilance. The First 75 Years Virginia Mason Medical Center 1920 – 1995.* page VIII. At https://vnet.vmmc.org/orgs/99580/documents/Vision_and_Vigilance.pdf; accessed 9/27/18.

21. 25th National Forum: "'Ah-Ha' Moment: It's About the Patients-Not Us". At: http://www.ihi.org/communities/blogs/_layouts/15/ihi/community/blog/itemview.aspx?List=81ca4a47-4ccd-4e9e-89d9-14d88ec59e8d&ID=38; accessed 7/3/18.

22. Kenney C. *Transforming Health Care. Virginia Mason Medical Center's Pursuit of the Perfect Patient Experience.* Boca Raton: FL, CRC Press; 2011, pages 4-5.

23. Steenrod W. "Interview with Dr. Hugh Jones, 6/13/90." Virginia Mason Historical Archives.

24. Bush RW. E-Mail to Dr. James Simmons on 2/13/16 in response to questions.

25. "Judith L. Bowen", OHSU website, at: https://www.ohsu.edu/people/judith-bowen/1F011C1AAC474528A79D978FA11A0430; Accessed 1/27/19.

26. Ross A. *Visions and Vigilance. The First 75 Years Virginia Mason Medical Center 1920 –1995*. Page 15. At: https://vnet.vmmc.org/orgs/99580/documents/Vision_and_Vigilance.pdf; accessed 9/27/18.

27. Simmons J. Presentation to the Executive Committee May 8, 1984. Private papers.

28. Ross A. *Visions and Vigilance. The First 75 Years Virginia Mason Medical Center 1920 – 1995*, pages 79-80. At: https://vnet.vmmc.org/orgs/99580/documents/Vision_and_Vigilance.pdf; accessed 9/27/18.

29. Hanson DE. E-Mail to Dr. James Simmons on 2/9/2016 in response to questions.

30. Aaronson B. Comment on Dan Hanson's 2/9/16 E-mail to Dr. James Simmons.

31. Kenney C. *Transforming Health Care. Virginia Mason Medical Center's Pursuit of the Perfect Patient Experience.* Boca Raton: FL, CRC Press; 2011, page 1.

32. "Q&A: Top Doctor Carrie Horwitch on Being an HIV Care Specialist and Why American Needs Universal Health Care." *Seattle Magazine*, at: https://www.seattlemag.com/top-doctors/qa-top-doctor-carrie-horwitch-being-hiv-care-specialist-and-why-america-needs-universal; last accessed 1/27/19.

33. "Carrie A. Horwitch, MD" at: https://www.virginiamason.org/carrie-a-horwitch-md. Last accessed 1/27/19.

34. Kenney C. *Transforming Health Care. Virginia Mason Medical Center's Pursuit of the Perfect Patient Experience.* Boca Raton: FL, CRC Press; 2011, page 6.

35. Ibid pages 1-2.

36. Ibid page 200.

37. Eintracht J. E-mail to Dr. Simmons responding to questions 3/11/14.

38. Gunby TC. E-mail of 3/4/16 responding to Dan Hanson's E-mail of 2/9/16 to Dr. James Simmons.

39. Kenney C. *Transforming Health Care. Virginia Mason Medical Center's Pursuit of the Perfect Patient Experience.* Boca Raton: FL, CRC Press; 2011, page 10.

40. Ibid, page 10-11.

41. Ibid, page22-24.

42. Ibid, page 22.

43. Ibid, pages 75-76.

44. Ibid, page 77-79.

45. Ibid, page 83.

46. Ibid, page 200.

47. Ibid, page 206.

48. Eintracht J. E-mail to Dr. James Simmons responding to questions 3/11/19.

49. Soung M. E-mail to Dr. Simmons responding to questions 7/16/18.

50. Witcher L. E-mail to Dr. Simmons 2/18/19.

51. Eintracht J. E-mail to Dr. Simmons 3/14/2019.

52. VMMC Forms with Providers Information printed between 9/2014 and 11/2015 and collected from Buck South Pavilion patient waiting room by Dr. Simmons in approximately 2017.

53. "Doctor" definition at: https://www.merriam-webster.com/dictionary/doctor; accessed 2/18/19.

54. "History and Etymology for hysteria." At: https://www.merriam-webster.com/dictionary/hysteria; Accessed 2/8/19.

55. Sutphen LR. E-mail to Dr. Simmons 6/24/16.

56. Lemcke D, Pattison J, Marshall L, et al. *Primary Care of Women, A Lange Medical Book.* NY: NY, McGraw-Hill: 1995.

57. Ibid, pages v-vii.

58. Pattison J. E-mail to Dr. Simmons 2/9/16.

59. Bucher J. E-mail to Dr. James Simmons responding to questions on 10/3/2019.

60. Smith P. E-mail to Dr. Simmons 5/24/16.

61. Frechette E. Conversation with Dr. Simmons 3/11/16.

62. Gortner DA. Notes on "GIM History 1973 -", ending with 2003.

63. Mecklenburg R. Talk to Virginia Mason Retirees' Association, January 31, 2018.

64. Moy N. E-mail to Dr. James Simmons responding to question on 10/3/2019.

65. "Congratulations to our New Master and Fellows." At: https://www.acponline.org/system/files/documents/about_acp/chapters/wa/winter_newsletter_2018.pdf; accessed 2/18/19.

66. "Laureate Award." At: https://www.acponline.org/system/files/documents/about_acp/chapters/nv/nvlaureate415.pdf; accessed 2/18/19.

67. "Community Service Award." At: https://www.acponline.org/about-acp/chapters-regions/united-states/washington-chapter/community-service-award; accessed 2/18/19.

68. "Top Doctors 2018: Internal Medicine." *Seattle Magazine.* At: http://www.seattlemag.com/top-doctors/top-doctors-2019-internal-medicine; accessed 12/13/19

69. "Seattle Met, Find a Doctor." At: https://www.seattlemet.com/doctors#?page=2&doctor_types=Internal%20Medicine; accessed 12/13/19.

70. Kirkpatrick JN. Email to Dr. Simmons 12/5/19.

71. "Astrid Pujari, MD." At: https://www.astridpujarimd.com/more-about; accessed 10/19/2019.

72. "CSS." At: https://www.cssresearch.org/servicesForHealthCareProviders; accessed 12/5/19.

73. "Carrie A. Horwitch, MD, MPH '83, FACP." *Berkeley Health Online.* At: http://berkeleyhealth.berkeley.edu/2014/03/carrie-a-horwitch-md-mph-83-facp/; accessed 3/19/19.

74. "Recipients of Mastership in the American College of Physicians." At: https://www.acponline.org/system/files/documents/about_acp/awards_ masterships/masters.pdf; accessed 3/19/19.

75. "President Clinton convenes APEC summit on Blake Island on November 20, 1993." At: https://historylink.org/File/5333; accessed 4/29/19.

76. Kirkpatrick J. E-mail to Dr. Simmons, 4/18/19.

General Internal Medicine, circa mid- to late 1980s
Standing L to R: Julie Pattison, Jim Simmons, John Kirkpatrick, Lucy Sutphen,
Deborah Fetherston, Paul Smith, Dave Gortner, Jim Bender
Kneeling L to R: Lesley Althouse, Roger Bush, Judy Bowen (PH 1936, VMHA)

General Internal Medicine 2005
Standing L to R: Julie Pattison, Lindsey McKeen, Joyce Lammert,
Tom Gunby, Keith Dipboye, Kirsten Hohmann, Dave Gortner, Tammira Price,
Maggie Adam, Kathy Kundert, Terry Cunningham, Leslie Lu
Seated L to R: Jason Eintracht, Lee Burnside, Cindy Rockfeld,
Jim Bender (kneeling), Cathrine Wheeler, Gail Gregerich, Karen Ting,
Alisse Ryan, Paul Smith, Jim Simmons (PH 9133, VMHA)

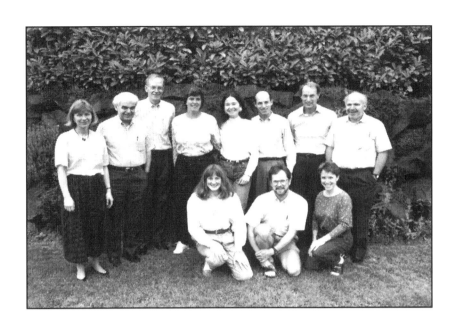

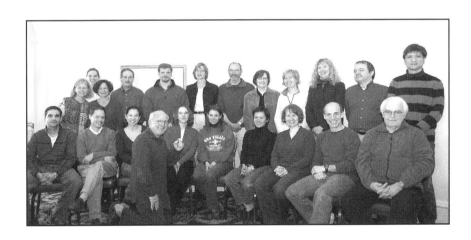

21

Integrative Medicine

by John Kirkpatrick, MD, and Astrid Pujari, MD

Virginia Mason first began to look into offering "alternative" or "complementary" medicine options for its patients when then State Insurance Commissioner Deborah Senn ruled that insurances had to offer these benefits for their subscribers. The Washington State Legislature then passed a statute in 1995 known as the "Every Category of Provider" law. It was the first in the nation to mandate insurance coverage for alternative medicine, and included acupuncturists, chiropractors, naturopaths, massage therapists and others. Virginia Mason had two physiatrists, **Arnel Brion, MD,** and **Ty Hongladarom, MD**, who had completed the required 200 hours of acupuncture training, but deferred offering these services in-house due to their controversial nature and lack of convincing evidence. In the late 1990s, anesthesiologist **Karen Roetman, MD**, and **Barb Hamil, CRNA,** did the obligatory acupuncture training and combined their knowledge of anesthesia with this method to treat approved conditions. However, because of low reimbursement for acupuncture, the anesthesiologists went back to doing just anesthesia, and management also declined to offer naturopathic or chiropractic care or massage therapy onsite, despite some requests from patients.

Astrid Pujari, MD, is board-certified in internal medicine and had a special interest in integrative Holistic Medicine, in which she was also board-certified. She was in the Section of General Internal Medicine from 2001-2005 and was known for her extensive breadth of knowledge in both traditional and alternative medicine and her kind, caring bedside manner. Dr. Pujari was particularly helpful to unsuspecting VM oncologists whose patients sometimes added extra "medications" on their own in an effort to combat their cancer, but never informed their doctor. With her expertise, she often figured out the puzzling, previously unknown side effect they were experiencing that turned out to be an herbal drug interaction. Dr. Pujari left Virginia Mason in 2005 to set up her own practice, "The Pujari Center." However, she maintained a special relationship with VM's oncology section, working one day per week for three years from 2005-2008 seeing individual cancer patients interested in exploring integrative medicine, and once a month seeing patients in a group setting. During that time, in conjunction with the Cancer Institute, she also created a "Healing from Within" course focusing on stress reduction and mind-body medicine, providing cancer patients and their loved ones with tools for stress reduction before, during and after treatment. These classes were very well received by patients and eventually the Cancer Institute added other similar classes for patients by developing a relationship with Cancer Lifeline.

In 2017, CEO Gary Kaplan, MD, reached out to Dr. Pujari because he felt the time was right for integrative medicine. Late that year she began consulting with Virginia Mason to develop an integrative medicine program, and in the spring of 2018 she started as medical director for the new program entitled, "The Center for Integrative Medicine at Virginia Mason." **Kevin Connor, ND,** who had been working in the Physical Medicine and Rehabilitation section, joined the center in November 2018, along with **Jacci Mahrt, COTA, LMT,** a massage therapist. Naturopath and acupuncturist **Lela Altman, MD, Lac,** began in spring 2019.

A formal "Center for Integrative Medicine" was added to the Department of Primary Care in 2019, providing a balanced, holistic approach to health. Partnering with Bastyr Center for Natural Health, the latest breakthroughs in Western medicine are combined with the centuries-old wisdom of natural therapies to provide safe, appropriate and effective care.

Services include diet modification, advice on nutritional supplements, botanical medicine (herbal therapy), mind-body techniques (meditation, guided imagery and visualization), acupuncture and therapeutic massage. Appointments are available at both Bainbridge Island and downtown Seattle locations.

22

The Development of the
Satellite System

by David Wilma and Katherine Galagan, MD,
with contributions from Gary Kaplan, MD, & Ingrid Gerbino, MD

The Mason Clinic was established on the model of a team of specialists who welcomed complex cases from community practitioners. The founders drove all over Washington State promoting relationships with local physicians who could refer patients. Alaska was another source of patients since Seattle was the gateway to the Far North. Informal visits by James Tate Mason, Sr., MD, and John Blackford, MD, with hospital interns or family in tow provided county medical societies with training and raised the visibility of the clinic. In 1937, to remember Dr. Mason after his death, Mason Clinic Day was held every spring as a way to bring community physicians to The Mason Clinic to attend lectures and demonstrations and to build a sense of fellowship. The model served to ensure an adequate referral base and interesting cases well into the 1970s.

In the 1970s, new players entered the health care field. Corporate interests bought up hospitals forming them into chains. They focused on health care profit margins and did not attempt to provide education or research. Not-for-profit hospitals banded into coalitions to effectively compete. Physicians formed preferred provider organizations to offer discounts to employers and insurance carriers, Dr. Mason's contract medicine idea from the 1920s. Insurance carriers pressed providers for discounts. Medic-

348

aid and Medicare reimbursements did not keep up with inflation and the rising costs to deliver care.

The first proposal for a satellite clinic came in 1970 from the Weyerhaeuser Company. The forest products giant wanted a Virginia Mason presence near their corporate headquarters in Federal Way. This was during the Boeing Bust and Administrator John Dare took a hard look. The idea did not make financial sense given the population there and the practitioners in place. The idea was set aside.

By 1980, the growth of communities east of Lake Washington and north and south of Seattle made the clinic's location on First Hill—Pill Hill—less convenient than before. Many Mason Clinic patients lived on the east side and regarded their specialists as their primary care physicians. Patients at The Mason Clinic waited longer for appointments. Physicians considered full appointment books a good thing, but patients did not. More specialists were moving to the region, many being trained locally at the University of Washington and The Mason Clinic, and setting up practices in suburban cities. The Henry Ford Clinic in Detroit eventually established the template of a central clinic of specialists and satellites with primary care, which came to be known as a "hub and spoke system". After much discussion and study by the clinic partners (and not a small amount of resistance), Clinic Chairman **Roger Lindeman, MD**, modified the clinic's mission statement to include primary care and went to find patients. He wrote, "The downtown campus concept has become a downtown nucleus with an outreach program." [1] In August 1980, The Mason Clinic purchased land in Kirkland across the street from Evergreen Hospital for a primary care clinic.

In November 1980, the first effort at affiliation began with a family practice in West Seattle constituted of recent residents and interns as partners. A similar arrangement was established at a clinic in Friday Harbor.

In January 1981, an affiliation with management by The Mason Clinic was established with Seatac Family Medical in Seatac. This was the practice of Drs. Don and **West McElroy** who had a long history of referrals to the downtown campus. Don retired and family practitioner

Ed Myer, MD, joined West and became the first Mason Clinic physician to be employed in a peripheral setting. In July, the Phillips Clinic in Mountlake Terrace became affiliated and there was some controversy as to branding. Was the Mason name to appear in place of the name familiar to the community? This eventually became The Mason Clinic Mountlake Terrace. In November, **Clayton Erickson, MD**, in North Bend joined The Mason Clinic system. Internist **Robert Webb, MD**, became the lead in convincing the partners of the wisdom of a clinic in Kirkland. At a special meeting in March the partners overwhelmingly approved the plan to establish Mason Clinic East.

The announcement of the plans for Kirkland was met with a request from local practitioners for a meeting in a conference room at Evergreen Hospital. When Lindeman and Administrator **Austin Ross** arrived, the meeting had moved to the hospital cafeteria to accommodate all the doctors worried about their own practices. Lindeman described the event more than twenty years later:

"This was a tough meeting. There was deep concern about competition. Many claimed to have appointment books that were only half full. Where were all the patients going to come from? Several physicians suggested rather bluntly that Virginia Mason stay downtown where you belong.

"I responded by saying that we had already purchased the property and that we were there to stay. I emphasized the rapid growth that Kirkland was experiencing and reiterated our intent to work together with them to make their medical center even bigger and better than it already was. Over time, things improved and we did indeed begin to work cooperatively and effectively together." [2]

Virginia Mason East opened on August 9, 1982 in a 20,000-square-feet, two-story building on time and under budget at $1.3 million. Dr. Webb was the first partner physician to practice there and he was joined by **Gary Kaplan, MD; Delbert D. Morris, MD,** and **David S. Paplow, MD**. Administrator Bob Boyle initially managed the satellites overall. Patient volume grew and another physician was added the following year.

The clinic attracted patients who had received specialty care downtown and desired primary care through the same system. They also began to attract many patients who were new to the system.

The Seatac clinic provided important lessons. Its location near the airport and the poor condition of the physical plant, free care, occupational injuries, and drug-seeking behaviors all contributed to the clinic never becoming profitable. The affiliation ended within two years.

In September 1983, the Fourth Avenue Clinic opened in the Unigard Financial Center to better serve a population of 150,000 working downtown as an urgent care clinic. **Bruce Stevenson, MD**, and **William Crounse, MD,** headed the staff there and patient visits quickly exceeded projections. To accommodate an increasingly athletic population the Sports Medicine Center opened in February 1984. This clinic was organized under the satellite system rather than the Orthopaedics Section of the main clinic, but still referred six to eight cases a month to Orthopaedics. Sports medicine-trained orthopaedic physicians saw patients of all ages with athletic-related concerns.

Expansion to the south was shifted to Federal Way where the clinic purchased seven acres of land for Mason Clinic South. The partners also secured 1.8 acres of land adjacent to Mason Clinic East to guarantee room for expansion.

Chairman Lindeman asked Dr. Kaplan of the Kirkland clinic to assume leadership over the expansion to Federal Way, but not to move his practice there. Dr. Kaplan learned that internist **Brian McDonald, MD,** referred many cases to the main clinic and recruited him to lead the new clinic. In July 1985, Mason Clinic Federal Way opened in rented space in the All Services Building while the new clinic was being constructed. The Children's Clinic was the premier children's practice in the South End, located in Federal Way. Kaplan and Administrator **Sandy Novak** spent a year developing relationships with the pediatricians including pizza dinners on Tuesdays. **Jon Almquist, MD**, recalled more than thirty years later:

"There were a couple of things that made us comfortable. Virginia Mason's willingness to basically take our staff, the fact that Virginia

Mason had several of the pediatric specialists that we respected and used ... (neurology, gastro-intestinal, allergy, as well as endocrinology) ... and the fact that Virginia Mason wasn't trying to become a competitive hospital with Children's Hospital and Regional Medical Center. I personally think the most important part time-wise was the staff question. We knew our staff was great and liked by our patients and Virginia Mason was smart to recognize that fact. I know that the fact that Gary Kaplan listened when I suggested practices to approach for other good pediatricians gave Virginia Mason an exceptional group of pediatricians." [3]

The two internists in Auburn Internal Medicine's group were added to the plan. By the time the clinic moved into its own space in October 1987 there were thirteen physicians.

In October 1985, The Issaquah Clinic merged with The Mason Clinic under the leadership of **Albert Einstein, MD**, and Administrator **George Auld**.

By 1987, Dr. Kaplan had been appointed Chief of the Satellite Clinics; patient visits to the main clinic rose just 1.5 percent while satellite visits were up 62 percent over the prior year. The satellite clinics were becoming a significant source of growth and new patients to the system. That year, the Washington Industrial and Occupational Medical Centers in Riverton, Bellevue, and Harbor Island were acquired. The Harbor Island clinic moved to First Avenue South and the Bellevue clinic got a better location. The Prompt Care Clinic at Alderwood Mall in Lynnwood and its three physicians became the anchor of a new north satellite until new construction there was complete.

The satellite clinics grew in size and volume. In 1991, the Mountlake Terrace clinic folded into the Alderwood Mall operation in Lynnwood as Virginia Mason North. In 1993, the Issaquah clinic moved into new space and a practice on Mercer Island was acquired with two internists. The year 1994 saw two expansion templates for the satellite program. New clinics were opened in Redmond and Bellevue (December 1993). Mercer Island Pediatrics Group joined the Mercer Island clinic, the Edmonds OB/GYN group moved in with Virginia Mason North, and the Winslow Clinic—later Bainbridge Island Clinic—joined the satellite system on January 1, 1995. Primary care at the downtown clinic expanded to accomodate new patients there. The Port Angeles Clinic and Fidalgo Medical Associates in Anacortes, and Sand Point Pediatrics became part of the Virginia Mason family in 1995.

The alliance with Group Health resulted in joint clinics in Kent (1995), and West Seattle and Monroe (1996). When these clinics proved challenging to manage and operate, Group Health purchased Virginia Mason's interest in the clinics. Additional clinics opened in Enumclaw and Sequim.

The rapid satellite expansion of the 90s was driven by Washington state's adoption of heath care reform modeled on the Clinton Health Plan. The prevailing wisdom was that managed care would soon become the predominant model of care with providers assuming total risk and capitation payments as the dominant payment mode. Primary care sites and a distribution system was critical. By the mid to late 1990s it became apparent that this would not be coming to fruition and the Washington health care reform legislation was repealed. The "old economy" was alive and well.

In 1998 and 1999, Virginia Mason Medical Center expenses exceeded revenues and financial changes were required. Smaller practices proved to be unprofitable and were consolidated into larger regional clinics, sold, or closed. The number of clinics shrunk from twenty-one in 1997 to fifteen in 1999. By 2004 there were nine:

Bellevue	Federal Way
Issaquah	Kirkland
Lynnwood	Port Angeles
Sand Point Pediatrics	Sports Medicine
Winslow	

The Sports Medicine clinic moved downtown to the 2nd floor of Lindeman Pavilion by 2008, although Sports Medicine providers are available in several of the satellites as well. The Port Angeles clinic was no longer a part of VM by 2006, and therefore by 2008 there were only 7 satellite clinics left, each with a large regional presence including primary care and selected specialty and procedural services.

In 2013, Bainbridge Island, Bellevue, Federal Way, Issaquah, Kirkland, Lynnwood, and University Village clinics became known as regional medical centers, acknowledging the expanded range of services available tied together electronically with the main campus in Seattle.

In 2018, the physicians of Edmonds Family Medicine had many acquisition offers and chose to join the Virginia Mason Health System as Virginia Mason Edmonds Family Medicine, bringing the total number of regional medical centers to 9 including the downtown campus:

Bainbridge Island	Bellevue
Edmonds	Federal Way
Issaquah	Kirkland
Lynnwood	Seattle
University Village	

Over the years, a model developed where the core group of physicians at the clinic, usually primary care providers including internists, family medicine practitioners, and pediatrics, had full-time practices at these locations, often in concert with physician assistants, Advanced Registered Nurse Practitioners, and others. Specialty care was occasionally given by full-time practitioners, but more often was provided by specialists rotating on a part-time basis to one or more of the satellite locations.

In addition to Dr. Gary Kaplan who was the first Chief of Satellites, subsequent Satellite Department Chiefs included **Brian McDonald, MD, Catherine Potts, MD,** and the current Chief, **Ingrid Gerbino, MD**. Their administrative partners included **Sandy Novak, Sarah Patterson, Marnee Iseman** and **Shelly Powell.** During Dr. Potts' tenure the Satellite Department evolved into the Department of Primary Care including the downtown sections of General Internal Medicine and Concierge Medicine, as well as all satellite primary care physicians (including the division of Pediatrics) and advanced practitioners.

The following is a list of physicians who practiced in the satellites and became members, with their tenure and specialty when known, in the order in which the satellites opened. The information is only as accurate as the rather limited sources that are available. Because space is limited and records are incomplete, the many excellent nurse practitioners and PAs are not listed.

West Seattle clinic (first effort at affiliation, with similar arrangement in Friday Harbor): Nov. 1980

SeaTac Medical Clinic (first clinic managed by VM): January 1981
West G. McElroy, MD (1981 - 1983)
> R. Ed Myer, MD (first VM physician to be employed in a peripheral setting, 1981 - 1983): Family Medicine

Phillips Clinic (The Mason Clinic Mountlake Terrace, merged with VM North/Lynnwood): 1981–1990; now **Virginia Mason Lynnwood**)
> Clifford Phillips, MD (July – Dec. 1981)
> Patricia L. Clayton, MD (1981–90; to North 1991–94): Family Med.
> Leonard C. Cobb, MD (1981 – 1982)
> Peter J. Dillon, MD (1981 – 1983): Family Medicine
> Bruce R. Gilbert, MD (1981 – 1982): Internal Medicine
> David J. Yonkers, MD (1981 – 1990): Family Medicine
> David Huntington, MD (1984 – 1991): Family Medicine
> Christine M. Adams, MD (1984 – 1990; moved to North 1991 only): Family Medicine
> Robert A. Scarr, MD (1987; moved to VM North in 1988 – 2005): Internal Medicine
> Kelvie Johnson, MD (1988 - 1993): Pediatrics
> Howard Uman, MD (1988 - 2000): Pediatrics
> Keith S. Graham, MD (1990; moved to VM North 1991 – 1993): Internal Medicine
> Henry G. Coit, MD (1992 - 2000): Pediatrics
> Alka Mehta, MD (1994 – 2000; moved to Winslow for 1 year when Pediatrics at North was discontinued; Winslow 2000 - 2001): Pediatrics
> Jill Sells, MD (1998 - moved to Winslow for one year when Pediatrics at North was discontinued; Winslow 2000 - 2001): Pediatrics

Mark O. Todd, MD (1988 – 1997): Internal Medicine

Naheed P. Esmail, DO (1992 – 1997): Family Medicine

Rory M. Laughery, MD (1992 – 1995): Family Medicine

Kathryn A. Zufall-Larson, MD (1994 – 2000): Internal Medicine

Kathryn L. Ponto, MD (1994 – 2000): Ob/Gyn

Ingrid Fuss Gerbino, MD (1995 – present): Internal Medicine

Derek Q. Schroder, MD (1996 – 2000): Internal Medicine

Kimberly J. Dickey, DO (1998 – 2000): Ob/Gyn

Sundance L. Rogers, MD (1998 – 2003; moved to Winslow in 2004 present): Internal Medicine

Elizabeth M. White, MD (1999 – 2003): Internal Medicine

Tom T. Nguyen, MD (2001 - 2005): Internal Medicine

Sue-Hui J. Paik, MD (2002 – 2007): Internal Medicine

John Y. Peng, MD (2001 – present): Internal Medicine

Erane Myint, MD (2002 – 2007): Internal Medicine

C. Vicky Beer, MD (2006 – present): Internal Medicine

Jimy E. Gillette, MD (2006 – present): Internal Medicine

Shelly K. Khurana, MD (2006 – present): Internal Medicine

Kristie Blade, MD, PhD, (2007 – present): Internal Medicine

Nancy Connolly, MD, MPH (2007 – 2018): Internal Medicine

Christian Herter, MD (2008 – 2012): Internal Medicine

Christine Pineda-Liu, MD (2008 – 2013; moved to Bellevue 2014 - present): Internal Medicine

Robin Atkinson, DO (2011 – present): Internal Medicine

Linda M. Kampp, MD (2015 – present): Internal Medicine

Ananth K. Shenoy, MD (2015 – present): Internal Medicine

Aerin K. Sembhi, MD (2016 – present): Internal Medicine

Amy Thomson, MD (2017 - present): Internal Medicine

North Bend Family Medical Clinic (became **Virginia Mason North Bend**): 1981 - 1997

Clayton Erickson, MD (became affiliated with VM in November 1981

William B. Kirshner, MD (1982 – 1997; moved to Issaquah by 1998;

retired 2019): Family Medicine

Mary E. Lambe, MD (1984 – 1990; moved to Issaquah 1991 - 1999): Family Medicine

Henry H. Hochberg, MD (1988 – 1990): Family Medicine

Jennifer Rowe, MD (1996 – 1998)

Virginia Mason East (now **Virginia Mason Kirkland**): Aug. 9, 1982 - present

D. Robert Webb, MD (1972 – 1989): Internal Medicine

Gary S. Kaplan, MD (1982–present); CEO: 2000-present: Internal Medicine

Delbert D. Morris, MD (1982 – 1991): Family Medicine

David S. Paplow, MD (1982 – 2018): Family Medicine

Sandra J. DiAngi, MD (1983 – 2016): Internal Medicine

James A. Lusk, MD (approximately 1985 – 1989): Internal Medicine

Kim R. Pittenger, MD (1985 – 2018): Family Medicine; **James Tate Mason Award** winner in 2006

Daniel R. Szekely, MD (1985 – 1997, moved to Port Angeles 1997 – 1999): Ob/Gyn

Dianne M. Glover, MD (1985 – 1998): Pediatrics

Ruth Ann Parish, MD (1987 – 1995): Pediatrics

Russell S. Goldberg, MD (1987 – 2018): Internal Medicine

Karen L. Ilika, MD (1988 – 2000): Ob/Gyn

Diane M. Yahn, MD (1988 – 2000): Internal Medicine

Alice M. Ormsby, MD (1989 – 2002): Dermatology

Katherine Grishaw-Jones, MD (1991 – 1993): Pediatrics

Richard M. Furlong, MD (1989 – present): Internal Medicine

Mary N. Brumfiel, MD (1990 – 2001): Ob/Gyn

Roland V. Feltner, MD (1993 - 1995): Family Medicine

Catherine Meltzer, MD (1992 – 1997): Pediatrics

Linda Warren, MD (1995 – 1999; moved to Winslow in 1999 when Pediatrics discontinued - 2006): Pediatrics

Lori Walund, MD (1994 – 2005), started at VM Redmond in 1994, moved to Kirkland in 1997: Internal Medicine

Laurel Morrison MD (1998 - present): Family Medicine

John Girard, MD (1998 – 2001) Kirkland, then Issaquah: Pediatrics

Kathleen A. Hughes, MD (1999 – 2006): Internal Medicine

Heidi T. Rogers, MD (2000 - present): Family Medicine

Yun Suhr, MD (2000 - present): Internal Medicine

Renata M. Jenkin, MD (2002 – 2012): Dermatology

Esther J. Park, MD (2006 – 2008): Internal Medicine

Sarah Dick, MD (2007 – 2015); Dermatology

Laine M. Gawthrop, MD (2009 – 2012): Internal Medicine

Lars P. Kaine, MD (2010 - present): Family Medicine

Kavita P. Chawla, MD, MHA (2013 - present): Internal Medicine

Helen N. Gray, MD (2015 – present): Family Medicine

Laura Popko, MD (2016 – present): Internal Medicine

Monika Wells, MD, MPH (2017 – present): Internal Medicine

Orion B. Wells, MD (2017 – present): Family Medicine

Fourth Avenue Clinic: September 1983 - 1998

Bruce E. Stevenson, MD (1975 in ED; total tenure until 2002): Internal Medicine

William E. Crounse, MD (1983 – 1988): Family Medicine

G. David Austin, MD (1987 – 1988): Internal Medicine; then did Pathology residency and now works as a pathologist in Tacoma

Cynthia G. Ferrucci, MD (1988 – 1999): Internal Medicine

David Frank, MD (1988 – present): 4th Ave and Downtown; Internal Medicine; Emergency Medicine

Sports Medicine Center: February 1984 - present

These physicians are discussed in the Orthopaedics Chapter in volume 2

Virginia Mason South (now **Virginia Mason Federal Way**): July 1985 in rented space; new building opened in October 1987 - present

Brian L. McDonald, MD (1985 - 2018): Internal Medicine

Thomas C. Gunby, MD (1985 – present; transfer to GIM downtown in 1997/8 and then hospitalist program): Internal Medicine

Curtis S. Endow, MD (1985 - 2018): Internal Medicine

Jon R. Almquist, MD (1986 – 2011): Pediatrics

Michael R. Anderson, MD (1986 – 1988): Pediatrics

Richard K. Gould, MD (1986 - present): Pediatrics

James E. Rogers, MD (1986 - 2002): Pediatrics and Sports Medicine; split time between downtown and Federal Way

Karen C. Smith, MD (1987 - 2016): Internal Medicine

Todd. D. Pearson, MD (1987 - 1995): Pediatrics

Dennis Hansen, MD (1987 – 2002): Cardiology

Barbara J. Gehrett, MD (in 1987 became affiliate at Auburn IM Assoc.; 1988 - 1998): Internal Medicine

Joseph O. Gehrett, MD (in 1987 became affiliate at Auburn IM Assoc.; 1988 - 1998): Internal Medicine

William H. Deschner, MD (1988 - 1995): Ob/Gyn

Jeffrey A. Hunter, MD (1988 - present); Surgery

Michael Ruthrauff, MD (1988 – 2000; rejoined VM at Edmonds in 2018): Psychiatry

Jeannie Larsen, MD (1989 – 2005): Pediatrics

Jill Turner, MD (1989 – 2000); Internal Medicine

Michael Wukelic, MD (1989 – 1995); Internal Medicine

David C. Beaudry, MD (1989 – 2019); Ophthalmology

Denise Wells, MD (1989 – 2000); Orthopaedics

Kelli R. Arntzen, MD (1990 – 2006); Dermatology

David Kieras, MD (1990 – present); Orthopaedics

Anthony W. Kiriluk, MD (1990 – 2005); Family Medicine

Kevin W. Judge, MD (1990 – 1998); Cardiology

Carl Wyman, MD (1991 - 1999)

Mary Lee Colter, MD (1992 - 2006); Internal Medicine

Anne E. Phalen, MD (1992 - 2005): Pediatrics

Joan Shen, MD (1992 - 2002): Ob/Gyn

Brian H. Kumasaka, MD (1993 - 2001): Dermatology

Gordon Naylor, MD (1993 - present): Pediatrics

Kimberly Witkop, MD (1994 - 1996): Internal Medicine

Susanne Purnell, MD (1994 - 2000): Pediatrics

Cynthia J. Goldor, MD (1994 - 1998): Ob/Gyn

Lee Carlisle, MD (1995 - 1999): Psychiatry

Yoo Jin Chong, MD (1996 - 2003): Internal Medicine

Maribeth Chong, MD (1996 - 2003): Internal Medicine

Richard Ling, MD (1996 - 1998): Internal Medicine

Matthew Eisenberg, MD (1996 - 2003): Pediatrics

William Cray, MD (1997 - 2008): Surgery

Jessica B. Richmond, MD (1997 - 2009): Internal Medicine

Paul Cummings, MD (1998 - 2001): Internal Medicine

Stephen Poore, MD (1998 - 2009): Ob/Gyn

Andrea Maynard Fasullo, MD (1998 - present): Pediatrics

Patrick J. Reagan, MD (1998 – 2008): Cardiology

Pepper Toomey, MD (1999 - 2000): Orthopaedics

Mahmuda Tasneem, MD (2000 – present; also works at Lynnwood):
    Internal Medicine

Mary H. Czuk, MD (1999 - 2009): Ob/Gyn

Douglas G. Merrill, MD (2000 - 2006): Anesthesiology

Gaston R. Deysine, MD (2000 - present): Orthopaedics

Jonathan R. Fox, MD (2000 - present): Pediatrics

Maureen G. Stevenson, MD (2000 - 2005): Internal Medicine

Gregory E. Chow, MD (2000 – 2004); Ob/Gyn

Suseela V. Narra, MD (2001 - 2011): Dermatology

Jane S. Dunham, MD (2001 – 2005; 2013- present): Internal Medicine

Karri K. Chinn, MD (2001 - 2005): Internal Medicine

Chi-Hyun Kim, MD (2003 - 2009): Internal Medicine

Steven J. Kao, MD (2003 - 2014): Internal Medicine

Kennard D. McNichols, MD (2003 - 2010): Family Medicine

Joseph I. Lee, MD (2004 - 2006): Internal Medicine

Vallikannu Muthiah, MD (2005 - 2007): Internal Medicine

Christine D. Ambro, MD (2005 – 2006): Dermatology

Linda Pourmassina Abraham, MD (2006 - 2011): Internal Medicine

Megan B. Ellingsen, MD, MPH (2006 - 2010): Internal Medicine

Elizabeth E. Jernberg, (2006 – present): Rheumatology

Corrie L. Takahashi, MD (2006 – currently working as locums): Pediatrics

Laura G. Sporl, MD (2007 - 2009): Ob/Gyn

Jenny L. Lobo, MD (2007 - 2012): Pediatrics

John T. Frederick, MD (2007 - 2015): Psychiatry

Dennis Rochier, MD (2007 - 2013): Internal Medicine

Betsy Alley, MD (2007 - present): Anesthesiology

William Callahan, MD (2008 - present): Orthopaedics/Sports Medicine

James Lee, MD (2008 - 2011): Cardiology

Amy Stepan, MD (2008 - present): Surgery

Anja B. Crider, MD (2009 - 2011): Ob/Gyn

Jordan Chun, MD (2009 – 2018): Orthopaedics/Sports Medicine

Alice Kim, MD (2010 – 2014): Internal Medicine

Robert M. Eager, MD (2011 – 2015): Internal Medicine

Jessica L. Ebberson, MD (2012 – present): Pediatrics

Marisa Dahlman, MD, MPH (2012 – present), also downtown: Ob/Gyn

Duc Ngo, MD (2012- present): Internal Medicine

Delia Viisoreanu, MD, MS (2012 - present): Internal Medicine

Christine Palermo, MD (2012 – present; now working as physician advisor); Internal Medicine

Lauren Athay, MD (2013 – present): Pediatrics

Christine Nguyen, MD (2013 – 2017): Internal Medicine

Shirley S. Koon, MD (2013 – 2016): Internal Medicine

Mary N. Morcos, MD (2014 – 2016): Internal Medicine

Elly Patterson Bhatraju, MD (2015 - 2019): Internal Medicine

Erika Cunningham, MD (2016 - present): Internal Medicine

Puneet Kakkar, MD (2017 - present): Family Medicine

Megha V. Rao, MD, MHA (2018 - present): Internal Medicine

Hong Ren, MD, MD (2018- present): Internal Medicine

Diana Revenco, MD, MPVI (2017 - present): Cardiology

Irina Triska, MD (2016 - present): Internal Medicine

Bryan N. Truong, MD (2015 - present): Internal Medicine

Issaquah Clinic (Virginia Mason Issaquah): October 1985 - present

William H. Kinnish, MD (1986 - 2005): Family Medicine

Jerome L. Bushnell, MD (1986 – 2018): Family Medicine

Jark R. Jabbusch, MD (1986 - 2005): Family Medicine

Elizabeth Lehmann, MD (1986 - 1988)

Mark R. Levy, MD (1985 - present): Family Medicine

John W. Tooley, MD (1986 - 1990)

Bruce C. Smith, MD (1987 – 1998): Internal Medicine

Fredric A. Stern, MD (1987 – 2000): Ophthalmology

Mary E. Lambe, MD (moved from North Bend, at Issaquah 1991 - 1999): Family Medicine

Kenneth L. Kay, MD (1992 – present): Internal Medicine

Kathleen Preciado-Partida, MD (1992 – 1999; moved to Bellevue when OB discontinued in Issaquah 1999 – 2001): Ob/Gyn

Susan S. Block, MD (1993 – 1999; moved to Bellevue when OB discontinued in Issaquah 1999 – 2001): Ob/Gyn

Stacie E. Maurer, MD (1993 – 2000): Internal Medicine

Monica Richter, MD (1993 - 1999): Pediatrics

Usha Sankrithi, MD (1993 – 1997): Pediatrics

Merrill S. Lewen, MD (1994 – 2001, also at Mercer Island and Bellevue): Ob/Gyn

Lance C. Larson, MD (1994; moved to Bellevue 1994 – present): Internal Medicine

Rebecca L. Smith, MD (1995 – 1999): Dermatology

Thomas D. Lindquist, MD, PhD, (1996 – 2005): Ophthalmology

Ann E. Sneiders, MD (1997 – 2008): Pediatrics

Robin D. Ifft, MD (1997 –2018): Pediatrics

Laurel Morrison, MD (1998 - 2010): Family Medicine

William B. Kirshner, MD (1982 – 1997 at North Bend; moved to Issaquah by 1998; retired 2019): Family Medicine

Janet L. Barrall, MD (1998 – 2013); Ophthalmology

John Girard, MD (1998–2001) Kirkland for one year, then Issaquah: Pediatrics

DeEtta M. Gray, MD (1999 – 2001; moved to Bellevue til 2004): Dermatology

Robert A. Miller-Cassman, MD (1999 – 2006): Internal Medicine

Kimberly M. Schrier, MD (2001 – 2018): Pediatrics

Sofia T. Bayfield, MD (2001 – 2005): Family Medicine

Nasima K. Vira, MD (2001 - present): Internal Medicine

Theodore S. Naiman, MD (2006–present; started 2005 at Winslow): Family Practice

Allison L. Hughes, MD (2006 – 2007): Dermatology

Sashi Amara, MD (2006 - 2010): Internal Medicine

Mei Lu, MD, MS (2006 - present): Family Medicine

Anika L. Sanda, MD (2008 – 2012): Pediatrics

Alice Kim, MD (2009 - present): Internal Medicine

Amy S. Cheng, MD (2009 – 2010): Dermatology

Arlo J. Miller, MD (2010 – 2012): Dermatology

Rebecca Partridge, MD (2012 – present): Pediatrics

Sara May, MD (2014 - present): Internal Medicine

Derrick L. Soong, MD (2017 – present): Pediatrics

David Schneider, MD (2019 – present; primarily in Bellevue): Pediatrics

Virginia Mason Occupational Medicine: 1987 – 2003

Susan L. Berg, MD (1987 – 1993)

John P. Holland, MD (1987 – 1991)

H. Doyle Perkins, MD (1987 – 1991)

Robert D. Petrie, MD (1987 – 1999)

Eric S. Smith, MD (1987 – 1992)

James E. Manning, MD (1989 - 2002)

Jay A. Brown, MD (1990 - 1993)

Calvin Jones, MD, MPH (1991 - 2002)

Samuel Strauss, DO, MP (1992 - 2001)

James Kunkler, MD (1993 – 2001)

Susan A. Bick, MD (1994 – 2000)

Clyde Wilson, MD (1995 – 2002)

John Lazzaretti, MD (1996 - 2001)

James Nelson, MD (1996 - 2001)

Virginia Mason Mercer Island: 1993 – 2003

Christine Robertson, MD (1993 - 1997): Internal Medicine

Chancey Paxson, MD (1993 - 1996): Internal Medicine

Julie Ellner, MD (1994 - 2000): Pediatrics

Danette Glassy, MD (1994 - 2000): Pediatrics

Ted Mandelkom, MD (1994 - 2000): Pediatrics

Hal Quinn, MD (1994 - 2000): Pediatrics

Janice Woolley, MD (1994 - 2000): Pediatrics

Hope L. Druckman, MD (1996 – 2002; then to Bellevue til 2006):
    Internal Medicine

Julia R. Smith, MD (1996 - 2000): Internal Medicine

Merrill Sue Lewen, MD (1996–2001; also at Issaquah and Bellevue):
    Ob/Gyn

Douglas Trigg, MD (1993 – 2002; then to Bellevue til 2019): Internal
    Medicine

John A. Addison, MD (1997 - 2002): Internal Medicine and Geriatrics

Linda Fairchild, MD (first at Redmond 1994–1997; then Mercer Is-
    land 1997–2002; then to Bellevue 2002-present): Internal Medicine

Suzanne Cosette, MD (1998 - 2001): Internal Medicine

Anne E. Tuttle, MD (2002; then to Bellevue 2002 - present): Internal
    Medicine

Virginia Mason Redmond: 1994 – 1997

David Pomeroy, MD (1994 – 1997): Family Practice

Linda Fairchild, MD (1994 – 1997; then Mercer Island 1997 – 2002; then Bellevue 2002 - present): Internal Medicine

Lori Walund, MD (1994–1997; then to Kirkland until 2005): Internal Medicine

Virginia Mason Bellevue: 1993 - present

Catherine J. Potts, MD (1993 - present): Internal Medicine

Joan E. Miller, MD (1993 – 1997; also downtown): Internal Medicine

Lance Larson, MD (1994 - present): Internal Medicine

Merrill Sue Lewen, MD (1996 – 2001; also at Mercer Island and Issaquah): Ob/Gyn

Frank Baron, MD (1998 – 2001): Dermatology

DeEtta M. Gray, MD (1999–2004; moved to Bellevue from Issaquah in 2001): Dermatology

Kathleen Preciado-Partida, MD (1999 – 2001; at Issaquah 1992 – 1999 until OB discontinued): Ob/Gyn

Susan S. Block, MD (1999 – 2001; at Issaquah 1993 – 1999 until OB discontinued): Ob/Gyn

Alan B. Rothblatt, MD (1999 – present): Gynecology

Lora Pelligrini, MD (2000 - 2003): Internal Medicine

Leland N. Teng, MD (2002 – present): Dare Center (Concierge Medicine)

Peter J. Jenkin, MD (2002 – 2012): Dermatology

Hope L. Druckman, MD (2002 – 2006; at Mercer Island 1996 – 2002): Internal Medicine, Dare Center

Jason P. Norsen, MD (2003 – present): Internal Medicine

Douglas Trigg, MD (2002 – 2019; at Mercer Island 1997 – 2002): Internal Medicine

Anne E. Tuttle, MD (2002 – present; at Mercer Island 2002): Internal Medicine

Linda Fairchild, MD (2002 – present; at Mercer Island 1997 – 2002; at Redmond 1994 - 1997): Internal Medicine

Patricia Auerbach, MD (2008 - 2010): Internal Medicine (Concierge

Medicine)

Janie M. Leonhardt, MD (2010 – 2014): Dermatology

Edward M. Esparza, MD, PhD, (2011 – present; also at Federal Way and downtown): Dermatology

Spoorthi Velagapalli, MD (2012 - 2015); Internal Medicine

Christine Pineda-Liu, MD (2008 - 2013 at Lynnwood; 2014-present): Internal Medicine

Helen (Wan Hua) Shih, MD (2014 - present): Internal Medicine

Kaori Yoshida, MD (2016 - present): Internal Medicine

David Schneider, MD (2019 – present; primarily in Bellevue): Pediatrics

Winslow (now **Virginia Mason Bainbridge Island**): 1995 - present

Thomas D. Haggar, MD (1995 - 2005): Family Medicine

Gregory E. Keyes, MD (1995 - 2002): Family Medicine

Kim Leatham, MD (1995 – 2017): Family Medicine

William V. Toth, MD (1995 - 2002): Family Medicine

Jeffrey S. Young, MD (1995 - 1997): Family Medicine

Bruce A. Nitsche, MD (1995 - present): Internal Medicine

Piero F. Sandri, MD (1995 - 2002): Internal Medicine

Diane E. Fuquay, MD (1995 - 2004): Pediatrics

Thomas R. Monk, MD (1995 - 2007): Pediatrics

David B. Cowan, MD (1996 - present): Family Medicine

Maureen Koval, MD (1998 - 2007): Family Medicine

Linda Warren, MD (1999 – 2006; at VM East 1995 – 1999): Pediatrics

Kris I. Colletto, MD (2000 - 2002): Pediatrics

Jillian E. Worth, MD (2001 - present): Family Medicine

Judith Rayl, MD (2002 - 2006): Family Medicine

Sundance L. Rogers, MD (2003 – present; VM Lynnwood 1998 – 2003): Internal Medicine

Charles V. Helming, MD (2003 - 2017): Orthopaedics

Frederick C. Walters, MD (2003 - 2006): Pediatrics

Richard Baker, MD (2003 - 2007): Urgent Care

Reuben M. Anders, MD (2006 – 2007): Dermatology

David Feig, MD (2007 – 2010): Family Medicine

Catherine Edwards, MD (2008 - present): Family Medicine

Simone Ince, MD (2009 – 2016): Dermatology

Michael Tomberg, MD (2012 - present): Family Medicine

Perry D. Mostov, DO (2016 - present): Family Medicine

Shannon H. Phibbs, MD (2016 - present): Family Medicine

Eric Bramwell, MD (2017 – present): Dermatology

John D. Osland, MD (2018 - present): Orthopaedics

Virginia Mason Port Angeles: 1995 – 2005

Elizabeth E. Christian, MD (1995 - 2005): Family Medicine

Peter J. Erickson, MD (1995 - 1997): Family Medicine

Larry A. Gordon, MD (1995 - 2005): Family Medicine

Edward A. Hapfner, MD (1995 - 1997): Family Medicine

R. Scott Kennedy, MD (1995 - 2002): Family Medicine

William R. Kintner, MD (1995 - 2005): Family Medicine

Roger M. Oakes, MD (1995 - 2005): Family Medicine

Mark S. Redlin, MD (1995 - 2005): Family Medicine

Marianne J. Ude, MD (1995 - 2005): Family Medicine

Richard J. VanCalcar, MD (1995 - 2005): Family Medicine

Michael F. McCool, MD (1995 - 1999): Gastroenterology

Robert S. Crist, MD (1995 - 2001): Internal Medicine

Mark D. Fischer, MD (1995 - 2005): Internal Medicine

Paul E. Pederson, MD (1995 - 2005): Internal Medicine

Kara Kurtz Urnes, MD (1995 - 2002): Internal Medicine

John Burkhardt, MD (1995 - 1998): Ob/Gyn

Margaret Baker, MD (1995 - 1999): Orthopaedic Surgery

Daniel Hudgings, MD (1998 - 2005): Family Medicine

Jim Geren, MD (1998 - 2001): Internal Medicine

Rob Gipe, MD (1998 - 2005): Internal Medicine

Daniel Szekely, MD (1997 - 1999; Seattle 1985-1997): Ob/Gyn

Stephen D. Bush, MD (2001 - 2004): Ob/Gyn

Michael E. Epler, MD (2003 - 2005): Family Medicine

Joseph F. Knapp, MD (2003 – 2005): Cardiology

Virginia Mason Fidalgo: 1995 – 2001

Mark S. Backman, MD (1995 - 2001): Family Medicine

Harold R. Clure, MD (1995 - 2001): Family Medicine

C. Les Conway, MD (1995 - 2001): Family Medicine

Gavin I. Gordon, MD (1995 - 2001): Family Medicine

Harold L. Eisland, MD (1995 - 2001): Internal Medicine

Nancy H. Llewellyn, MD (1995 - 2001): Internal Medicine

John R. Mathis, MD (1995 - 2001): Internal Medicine

R. Kevin Connor, MD (1995 - 2001): Neurology

Robert P. Prins, MD (1995 - 2001): Ob/Gyn

Jeanne B. Olmsted, MD (1995 - 2001): Pediatrics

Les Richards, MD (1995 - 2001): Pediatrics

Shawna Laursen, MD (1998 – 2001): Family Medicine

Sand Point Pediatrics: 1995; moved and became **Virginia Mason University Village**: 2014

Ann N. Champoux, MD (1995 - 2018): Pediatrics

Steven W. Dassel, MD (1995 - 2012): Pediatrics

Leslie Mackoff, MD (1995 - 1997): Pediatrics

Donnal L. Smith, MD (1995 - present): Pediatrics

Margaret A. Wheeler, MD (1995 - 2014): Pediatrics

Peggy Sarjeant, MD (1997 - 2009): Pediatrics

Tao Kwan-Gett, MD (1998 – 2006, 2017 - present): Pediatrics

Kathy A. Risse, MD (2001 - present): Pediatrics

Thomas E. Numrych, MD (2003 - present): Pediatrics

Merrill T. Wiseman, MD (2003 – 2009): Pediatrics

Whitney R. Anderson, MD (2004 - 2005): Pediatrics

Michael Dudas, MD (2006) (2007 – present): Pediatrics

Kristin Nyweide White, MD (2007 - present): Pediatrics

Benjamin Jackson, MD (2009 - present): Pediatrics

Ruth A. Conn, MD (2010 – 2016; practiced downtown 1987 – 2010): Pediatrics

Robert T. Fukura, MD (2010 – 2015; practiced downtown 1991 – 2010): Pediatrics

Kathy Rosen, MD (2012 - present): Pediatrics

Liana K. McCabe, MD (2014 - present): Pediatrics

Alejandro J. Candelario, MD (2015 - present): Pediatrics

Traci L. McDermott, MD (2016 - present): Pediatrics

Elizabeth S. Cochrane, MD (2017 - present): Pediatrics

Virginia Mason Enumclaw: 1996 – 1999

Deidre Feeney, MD (1996 – 1999): Family Medicine

Joel Finman, MD (1996 – 1999): Family Medicine

Mary Ellen Maccio, MD (1996 – 1999): Family Medicine

Virginia Mason Sequim: 1996 – 2002

Michael W. Crim, MD (1997 - 2002): Family Medicine

Kari D. Olsen, MD (1997 - 2002): Family Medicine

Roger D. Olsen, MD (1997 - 2002): Family Medicine

Charles Sullivan, MD (1997 - 2002): Family Medicine

Claire Haycox, MD, PhD, (1999 – 2002): Dermatology

Joel R. Finman, MD (1999 - 2002): Family Medicine

Rebecca Corley, MD (1999 - 2002): Internal Medicine

Virginia Mason Edmonds: 2018 - present

Ann K. Begert, MD (2018 – present): Family Medicine

Ginger J. Blakeney, MD (2018 – present): Family Medicine

Amy E. Bredenberg, MD (2018 – present): Family Medicine

Ross G. Carey, MD (2018 – present): Family Medicine

Stephen T. Carter, MD (2018 – present): Family Medicine

Brittany N. Gallaher, DO (2018 – present): Family Medicine

Myra G. Horiuchi, MD (2018 – present): Family Medicine

Joseph G. Petrin, MD (2018 – present): Family Medicine

Marc S. Rosenshein, MD (2018 – present): Hematology/Oncology

Christopher J. Sargent, MD (2018 – present): Family Medicine

Martha A. Shilling Bennett, MD (2018 – present): Family Medicine

Jae H. Sim, MD (2018 – present): Family Medicine

Barton E. Smith, MD (2018 – present): Family Medicine

David E. Taibleson, MD (2018 – present): Family Medicine

Donald J. Tesch, MD (2018 – present): Family Medicine

Susan B. Thomason, MD (2018 – present): Family Medicine

Andrew F. Thurman, MD (2018 – present): Family Medicine

Mary E. Tolberg, MD (2018 – present): Family Medicine

Ingrid E. Van Swearingen, MD (2018 – present): Family Medicine

Biography of Gary S. Kaplan, MD

Gary Kaplan attended the University of Michigan Medical School, graduating in 1978. He did his residency in internal medicine at Virginia Mason and served as chief resident in 1980 – 81. He helped establish Virginia Mason East (Kirkland) with Drs. Morris, Paplow and Webb in the summer of 1982.

A year later, Dr. Lindeman asked him to lead the expansion in Federal Way, which opened in rented space in July 1985 and later moved into a new building in October 1987. At this point, Dr. Kaplan had been appointed Chief of the Satellite Clinics, and the next 10 years saw a significant expansion of the satellite system into communities both near and far. By 1997, there were 21 satellites; however, economic considerations resulted in the closure of some of the smaller, less profitable clinics so that by 1999, there were 15.

It was at this point that Dr. Lindeman announced his retirement, and Gary was elected as Chairman in 2000. Not long after, he was appointed as CEO by the board of directors when they discontinued the election process for leadership positions. During the 2000s, he worked with his administrative partner, Mike Rona, President, to establish the LEAN philosophy of quality improvement (as manifested by the Toyota Production System), as the management method at Virginia Mason. This was a quantum shift in thinking for the medical center and eventually led to the establishment of the Virginia Mason Production System.

Dr. Kaplan has been a regional and national leader in safety and quality improvement efforts in health care and a strong proponent of the Virginia Mason Production System. This has led to many awards and accolades for the medical center, Dr. Kaplan, and other leaders at Virginia Mason.

References:

1. Lindeman RC. "Annual Report of the Chairman." 1980, p. 4; VM Archives.

2. Lindeman RC. "Personal History." 2005, p. 7, VM Archives.

3. Almquist J to Sandy Novak, email dated January 13, 2019.

23

Pediatrics / Adolescent Medicine

by F. Richard Dion, MD

The beginnings and growth of the Pediatric Section: 1962 – 1984

Some 35 years after its founding in 1920, The Mason Clinic decided to expand, build a new building on Ninth and Seneca, and add a number of specialties to their basic medical surgical staff. The family-oriented specialties of obstetrics and pediatrics were to be included. Although Virginia Mason Hospital had had an Obstetrics Department from its early years with a Labor and Delivery suite and newborn nursery, it had been staffed by outside physicians on the hospital staff, including Robert Rutherford, MD (Ob/Gyn) and his group, and **Fred Rutherford, MD** (pediatrician). Fred Rutherford was Chief of Pediatrics during this time and remained in that position for several years.

The new clinic building, which opened in 1954, soon added a dedicated pediatric office area on the second floor with its own waiting room, complete with blackboard and play table, four exam rooms and an office. This would remain the focus of the growing department for the next 40 years until they moved to the eighth floor of the Lindeman Pavilion. A few years later, the group moved to the first floor of Lindeman into a space designed using Lean principles.

Glen Hayden, MD, became the first obstetrician to join the Clinic in 1959 from the faculty of the University of Chicago. **F. Richard Dion, MD**, who was completing an extra year of training in pediatric endocrinology at the Mayo Clinic, was advised by his friend Pat Ragen, MD, that The Mason Clinic was looking for a pediatrician. Letters were exchanged with Joel Baker, MD, Chairman, and subsequently Luke Hill, MD, personnel committee chair, and Bill Crenshaw, MD, who made a visit to Mayo for an interview. Arrangements were made for a trip to Seattle in June 1961, which resulted in Dr. Dion starting practice in January 1962.

Within the first two weeks, Dr. Dion was welcomed to the staff of Children's Orthopedic Hospital by Jack Docter, MD, and also to the clinical faculty of the University of Washington Pediatric Department by Robert Aldrich, MD. Both Dr. Aldrich and his father had spent time on the staff at the Mayo Clinic.

The practice grew slowly since this was a time when families were moving from the inner city to the suburbs, but soon there was a foundation of primary care and patients seeking consultation from the WAMI (Washington, Alaska, Montana, Idaho) area. In addition, adult members of families who were receiving care at the Clinic started bringing their children to Dr. Dion, as well as children of the professional staff and the house staff who were always welcome as patients.

Patients were hospitalized at Children's Hospital when necessary and Dr. Dion participated in the teaching program on the wards and in the Endocrine Clinic there. There were no emergency room physicians for a number of years, so if a pediatric patient needed care in the ER, the pediatrician went in to see them at whatever hour. Likewise on the ward, the house staff was inexperienced with pediatric diseases, so inpatients often needed the pediatrician's presence. House calls were also a definite part of the early practice years. The pediatric office nurse for the first 12 years was **Marge McQuillan, RN**, who not only gave wonderful care and advice to patients but kept a shadow card file on her desk listing shot records and notes to supplement her excellent memory. This proved essential when children went off to school and those records taken home from the office had gone missing.

Immediate neighbors on the second floor included ophthalmologist Louis Hungerford, MD, who was always swamped with patients (as well as with charts and records) and, on the Ninth Avenue side, the Section of Endocrinology. This was one of the largest sections in the Department of Medicine. One of their daily activities occurred around 4 p.m., when diabetic class patients would gather in the hall outside the bathroom for their "cocktail hour." Twenty-some diabetics, each holding their plastic specimen cup, awaited instructions on how to do a Benedict's test for sugar. Bob Nielson, MD (one of the endocrinologists), loved to take a little break either lounging in the pediatric waiting room or provoking Dr. Hungerford. Nurse McQuillan tried to keep the waiting area picked up and clean – one day she was alarmed when Dr. Nielson said, "What's this brown lump on the floor?" She screamed and leapt to clean it up only to have him pop the piece of fudge he had planted into his mouth.

Patrick Mahoney, MD, joined the Clinic in 1968 from his position as Associate Professor of Pediatric Endocrinology at the University of Washington. He soon had a large number of juvenile diabetics in his practice as well as patients suffering from diseases related to his other interests including cystinosis, Vitamin D-resistant rickets and thyroidology. In 1968 the section sponsored the first postgraduate course in pediatrics, which became an almost annual affair that was held 27 times over 35 years, registering as many as 150 participants.

The Pediatric Section aligned itself with the model adopted for Adult Medicine at The Mason Clinic. Although the vast majority of the physicians practiced routine patient care, most were specialists and excelled in the complex problems that often presented themselves, utilizing the concept of "team medicine" from the start. In pediatrics, both Drs. Dion and Mahoney had specialty training in endocrinology, and the third pediatrician to join their group in 1977, **Dennis Christie, MD**, had a specialty interest in gastroenterology. **David Stempel, MD,** with his training in pediatric allergy and pulmonary disease, was the next member of the section in 1980. At that point, Dr. Dion suggested that the role of section head, which he had held since his arrival, should be rotated annually amongst the members of the section, to allow all members to be familiarized with other specialties and the overall administration of the clinic and hospital. **Steven Glass, MD**, began the new Subsection of Pediatric Neurology in 1982, with **Brien Vlcek, MD,** joining him in the subsection two years later.

It wasn't until July 1984 that the section hired a general pediatrician (who also focused on newborn care) - **Kyle Yasuda, MD**. The section of adult general internal medicine had been established in the 1970s after considerable debate, and took the specialty-oriented Mason Clinic in new directions. In 1980, "land was acquired adjacent to Evergreen (hospital) in Kirkland for a new clinic to be called Mason Clinic East" [1], which opened in 1982. These decisions began an expansion into primary care both downtown and at the satellites, which was mirrored in pediatrics over the next 20 years.

Pediatrics Expansion (and Contraction) in the Satellites: 1985 – 2001

In September 1985, **Dianne M. Glover, MD** (1985 – 1998) was welcomed as the first pediatrician in the satellites at Mason Clinic East. In October of this year, The Issaquah Clinic merged with The Mason Clinic, establishing a satellite in that area, and they would welcome their first pediatrician, **Monica Richter, MD**, to their practice in 1993; she was joined a few months later by **Usha Sankrithi, MD** (1993 – 1997). An existing pediatric practice in Federal Way joined Virginia Mason in 1986 and moved into the newly established Mason Clinic Federal Way in 1987, consisting of four pediatricians: **Jon Almquist, MD** (served as Chief of Pediatrics for several years before retiring in 2011, and was recipient of the **James Tate Mason Award** in 2002); **Michael R. Anderson, MD** (left in 1988 and now practicing at Valley Children's Clinic in Renton); **Richard K. Gould, MD** (still working as of March 2019); and **James E. Rogers, MD** (retired in 2002). **Todd D. Pearson, MD**, also joined the group (left in 1995), followed by **Jeannie Larsen, MD** (1989 – 2005) after

Dr. Anderson left; **Ann Maza, MD** (1989 - 1990) and **Lorin Solnit, MD** (1991 – 1992) joined VM South for a year or two during that time as well.

In 1987, **Ruth A. Parish, MD**, joined Dr. Glover at Virginia Mason East as a practicing general pediatrician (left in 1995); in 1991, **Katherine Grishaw-Jones, MD**, was practicing there as well (left by 1993); and **Catherine Meltzer, MD** (1992 – 1997) joined the group when Dr. Grishaw-Jones left. **Linda Warren, MD** (1995 – 2006) replaced Dr. Parish in 1995; she moved to Winslow in 1999 when pediatrics was dissolved as a section at VM East. **John Girard, MD**, joined the group in 1998, and then moved to the Issaquah Clinic for a few years before leaving VM in 2001.

The downtown group also grew with the addition of **Ruth A. Conn, MD**, in 1987 as a general pediatrician (she moved to Sand Point in 2010 when downtown pediatrics closed, and subsequently retired in 2016). **Richard O. Gode, MD**, joined the section of Psychiatry in that same year as the first child psychiatrist (retired in 1996) and was soon followed by **Jim McKeever, PhD**, a child psychologist, in 1988 (both of these gentlemen are described in the chapter on Psychiatry in this volume). Dr. Christie left VM that year to take a position as Chief of Gastroenterology at Children's Orthopedic Hospital in Seattle. **Robert T. Fukura, MD**, joined the downtown practice in 1991 as a general practitioner, coming from his practice in Yakima. Dr. Fukura also joined the Sand Point group in 2010, and retired in 2015. **Roberta L. Winch, MD**, joined the downtown practice in 1993 (left in 2006); Dr. Mahoney retired from VM in 1993, and took a position as Chief of Endocrinology at Children's Orthopedic Hospital.

Howard Uman, MD (1988 – 2000), and **Kelvie Johnson, MD** (1988 - 1993), became part of The Mason Clinic at its new Lynnwood location, Virginia Mason North, in 1988. In 1992, **Henry G. Coit, Jr, MD**, joined their practice, where he also served as satellite head. **Alka Mehta, MD**, joined the group in 1994 and **Jill Sells, MD,** joined in 1998. Drs. Uman and Coit left at the beginning of 2000 when the Lynnwood pediatrics group was closed because of contractual issues. Dr. Coit served as the Medical Director of Regence BlueShield for one year and then was appointed as the new Chief Operating Officer for the UW Physicians Neighborhood Clinics in 2001. [2] Both Drs. Mehta and Sells moved to VM Winslow for one year in 2000 after the North pediatrics group was discontinued, after which they left VM.

Meanwhile, **Anne E. Phalen, MD**, joined VM South in 1992 (left in 2005); **Gordon S. Naylor, MD**, in 1993 (still in practice there); **Susanne Purnell, MD,** in 1994 (left in 2000); and **Matthew Eisenberg, MD**, in 1996 (left in 2003).

Satellite expansion continued over the next two years at a rapid pace. The Mercer Island Pediatrics Group joined VM in 1994, which included five pediatricians: **Julie Ellner, MD; Danette S. Glassy, MD; Theodore D. Mandelkorn, MD; Hal C. Quinn, MD**, and **Janice W. Woolley, MD.** The Winslow Clinic (later Bainbridge Island) was opened in 1995 with pediatricians **Diane E. Fuquay, MD** (retired in 2004) and **Thomas R. Monk, MD** (left/retired in 2007), who were joined by Dr. Warren in 1999 when pediatrics was discontinued at VM East, and Drs. Mehta and Sells for one year in 2000 when the Lynnwood clinic discontinued pediatrics.

Dr. Dion retired at the end of 1995, and the Sand Point Pediatrics Group was acquired that year with pediatricians **Ann N. Champoux, MD** (recently retired but working as locum); **Steve W. Dassel, MD** (left in 2012); **Leslie Mackoff, MD** (left in 1997) **Donna L. Smith, MD** (who served as Chief of Pediatrics from 2002 – 2007 and is currently Medical Director of VM Clinics as of Spring 2019); and **Margaret A. Wheeler, MD** (retired in 2014).

The Fidalgo Clinic opened in 1996 with pediatricians **Jeanne Olmsted, MD** (1996 – 2001), and **M. Lester Richards, MD** (1996 – 2001). Unfortunately, the Mercer Island and Fidalgo satellites left Virginia Mason in 2001 when the fortunes of the medical center required a closer look at these investments.

Over the next several years, several pediatricians were hired at various satellites: **Peggy J. Sarjeant-Tuggy, MD** (1997 – 2009) and **Tao Sheng Kwan-Gett, MD** (1998 – 2006, 2017 - present) at Sand Point;

Ann E. Sneiders, MD, at Issaquah (1997 – 2008); Robin D. Ifft, MD, at Issaquah (1997 - 2018); Andrea M. Fasullo, MD (1998 – present); and Jonathan R. Fox, MD (2000 – present, at Federal Way. Kimberly M. Schrier, MD, joined the Issaquah group in 2001. She has recently left practice to take up her duties as a national Congresswoman for the 8th Congressional District of Washington state. Kathy A. Risse, MD (2001 – present) was hired the same year at Sand Point and is still working there.

Meanwhile, the Pediatrics Section at Virginia Mason East (now Kirkland) was dissolved in 1999, and the pediatric care was taken up by family medicine physicians, an ARNP (Kathy T. Daotay, ARNP) and a physician assistant (Amanda J. Heckman, PA-C), who see pediatric patients in varying amounts. The family practice physicians currently including Laurel Morrison, MD (1998 - present); Heidi Rogers, MD (2000 - present); Lars Kaine, MD (2010 - present); Helen N. Gray, MD (2015 – present); and Orion B. Wells, MD (2017 - present).

Dr. Yasuda left the downtown practice in July of 2001, and joined the faculty at the University of Washington. He became President of the American Academy of Pediatrics in 2019.

The New Millennium: 2002 – Present

The number of satellites diminished from 20 in 1997 to only nine by 2004. Family medicine practitioners also replaced the pediatricians at Winslow (now Bainbridge), who left between 2000 and 2007 (including Drs. Fuquay, Monk, Warren and Frederick C. Walters, MD, 2003 - 2006) and now include Jillian Worth, MD (2001 – present); Catherine Edwards, MD (2008 – present); and Michael Tomberg, MD (2012 – present); along with Ashley D. Calahan, PA-C, and Sydney E. Thompson, ARNP. Kris I. Colletto, MD, who holds board certifications in internal medicine and pediatrics, also saw patients there between the end of 2000 and 2002.

In 2010, the original downtown practice, at that time composed of Dr. Conn, Dr. Fukura, and Gabriel Berson, MD (2007 -2010), was closed, with Drs. Conn and Fukura moving their practices to the Sand Point Pediatrics Clinic. In 2013, the Sand Point clinic relocated to a new regional medical center at University Village.

In 2013, **Rebecca Partridge, MD** (2012-present) began the Virginia Mason Down Syndrome Clinic, the first comprehensive clinic for people with Down syndrome in the Northwest. This has grown and expanded to our University Village location, as well.

In February 2018, VM acquired the Edmonds Family Medicine group and a few of those family medicine physicians also practice pediatrics, including **Myra G. Horiuchi, MD**, and **Ingrid E. Van Swearingen, MD**.

In June 2019, our first new site in many years staffed by a pediatrician was opened at the Bellevue Regional Medical Center with the hiring of pediatrician, **David Schneider, MD** (2019-present), and support from the Issaquah pediatric group. Pediatricians now staff four locations (as of August 2019): University Village has 12 pediatricians, one pediatric ARNP, **Susie Paeth**, and one behavioral health ARNP, **Jason Law**; Federal Way has six; Issaquah has two and one ARNP, **Jenny Baker**; and Bellevue has Dr. Schneider. In total, pediatric care, either from a pediatrician or a family practitioner is now available at the following clinics as of August 2019: University Village, Federal Way, Kirkland, Issaquah, Bainbridge, Bellevue, and Edmonds.

Several pediatricians were hired in the satellites and downtown and subsequently left between 2002 and the present. These include:

Claire M. Hebner, MD – Federal Way (2002 – 2006)

Merrill T. Wiseman, MD – Sand Point (2003 – 2009)

Varun M. Jhaveri, MD – downtown Seattle (2003 – 2005)

Whitney R. Anderson, MD – Sand Point (2004 - 2005)

Corrie Takahashi, MD – Federal Way (2006; currently working as a locum)

Gabriel Berson, MD – downtown Seattle (2007 – 2010)

Jenny L. Lobo, MD – Federal Way (2007 – 2012)

Anika L. Sanda, MD – Issaquah (2008 – 2012)

The pediatricians currently providing care at the satellites (as of June 2019) mentioned above and the years they joined VM are listed as follows:

Sand Point

Alejandro J. Candelario, MD (2015)

Elizabeth S. Cochrane, MD (2017)

Michael Dudas, MD (2006) Chief 2007 - present

Benjamin Jackson, MD (2009)

Tao Shen Kwan-Gett, MD (1998, 2017)

Liana K. McCabe, MD (2014)

Traci L. McDermott, MD (2016)

Thomas E. Numrych, MD (2003)

Susie Paeth, ARNP (2000)

Kristin Nyweide White, MD (2007)

Kathy Risse, MD (2001)

Kathy Rosen, MD (2012)

Donna L. Smith, MD (1995) Chief 2002 - 2007

Federal Way

Lauren Athay, MD (2013)

Jessica L. Ebberson, MD (2012)

Andrea Fasullo, MD (1998)

Jonathan R. Fox, MD (2000)

Richard K. Gould, MD (1986)

Gordon S. Naylor, MD (1993)

Issaquah

Rebecca Partridge, MD (2012)

Derrick L. Soong, MD (2017)

Jenny Baker, ARNP (2019)

Bellevue

David Schneider, MD (2019)

Timeline for the Development of the VM Pediatric Department

1920: The Mason Clinic founded.

Mid-1950s: Decision to expand to other specialties and build a new clinic building.

1958: New building opens; planning for pediatric office suite on second floor of new clinic building.

1959: First Mason Clinic obstetrician, Glen Hayden, MD (1959 – 1986).

January 1962: First Mason Clinic pediatrician, F. Richard Dion, MD, starts (retired at the end of 1995).

Spring 1962: Conversion of small pediatric ward at VM hospital to the first Adult Intensive Care Unit under Leo Hughes, MD, cardiologist (1960 – 1985).

September 1968: Dr. C. Patrick Mahoney becomes the second pediatric practitioner with a specialty in endocrinology. (retired 1993).

December 1968: We put on our first Pediatric Postgraduate Course, which continues almost annually for 35 years.

July 1977: Dennis Christie, MD, becomes our third pediatrician with a specialty in gastroenterology (left in 1988).

September 1980: David Stempel, MD, begins his practice in pediatric allergy and pulmonary disease (retired 2002).

July 1982: Dr. Steven Glass (left in 1989) begins a new section of Pediatric Neurology and is joined in 1984 by Brien W. Vlcek, MD (left in 1989).

July 1984: Kyle E. Yasuda, MD, joins the section in General Pediatrics and Newborn Care (1984 – 2001).

September 1985: Pediatrics in the satellites begins with Dianne M. Glover, MD, at the Kirkland satellite (left 1998).

1986: An existing practice of four pediatricians in Federal Way joins VM including Jon Almquist, MD (retired 2011); Michael R. Anderson, MD (left in 1988); Richard K. Gould, MD (still in practice); James E. Rogers, MD (retired in 2002).

1987: Ruth A. Conn, MD, begins her practice downtown (retired in 2016); Ruth A Parish, MD, joins Dr. Glover (left 1995).

September 1987: Richard O. Gode, MD, joins as our first child psychiatrist joined by Jim McKeever, PhD, in child psychology in 1988.

1988: The Lynnwood Clinic opens with pediatricians Kelvie Johnson, MD, and Howard Uman, MD.

1991: Robert T. Fukura, MD, joins the downtown practice from Yakima (retired 2015).

1993: Monica Weitzer Richter, MD (left in 1999), joined a few months later by Usha M. Sankrithi, MD (left in 1997) brings pediatrics to the Issaquah Clinic.

1994: The Mercer Island Clinic is opened with the purchase of the Mercer Island Pediatric Group including Julie Ellner, MD; Danette S. Glassy, MD; Theodore D. Mandelkorn, MD; Hal C. Quinn, MD; and Janice W. Woolley, MD.

1995: The Sand Point Pediatric Group joins with five pediatricians: Ann N. Champoux, MD (recently retired but working locum for University Village); Steve W. Dassel, MD (left 2012); Leslie Mackoff, MD (left in 2001); Donna L. Smith, MD (still working at present); and Margaret A. Wheeler, MD (retired in 2014). In addition, the Winslow satellite begins with pediatricians Diane E. Fuquay, MD (retired in 2004), and Thomas R. Monk, MD (left/retired in 2007). Dr. Dion retired at the end of the year.

1996: The Fidalgo satellite begins with Jeanne Olmsted, MD, and M. Lester Richards, MD.

1999: The pediatrics section at VM East is dissolved with pediatricians moving to Winslow and the Issaquah Clinic. Family Medicine physicians take up the care of pediatric patients in varying amounts.

2000: The pediatric group at Lynnwood is discontinued, with Drs. Coit and Uman leaving VM, and Drs. Mehta and Sells taking positions at the Winslow Clinic for one year before leaving VM.

2001: The Fidalgo Clinic is closed.

2003: The Mercer Island Clinic is closed.

2004: As of 2004, there are nine satellite clinics left at VM. Pediatricians are practicing at four of these (Sand Point, Federal Way, Issaquah, Winslow), as well as downtown.

2007: The last pediatrician at Bainbridge leaves and all pediatrics care at the clinic is now done by family practitioners.

2013: The University Village Clinic is opened in December and Sand Point and downtown pediatricians move there.

2018: The Edmonds Family Medicine group is purchased in February and two of the family practitioners also include pediatrics in their practices: Drs. Horiuchi and Van Swearingen.

2019: Dr. Schneider, pediatrician, opens a pediatric practice at the Bellevue satellite. Pediatrics is available in seven locations: University Village; Federal Way, Issaquah, Kirkland, Bainbridge, Bellevue, and Edmonds.

References:

1. Ross A. *Vision and Vigilance: The First 75 Years, Virginia Mason Medical Center.* Virginia Mason Medical Center, Publisher, 1995, p.74.

2. "Coit Joins UWPN." *UW News, Health Sciences Brief News.* November 29, 2001. At:http://www.washington.edu/news/2001/11/29/health-sciences-brief-news-2/. Accessed March 23, 2019.

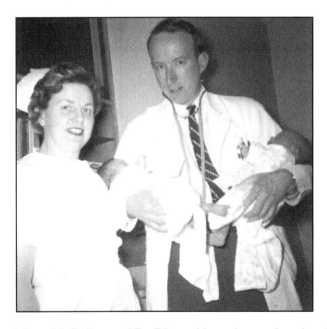

Nurse Marge McQuillan and Dr. Dion, with newborn twins, circa 1960
(PH 1309, VMHA)

24

History of the Lewis and John Dare Center and Concierge Medicine

by John Kirkpatrick, MD

In the mid 1990s marked changes were occurring at Virginia Mason. Reimbursement had declined to 50% (referred to as the "concession rate"), our urgent care clinics on 4th Avenue and in the emergency room had closed, and the Section of General Internal Medicine with 23 doctors, had been reduced to one phone line in a cost-saving measure. The 1000 plus phone calls coming in on this one line were answered by 5 moderately skilled operators. Personalized medical attention was just not possible. Many were frustrated as the hard economics of the day took their toll.

Just three blocks away from VM's hospital, a new concept in primary care and medicine was being born. "Concierge Medicine" (or as the founders Howard Maron, MD, and Scott Hall, MD, preferred to call it -"Highly Attentive Medicine") began in 1996 and would go on to become a national movement. Closely affiliated with competitor Swedish Hospital, the new program, called "MD-squared", limited its practice to 50 patients per doctor, promised 24/7 cell phone coverage directly to the doctor, performed house calls, and included laboratory tests and x-rays (all in lavish surroundings) for the all-inclusive price of $1000/month per person (discounted to $500 for the second family member). Several of Virginia Mason's important donors found this package so appealing that they left

VM, a critical factor since visit billings alone were not enough to balance expenses.

But several other extremely loyal patients thought VM should have a similar program, as did co-founding physicians **Bruce Nitsche, MD**, and **John Kirkpatrick, MD**. And thus, the Lewis and John Dare Center was conceived, although not without the considerable and agonizing debate that organizations are wont to experience when vetting new ideas. A core team of Drs. Nitsche and Kirkpatrick, Vice President of Marketing and Business Development **Darlene Corkrum**, Chief Nurse **Patti Crome**, patients **Nancy and Vic Parker, Jacki and Carl Meurk**, and administrative fellow **Danielle Smith** (with very able mentoring from President **Mike Rona**) was charged with making this happen. The 18-month process of seemingly endless meetings, focus groups, business case analysis, and Executive Committee debate culminated in the planned opening of the Dare Center in January of 2000. A "CAN-DO" team of Bruce and John, nurses **Nancy Lencioni** and **Katie Clack**, and medical assistant **Cathy Greenawalt** hammered out the details of how the Center would provide care, and everyone was primed for the quiet rollout of this low profile program until …

A reporter from the *Seattle Times* somehow obtained a brochure, and thinking that this was a newsworthy event, wrote an article that appeared in the Christmas Eve edition of the then evening paper headlined, "Hefty Fee Guarantees Access at Virginia Mason". Employees had not been informed, and the quiet planned debut immediately was replaced by an overwhelmingly negative rant. The cost per person was $250 per month, far below the Swedish MD^2 program, but that didn't matter. The "plush" un-air-conditioned surroundings of the defunct Center for Women's Health on the 2nd floor of the Buck Pavilion with a waiting area shared with Psychiatry didn't matter – it was the PRINCIPLE that for an extra fee, a certain population of patients could receive better SERVICE, implying that the service and possibly the care for the rest of the patients would be sub-standard. An immediate noon-time forum was held, where Drs. Nitsche and Kirkpatrick sat in front of the angry crowd to address their concerns, with support from President Mike Rona and CEO **Roger Lindeman, MD** (after all, it was THEIR PROGRAM), and within a short time, tempers subsided and the fledgling group set out on their journey to provide an uncommon level of service (and not better care, as the rest of the providers in the medical center would prove to be the case).

The initial Winslow space was in the basement of the satellite in the treadmill room, and the overflow exam room was the "chicken pox quarantine room". We started our downtown clinic on the second floor of the Buck Pavilion. As panels of patients filled, additional providers were added. **Lesley Althouse, MD,** and **Tammira Price, MD**, joined the downtown site, a Bellevue office was started, staffed by **Leland Teng, MD,** and **Greg Keyes, MD**, was added to the Winslow site to partner with Dr. Nitsche. The revenue was enough to balance the losses incurred in primary care and the group flourished. When space opened on the 2nd floor of Lindeman Pavilion, the team jumped at the chance to have air-conditioned surroundings. Several of their patients thought they deserved a nicer space, and one couple donated funds to upgrade the facilities. Just at that time, the fertility group vacated the space on the top floor of the Lindeman Pavilion, and the funds were sufficient to remodel the space into the premier location that had been desired from the outset. On Bainbridge, the small domain that housed the Humane Society became available and was remodeled to become the present day Winslow Dare Center.

Soon the Dare Center became the model for other medical centers around the country. Park Nicollet of Minneapolis, University of Alabama Birmingham, Scripps Clinic of La Jolla, Baylor, Henry Ford Hospital, the University of Nebraska and the Mayo Clinic of Scottsdale all sent representatives or teams to VM to learn how to put together a similar program at their institutions. The group also responded to requests for on-site consultations, and traveled to the Cleveland Clinic of Florida and the Carolinas Healthcare System in Charlotte, North Carolina. A national organization of "concierge" physicians was formed, initially called the American Society of Concierge Medicine, which morphed into the Society for Innovative Medical Practice Design, and then finally into the American Academy of Private Physicians (AAPP). VM physicians made presentations at these national meetings. In October of 2012, a separate track was set up for medical centers at the established AAPP meeting, which provided a wonderful sense of camaraderie that did not exist in the greater organization, leading to an agreement to meet separately thereafter. The Medical Centers Concierge Alliance was formed and held its inaugural meeting in Seattle in August of 2013, discussing common problems and solutions, and further enhancing a common network of similar programs.

The section was blessed with outstanding RN and MA staff from the beginning. Nancy Lencioni, Katie Clack and Cathy Greenawalt provided warm, friendly, extremely competent and caring help for this very special group of patients. There was nothing about customer service they didn't understand, and they were a prime reason that patient satisfaction was at the 99th percentile when compared nationally. They set the standard for those who followed in nursing: **Sandy Stevens, Sandy Weir, Loretta Lilly, Colleen Morgan, Karla Litzenberger, Maureen Grant, Janice Page**; and medical sssistants: **Heidi Manwaring, LaTonya Purnell, Kim Tossman, Sheri Chifulio** and **Cynthia Watson**. The section also had extremely capable administrative managers in **Amin Neghabat, Jim Bevier, Jennifer Graves** and **Theresa Shipley** (who came as a marketing specialist and wound up with over 10 years of amazingly competent managerial leadership). There was strong Department of Medicine support from Chief **Bob Mecklenburg, MD**, and, when the section became part of the Department of Primary Care, from Chief **Catherine Potts, MD**, and administrative VP **Mike Ondracek,** and Chief **Ingrid Gerbino, MD,** and administrative VP **Shelly Fagerland**.

Over the years, there was a lot of media inquiry and the group was extremely well coached by **Linda Stepanich**, who had joined Virginia Mason after a stint at the American Medical Association in Chicago. There wasn't a reporter she didn't know, and she had a talent for understanding the perspective of the questioner. She sat in at phone and in-person interviews, and would use a signal for answering the "difficult questions". The VM Communications department was also helpful, especially **Kathleen**

Paul. Robin Turner and **Lynne Chafetz** provided excellent legal support, especially during, and in preparation for hearings in Olympia where the Insurance Commissioner questioned the concepts of "concierge medicine".

The department has maintained 5 doctors in the three sites – downtown, Bellevue and Bainbridge Island. Upon the retirement of Section Head John Kirkpatrick, Leland Teng assumed his role. Executive Health 365, the combined product of a pre-determined health testing panel with the 24/7 "concierge medicine service" has grown under the leadership of Dr. Teng and Coordinator **Lynn Benedict**. Over 1200 patients enjoy the service and care of physicians Nitsche, Althouse, Teng, Price and recent additions **Paul Kassab, MD**, and **Eileen Bailey, MD.** The name of the Dare Center was changed to "Concierge Medicine" in 2017 to reflect current trends and the broader acceptance of the term "concierge". In 2020, the program will celebrate its 20th year of truly placing the patient at the top of VM's strategic plan pyramid.

Physician Biographies:

John Kirkpatrick, MD (1976 – 2013): Longview, WA native; UW Medical School/ Mayo Clinic internal medicine residency; 23 years in VM's GIM Department; Co-founder of Dare Center: 2000 – 2013

Bruce Nitsche, MD (1995 – present): Seattle, WA native; USC Medical School; Virginia Mason internal medicine residency; 15 years at VM Winslow; Co-founder of Dare Center: 2000 – present

Lesley Althouse MD (1985 – present): Manchester, England native; Oxford Medical School and internal medicine residency; geriatrics fellowship at Johns Hopkins; 15+ years in VM's GIM section; Dare Center: 2001 – present

Leland Teng, MD (2001 – present): Dallas, Texas native; UT Dallas Medical School; primary care internal medicine residency at UW; 15+

years in private practice in Bellevue; Dare Center: 2001 – present

Tammira Price, MD (1997 – present): Tacoma, WA native; Cornell Medical School; Virginia Mason internal medicine residency; 15 years in GIM at VMMC; Dare Center: 2011 – present

Paul Kassab, MD (2007 – present): American University of Beirut Medical School; University of Rochester internal medicine residency; private practice in Kansas; 8 years in Virginia Mason GIM; Dare Center: 2015 – present

Eileen Bailey, MD (2020 – present): California native; Creighton University School of Medicine; Virginia Mason internal medicine residency; 5 years in private practice in Redwood City, CA; 13 years in Virginia Mason GIM; Concierge Medicine 2020 - present

Other physicians who served shorter terms in the Dare Center include **Greg Keyes, MD** (Bainbridge); **Hope Druckman, MD** (Bellevue); **Patricia Auerbach, MD** (Bellevue), and **Christian Herter, MD** (Seattle).

25

The SENSE Program at Virginia Mason

by G. Ted Johnson, MD

This is a subjective history, long on impressions and trends, short on specific dates.

In the early 1980s, the Executive Health Program wanted to offer new products to businesses and their employees. One strategy adopted to that end was a health promotion/wellness program. "Health Promotion" was enjoying rising popularity across the nation at that time. Patients and providers alike were interested in going beyond disease recognition and treatment to disease prevention and even further to creation of a sense of overall wellness. There was also speculation and hope that the cost of health care would decrease as lifestyle-related illnesses were prevented.

Rather than develop its own, VM purchased an existing wellness program from the Park-Nicollet Clinic in Minnesota. It was called SHAPE, but the VM program was launched as SENSE, which was an acronym for the Satisfying Effects of Nutrition, Stress Management and Exercise. From SHAPE, VM received curricula and supporting materials for experiential and education programs in the areas mentioned in its name, as well as a smoking cessation program that had somehow escaped the acronym.

Having obtained the framework from Park-Nicollet, VM began to build its Health Promotion team. The first medical director was **Bill**

Crounse, MD, a physician at the VM 4th Avenue Urgent Care Center. He had local media experience and connections and it was felt he would be a good ambassador for the program. Additional physicians were recruited to the program including myself from the Emergency Department, **John Kirkpatrick, MD,** from General Internal Medicine, and **Carter Hill, MD,** another Emergency physician. The first administrative director was **Eve Stern**, an RN with management expertise. (She was incidentally married to Fred Stern, MD, an ophthalmologist at VM.) Eve was a bright and engaging person with boundless energy and creativity. She assembled a team of subject matter specialists from several VM departments. **Cyndi Welke, RD,** and **Judy Delgado, RD,** were registered dietitians who covered the area of healthy diet and weight management; **Kathe Wallace, PT,** was a physical therapist who addressed the benefits of exercise; and **Arden Snyder, PhD**, and **Bob Pogano, PhD**, were psychologists who gave presentations on mental health - specifically, the realm of stress management. **Judy Hansen, BA,** (in Speech and English), an experienced community presenter on life planning, was hired to help participants pull all the information together and address the reality of behavior change.

To launch the program and gain visibility, an intensive 4-day seminar at Rosario Resort on Orcas Island was offered to prominent local business leaders and their spouses. The guest list included many long-time VM supporters and donors as well as business owners and perceived opinion shapers. The weekend offered lectures, individual health assessments with physiologic measurements and blood tests, consultations on lifestyle and health, exercise sessions, and healthy meals prepared according to the recipes in the SENSE cookbook. In addition to the information and experiences, participants were provided with motivational presentations and practical tips for setting goals and changing their current lifestyle habits into healthier ones. AND, they each received a shiny polyester, navy blue exercise suit. It had a white stripe down the arms and legs and it became the work uniform for all SENSE staff.

By that time, for reasons that now escape me, I had replaced Bill Crounse as Medical Director of SENSE. In that role, I gave the introductory overview of the subject areas to be covered and the weekend schedule. It was a very energetic and well-received weekend but not without some challenges behind the scenes. One moment that sticks in my mind occurred at the first evening cocktail hour (responsible drinking strongly recommended and modeled by staff) when one of my colleagues gently interrupted me in conversation with a guest to tell me that one of our contract fitness consultants was regaling a small group of participants with the health benefits of drinking your own urine daily. I quickly joined his conversational group and gently but firmly made it clear that his views on urine were personal and not endorsed by the SENSE program. I shared a room that weekend with the same fitness consultant. On the second morning, I awoke to the sight of him standing on his head against a wall, naked. He told me that he routinely recommended this maneuver to clients to start their day with the most energy and mental clarity. We all kept a close eye on him during the rest of the weekend and his contract was terminated shortly after we returned to Seattle.

After the kick-off, we began marketing our menu of services. We had a 2-3 day comprehensive experiential seminar, similar in content and format to what we had provided at Rosario, only somewhat condensed and, of course, for a fee. It was intended for business leaders investigating SENSE for their companies, and by individuals and couples who were looking to improve their health. We also added a variety of lifestyle management courses to the quarterly calendar at VM's downtown campus. Each was a series of 4-6 weekly sessions. Our three primary programs were "Smoke Stoppers" for smoking cessation, "Be Trim" for nutritional and weight management, and a stress management course that didn't have a catchy name. All curricula had been purchased from the Park Nicollet Clinic but were gradually modified based on our experiences. We partnered with **Angela Peterson** in Executive Health to market health assessments that would summarize lifestyle-related risks and opportunities for improvement.

As we enhanced our program offerings, we also expanded our full-time staff. **Marilyn Guthrie, RD,** was hired to oversee the nutritional aspects of the program. Similarly, **Robyn Stuhr, MA**, was hired to manage the exercise/fitness component along with the Personal Health Assessment tool and process. **Judy Hansen** received an MA in Communications and she and I assumed responsibility for teaching the stress management courses. (The staff in the ED where I worked clinically were quite amused to learn that I was teaching stress management. Apparently, I didn't always present a calm and relaxed demeanor at work.) And we hired **Harry Franzheim** to market all of our programming, including custom-tailored programs, to businesses in the Puget Sound region. All of our specialists were available to Harry for consultation with prospective clients and presentations to leaders and their employees on their specific area of expertise – nutrition, fitness, mental health, habit change, smoking cessation, etc. Eve Stern, our Administrative Director, left to pursue other opportunities and was replaced by a series of directors - **Lori Lancaster, Cindy Dausman**, and Judy Hansen. Eventually, Marilyn Guthrie took on the responsibility of Administrative Director while continuing to manage the nutritional component of the program.

Surprisingly to me, I became a popular banquet speaker. My most popular presentation, unimaginatively entitled "Your Lifestyle and Your Health" was the same talk with which I began our seminars. As the title suggests, it was an overview of current knowledge about the lifestyle habits known to have an impact on health. I also offered presentations on "Stress Management" and "Humor and Health". In an attempt to retain audience attention, I used a fair amount of humor in these talks and as a result, I got a regional reputation for being entertaining. Organizations looking for an informative speaker who was also funny found me by word of mouth, and I ended up giving hundreds of presentations at conferences, professional organization meetings, service organization lunches and even at high schools. The latter audience required that I modify my approach to keep the kids interested. Soliciting questions from the students seemed to work best, but perhaps predictably, the nature of the questions shifted the content primarily to sex and I discovered just how little valid information teenagers had about sexual anatomy, physiology and disease. One young woman, during my presentation, asked if what her mother had told her was true, namely that teenage boys could have only one erection each day. The resulting outburst from the collective males in the audience was a clue to my correct response to her query. The fees generated by my presentations represented a small portion of our revenue, but the exposure often led to further programming and some individual enrollment in our various programs. And, I had a good time. Also, I ate a lot of mediocre banquet food. I don't miss that at all.

One of the most noteworthy projects during our robust period was our outreach to the Pacific Rim in partnership with the recently launched VM Center for Asian and International Medical Affairs (CAIMA). One of their goals was to encourage American corporations working in Asia to send their expat executives back to VM for routine and semi-acute care. To help meet that goal, I was sent to Korea, Japan and Taiwan to meet with American business leaders in Seoul, Tokyo and Taipei and sell our programming. I was accompanied by **Mike Ferris**, a multi-lingual VM employee who worked with clinicians to improve health care delivery to our local Asian-American and Asian immigrant populations. It was a busy, 6-day tour that resulted in contracts for Health Promotion programming in Tokyo and Taipei. Several weeks after my initial trip, Marilyn Guthrie, Robyn Stuhr, Judy Hansen and I set off for Asia, again ably shepherded by Mike Ferris who saw to all of the logistical arrangements and translational needs. We presented one-day programs for the Japanese-American club in Tokyo and the Taipei-American club in Taipei. In both cases, attendees were primarily American expats, so language was not an issue.

In Taipei, our program was attended by a Taiwanese business owner who was so inspired by the experience that he contracted with us for the same presentation to all of his employees 2 days later. He assured us that they all understood English. However, on the day of the seminar, as the participants assembled in the lecture room, it became apparent that he had over-estimated his employees' facility with our language. As we began our standard presentations, we quickly realized that despite their uniformly smiling faces, no one was understanding anything. Absolutely nothing was getting through. Each of us began to adapt our lectures while delivering them, simplifying our vocabularies and in some cases, adding gestures. When Judy Hansen, teaching stress management, waved her hands under her arms to signify the sweat that might be associated with the stress response, those of us observing in the back of the room pretty much lost it and had to step out to regain our professional demeanors while Judy soldiered on bravely to the end of her talk.

Over our approximately 10-year history at VM, we faced several challenges. We were never able to integrate well with primary care. We were viewed by some providers in General Internal Medicine as a fad only available to well-heeled patients. We were never successful at making the Personal Health Assessment part of the patient medical record (still a paper-based document at that time), which was another reason that Primary Providers had trouble working with us. And eventually, the medical center faced financial challenges that prompted them to reconsider the usefulness of supporting a Health Promotion and Wellness program.

As a result, in the early '90s, our program was severely pared and placed under the broad umbrella of Patient Education. I became Medical Director of Patient Education and chair of the associated committee. Marilyn Guthrie was retained as Manager of Patient Education and Health Promotion. Robyn Stuhr, our fitness coordinator, transferred to the Sports Medicine section, but continued to conduct health fitness assessments as part of the Executive Health program. The positions held by Judy Hansen and Harry Franzheim were eliminated.

For a time, we continued to try and offer as much of our previous programming as possible. Robyn continued to give presentations, but, given the responsibilities of her new position, she didn't have the time to oversee our Personal Health Assessment program, which atrophied and died. Judy provided services on a contract basis in the area of Stress Management, but without Harry Franzheim, new business slowly dried up leaving us with less demand. The behavior modification programs ("Be Trim", "Smoke Stoppers" and "Stress Management") were still offered periodically, but without money or other resources for advertising, attendance declined. When Marilyn accepted a position outside the medical center, most of the programming stopped. I continued to give occasional presentations and chair the Patient Education Committee, but, given limited resources, what we offered amounted to pamphlets and some free informational lectures. When I stepped down from the Patient Education Committee sometime in the mid '90s, the last vestige of the SENSE program disappeared.

Of interest to me at the time of this writing is the renewed interest in Health Promotion and Wellness, both nationally and on the part of VM. Presented to the public as a way to prevent illness and increase vitality, there is also a financial incentive. As the Health Care industry continues to struggle with rising costs, it is hoped that a healthier patient population will reduce the expensive care needed to deal with potentially preventable chronic conditions. Insurance companies and corporations are offering personal health risk assessments and financial incentives to adopt healthier lifestyle habits. The problem is that the benefits of a healthy lifestyle take decades to be realized. What remains to be seen is whether or not current efforts will be supported for long enough to see that sort of change.

26

Outpatient Nursing

by Rita Kelly, RN, and Nancy Lencioni, ARNP

Physicians have relied heavily on a variety of staff to ensure quality and complete care for patients. From medical assistants to transcriptionists, receptionists to technologists, the work of the physician is amplified and improved by these important professionals. This chapter is a small look at one of these important groups: nurses, and in this case, outpatient nurses, who work alongside the physicians to ensure high quality outcomes for their patients.

Nurses work in a variety of settings throughout the Medical Center, including the hospital, the clinics, administration, and procedural areas. One cannot begin to do justice to the contributions and accomplishments of nurses at Virginia Mason in one short chapter - from **Anna Fraser, RN,** who was present at the founding of The Mason Clinic, to **Marguerite Mansperger, RN; Pat Maguire, RN; Patti Chrome, RN,** and **Charlene Tachibana, RN**, to name but a few - another volume would be needed to relate this history.

These two short vignettes tell the stories of two nurses, **Rita Kelly, RN** and **Nancy Lencioni, ARNP**, and serve as a testimony to the work of many more. For the story of an outpatient team nursing approach, see the Gastroenterology chapter in this volume.

One Nurse's Outpatient Career at Virginia Mason
by Rita Kelly, RN

I moved to Seattle in Aug 1972 and began looking for a nursing job at the local hospitals. Normally that would have been a fairly easy task but it happened to be right in the middle of the Boeing economic slump. Many hospitals, including UW and Harborview, were not even accepting applications for RN jobs. VM Hospital had an opening for a RN in the Nursery on the night shift, which was not exactly my dream job. I met with the Hospital Personnel staff and happened to also inquire about RN jobs at The Mason Clinic, as it was called in those days. They told me that the clinic had a separate Personnel Department and I would need to check with them myself. Since I was already on campus, I walked across the street and filled out an application. As luck would have it they had an opening for a RN in the Nephrology section working with Dr. Paton. He had apparently called down to the Personnel Department the previous day informing them that he wanted to hire a second nurse to support his practice. In those days that was all that was required to add a position. How things have changed! I was hired and began working in late September.

Dr. Paton had one of the busiest practices in the Department of Medicine at that time. We saw patients with hypertension, kidney disease, and those on dialysis. Dialysis was very new at the time and due to federal government funding it had become more readily available to all those needing it. VM had done their first kidney transplant just a few months before I started working there. It was a very busy and challenging practice, and there was a lot that the nurses could do to support this patient population. We ran classes teaching patients how to take their own blood pressure readings at home, which allowed them to better manage their disease, and fielded many phone calls triaging their medical problems, refilling medications, and overall symptom management. This was all before computers.

Every phone call, medication refill request, etc., required a call to medical records to request their chart. The charts were in the basement of what is now Buck Pavilion, so it took time to get them and thus required calling patients or pharmacies back once the chart was received. To determine when a patient was last seen by the doctor, what meds they were taking, and when they were last refilled could only be determined by reviewing the chart. There were approximately 80 physicians at that time so you can imagine the number of phone calls generated every day to medical records just to do the basic day-to-day activities that are now done in a few seconds by accessing the electronic medical record. In addition, every lab test and radiology study required a paper requisition, often unique for each study. A patient coming in for their annual physical would often require 10-12 different requisition slips that needed the patient's name, medical record number, doctor's name and billing code, date, and the desired study filled in on each individual slip. This was all very time-consuming compared to how it is done now electronically.

At that time there were few RNs working in the clinic. Most were concentrated in the Injection Room and Allergy lab; the rest of the various clinics would have one RN, if any at all. Over time we were able to demonstrate the value of using RNs in the clinic to free up physicians from many support functions and phone calls that were necessary to run their practices but could be easily performed by a nurse. Gradually over the years there were more and more nurses added.

I worked in Nephrology for 8 years before transitioning to a new role as the Clinic Nursing Educator in 1980. This position was created to provide oversight of the training and orientation of new OA (office assistant) staff to the clinic. They were taught policies and procedures, how to complete all the forms and paperwork necessary for the day-to-day running of a practice, as well as CPR, sterile technique, etc. A typical class would have 8-10 students and would last 3-4 weeks. Towards the end of the class the student would begin to rotate through various clinics, applying what they had learned and honing their skills. When an opening occurred in one of the offices, the students would be assigned to cover the practice. This provided an opportunity to see if they were a good match for the demands of that particular physician and practice. We jokingly referred to this as the "dating game".

Gradually we moved away from this model and began hiring support staff directly into open positions. During this time we also began to hire RN managers (clinical coordinators) into the individual departments. This provided local management and clinical support, which had been centralized in prior years, and became more important as the clinic began to grow in size. Satellite clinics were coming on board as well. The first administrative nursing directors were added to support the Departments of Medicine and Surgery. Eventually I became the administrative director for the Department of Surgery. I worked closely with the Chiefs of Surgery, including Drs. Jolly, Yarington, and Ryan consecutively during my tenure. I stayed in this role until 1993 when the Medical Center went through one of its many "downsizing" events. The clinic administrator for Surgery and the hospital administrator for Surgery positions were combined into one job. I was given an interim assignment on the newly created Managed Care Task Force.

Health care was in a major transition at this time in the US and it looked like everything was headed toward a managed care model. VM had hired a team of consultants from Arthur Andersen to help assist with this change. They needed some VM staff to work closely with the consultants so they could better understand our current fee-for-service systems and help design new ones that would work in a managed care environment. Having been at VM for over 20 years, I had a good working knowledge of our systems and how they worked in the clinic setting. This was very challenging, and I equated changing physician behavior and expectations to "herding cats".

After 6 months on the Task Force there was a new opportunity to work in General Surgery with Drs. Thirlby and Wechter. I had missed taking care of patients and decided to take advantage of this opening. It turned out to be one of the most rewarding and challenging roles of my career. Neither physician had had a nurse work with them before in their clinic so it was fun to design a new role and look for ways to help care for the population of patients they served. Over time things evolved and eventually, as Dr. Wechter began to focus more and more on breast cancer patients, my role evolved as well, ultimately into that of breast cancer coordinator.

We set up a multidisciplinary clinic that served as a model for other cancer teams and included physicians from Breast Surgery, Radiology, Medical Oncology, Pathology, and Radiation Oncology, making it possible for the patient to see the members of the team in one visit. This made it easier for the physicians to come up with a comprehensive care plan for the patient in a very efficient time frame. This model was very satisfying to both providers and patients. The nurse cancer coordinator was usually the first person the patient contacted once they received a diagnosis of breast cancer. The coordinator was the main person talking to the patient and getting them set up with physician appointments and diagnostic studies necessary to come up with a care plan and to begin treatment. For me professionally, it was a great job, with lots of contact with patients and their families. You had the opportunity to offer clinical and emotional support to them at a time when they often felt overwhelmed and vulnerable. In all, I spent 23 years in the section of General Surgery and 43 years total at VMMC; it was a satisfying career and I retired in Aug. 2015.

The Diabetes Education Center: A Brief Personal Glimpse of the Program and Nursing in Endocrinology during these Years by Nancy Lencioni, ARNP

When I started at VM in 1972 the diabetes classes were already in high gear albeit small in size. The classes were held every week for 5 days in a small room close to the cafeteria. Three meals a day were provided and were used as a teaching tool. The average attendance was around 10-12 patients. **Tippy Hansen, RN,** was the instructor, and **June Holmes** was the dietitian. Both of these women had been there for many years. The doctors were Bob Nielsen, Bob Metz, Bill Steenrod and John Leonard. Classes had been going on for many years. Drs. Nielsen, Steenrod and Crampton (who I never met) were the ones responsible for formalizing the class and turning it into the success it became.

Carolyn Sannar and **Pat Brazel** (later, **Vinje**) were RNs working as office nurses. We all started working in the Endocrine Section within 3 years of each other. When Tippy retired, the physicians decided to use the three of us as teaching nurses for the class. Near the end of the 1970s the Director of Nursing, **Mary Jo Beeman**, set up an in-house formal curriculum to turn about six or seven RNs into "Nurse Clinicians". The Mason Clinic physicians were our instructors for both the classroom and the clinical settings. In the early 1980s, when the nationally-recognized Advanced Registered Nurse Practitioner (ARNP) came into being, we all took the exam and became nurse practitioners.

By this time Mary and Del Buse had donated a large amount of money to VM to create a larger, more efficient classroom setting. Our new setting could accommodate up to 20 patients and family members. The 3 meals a day were taken in the new setting, which was very convenient. We had one session a week from the Psychiatry Section, Physical Medicine and Pharmacy. I think that's when the program gained strength. We had many requests from hospitals around the country to come spend the week with us so they could set up their own programs.

In 1986 the Certified Diabetes Educator (CDE) was established and eventually we became part of it. I think either Pat or Carolyn or both were president of that organization.

Although our patients received excellent medical care and the best information available to live as well as possible with diabetes, I always thought the greatest gift was the knowledge and comfort of knowing they weren't alone. They learned diabetes did not discriminate. They shared stories and they made friends and many of those friendships were long lasting.

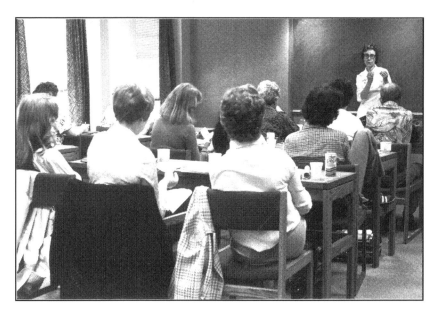

Pat Brazil, RN, teaching a class in the Buse Diabetes Teaching Center, 1979
(PH 1503, VMHA)

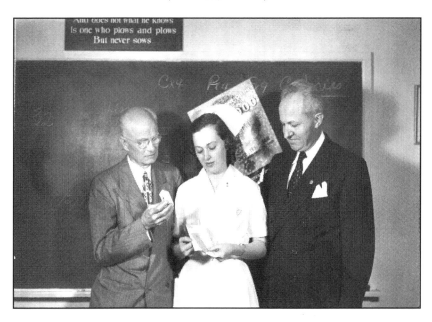

Dr. Lester Palmer (L), President of the Am. Diabetes Assoc. at the time with Nadine Yarwood, student president of the VM School of Nursing, & Art Longre, Executive Director of ER Squibb & Sons, Seattle Division, 1950 (PH 7094, VMHA)

27

The Department of Hospital Services: An Overview

by Joyce Lammert, MD, PhD

The last twenty years have seen dramatic changes in the care of hospitalized patients, fueled by technological advances, cultural shifts and healthcare policy directives.

Technological advances such as laparoscopic surgery, transcatheter aortic valve replacement (TAVR) and video-assisted thoracoscopic surgery (VATS) are just a few examples of advances that have resulted in patient-centered care with excellent outcomes and reduced hospital lengths of stay. Procedures such as hernia repairs, appendectomies, and cholecystectomies are now routinely done as outpatient procedures. Total joint replacements range from same day to a few days of hospitalization.

Changing outpatient care models that incorporate a care team (physician, care nurses, advanced practice providers, pharmacists, behavioral health specialists), have reduced the frequency of medical patients requiring hospitalization, much like the procedural advances for surgery. The result has been a shift in the type of patients cared for in the hospital. They are older, have multiple co-morbid conditions, their surgeries are more complex and their care requires careful coordination across different sections and departments.

In 2000, *To Err is Human* was published by the Institute of Medicine.

It was estimated that about 100,000 people died every year because of medical error in hospitals. The subsequent "100,000 Lives Campaign" set a national agenda to provide safer care by building safer care systems in hospitals. In 2004, Mary McClinton, a patient at Virginia Mason, died because of a medical error while in our care. In addition to the national agenda, it served as a very personal rallying cry for the organization. Over the last 16 years, the Virginia Mason Production System (VMPS) has been used to improve the systems of care in the hospital, with special attention to mistake-proofing and smoothing the patient's journey across the systems of care. With the increasing complexity of care, the hospital has developed additional behavioral health expertise and has added palliative care and bioethics expertise. VMPS has helped the organization focus on the journey of the patient across the acute care continuum (ED, ICU, medical-surgical floors, home).

The leadership at Virginia Mason Medical Center recognized early the value of grouping hospital-related care under one umbrella. In late 2002/early 2003, they named A. James Bender, MD, as Medical Director of Hospital Services, which was a loose group including Critical Care, Emergency Medicine, the Hospitalist Service and initially, Infectious Disease. Over the next four years, Dr. Bender looked for ways to build linkages between these groups to improve inpatient care. Within a few years, Infectious Disease returned to the Department of Medicine, and in 2007, Donna Smith, MD, became the Medical Director for the next six years. During her tenure, inpatient physical medical and rehabilitation (PM&R) and psychiatry were added to the group, and at some point, Critical Care became its own section and PM&R returned to the Medicine Department. Pulmonary Medicine no longer included Critical Care in its title by 2012, although some of its members still worked in the critical care arena.

In 2013, Joyce Lammert, MD, PhD, became the new Executive Medical Director of Hospital Services. In order to assure seamless, coordinated care for the patient across their journey in the hospital, in 2019 the decision was made to form a new department, the Department of Hospital Care Services, and Evan Coates, MD, was named Chief. As one department, hospital goals are shared by ED, ICU, hospitalists and other hospital clinicians. It improves care coordination and communication and helps establish a common direction for the teams. This is in stark contrast to many of the other organizations in the region, where the hospitalists and ED providers are often independent groups who contract with the organization and remain "siloed" in their work. Early data suggest it has already resulted in better care for patients (reduced length of stay and improved satisfaction) and better satisfaction for clinicians.

The following 3 chapters detail the history of these sections: hospital medicine, emergency medicine and critical care medicine. The inpatient psychiatric service is described by Scott Hansen, MD, Section Head of the Inpatient Psychiatry Consultative Service, in the chapter on Psychiatry and Psychology in this volume.

28

Hospital Medicine

by Barry Aaronson, MD, and Dan Hanson, MD,
with contributions from Stephanie Perry, MA

Historically, just as with most physician specialty groups, the hospitalist section was created to fully meet the needs of patients and the providers who serve them. The early vision of the potential role of hospitalists began to become apparent in the 5 to 7 years before the actual founding of the section.

In the early 1990s, physicians at VM were responsible for taking care of their own patients when they were in the hospital. Over time, a call system was arranged, where one physician would cover for their section's patients in the hospital, on a nightly or weekly basis. However, the coverage of unassigned admissions from the Emergency Department (ED) was an ongoing issue, so in 1993 a new process was arranged. The Graduate Medical Education (GME) department wanted to make the role of chief medical resident more appealing, so they increased the salary and asked the chief resident to take unassigned admissions from the ED and be their primary attending. The General Internal Medicine (GIM) providers would still be the primary attending for General Internal Medicine (GIM) patients who already had a primary care provider (PCP) in GIM, but the chief resident would take care of the unassigned and see them in follow up in their clinic. This was all negotiated by **Lance Larsen, MD,** who was recruited to be the chief medical resident for the 1993-94 academic year. Then, in 1994, when **Dan Hanson, MD**, became chief medical resident, he inherited the same process. The volume of unassigned patients became quite high however, and he typically had 6 patients in the hospital that he was caring for at any given time. Most of the patients he was caring for by himself without house staff and he was quite busy. He remembers feeling responsible to make sure it was a financially viable process for VM so that they would be able to continue supporting it.

Dr. Hanson was hired by GIM in July of 1995 - not long after, concerns started to arise about the challenges of being on-call for the GIM provider group. The GIM physician on-call for the week was challenged by the volume of work and in an effort to improve this, there was a trial period where the GIM on-call physician would not have clinic and would round all day covering all patients for the other GIM doctors. John Kirkpatrick, MD, was the first one to give it a try, as he was a big proponent of it. Dr. Hanson was also one of the first doctors to try it. However, the on-call physician could end up rounding on dozens of patients, so it was stopped after only a month.

Coverage reverted to the previous process for the next few years. In 1998, it was widely recognized that the hospitalized patient volumes and complexity were becoming challenging for the internal medicine residency teams and that the alternative staffing plan needed to be revisited. Residency teams continued to care for all non-surgical patients and **Roger Bush, MD**, the new Program Director was working hard to find support for house staff. Through his contacts as a Program Director, he became aware of hospitals around the country hiring internal medicine graduates to work as inpatient-only providers. The term "hospitalist," was not widely known. Dr. Bush then went to one of the first Society of Hospital Medicine conferences in San Francisco and met **Barry Aaronson, MD**, during a break. It happened that Barry was looking for a better job (he was working in Tacoma) and Roger was there to recruit someone to start a hospitalist program.

As with the beginning of any great endeavor, details of the events and personalities involved can provide interesting insights on how the character of individuals, organizational values, commitment, and some luck bring us to where we are today.

Barry's background made him well suited to a hospitalist position. His internal medicine residency at Walter Reed Army Medical Center from 1991-94 had been ward heavy. The wards at the tertiary care hospital were an exciting place to work and represented the breadth of *Harrison's Textbook of Internal Medicine*. Patients were sent there from all over the world for diagnosis and treatment. In contrast, his limited outpatient work had not been a good experience for him. His attraction to inpatient medicine made sense. After completing his residency, he became Chief Resident, which is a highly desirable position in military medicine since the Chief for the most part gets to decide where they want to be assigned at the end of that year, while their cohorts are sent off to undesirable locations. He chose to stay at Walter Reed as a ward attending instead of in clinic, working as a hospitalist before Bob Wachter coined the term "Hospitalist" in the *New England Journal of Medicine* in 1996.

Barry was set to leave the Army in 1997, but wanted to keep doing what he had been doing at Walter Reed as a civilian in Seattle, which was his home before leaving for medical school at George Washington University in 1987. While researching options in Seattle, he heard about the Group Health hospitalist program at Virginia Mason, but was not enthused about working only sporadically with family medicine residents so he decided to stay in the Army as a general internist and took a position at Madigan where he supervised internal medicine residents on the wards. It was not quite Seattle but close enough, he thought. Just as he was about to deploy to Madigan, he received a call from J.D. Fitz, MD, at Tacoma Family Medicine who made him an offer he could not refuse that involved supervising their family medicine residents at Tacoma General Hospital and also working in the internal medicine clinic. He took that position and moved to Tacoma from Washington, DC. Once there he quickly learned that his partners did not like their hospital attending rotation and since he did not enjoy clinic, they came up with the solution of Barry doing all the

410

hospital attending work (i.e. being a teaching hospitalist) while they did his clinic work. In that way, he gained the experience of initiating a hospitalist program and was the first full-time hospitalist at Tacoma General (TG) and Allenmore Hospitals.

About 6 months into his work at Tacoma General (1998) he saw an ad in the newsletter of the brand new National Association of Inpatient Physicians (NAIP) looking for someone to start the hospitalist program at VM. It looked attractive but he did not feel comfortable leaving TG so soon after arriving, so he passed up that opportunity. About 6 months later, at the second national meeting of NAIP (of which he later became a charter member before it changed its name to the Society of Hospital Medicine), he had the good fortune of running into Roger Bush and learned that the VM position was still open. At that point, he had had enough of Tacoma and was ready to make the transition to his original target of Seattle. He accepted the position. Kimberly Bell, MD (a VM residency graduate in 1994) was the other main candidate but she ended up going to Providence Cherry Hill. On the committee to create this new hospitalist service at VM were **Bob Mecklenburg, MD** (Endocrinology, not yet Chief of Medicine), **David Gortner, MD** (GIM Section Head), **John Holmes, MD** (Cardiology Section Head), **Roger Bush, MD** (GIM, Internal Medicine Residency Program Director), and **Jack Brandabur, MD** (GI Section Head).

David Gortner had been running what was called the non-house staff admitting service (NHAS), which was composed mainly of University of Washington locum providers. They worked at night from 10 p.m. to 7 a.m. and the plan was that Barry would take over in the morning for the patients they admitted at night. These patients had previously been going to house staff, but this was causing them to go over their Residency Review Committee work hours' limit, so having him accept these patients allowed the house staff to remain within their limit.

During his interviews, he made it very clear that he wanted to work with the medicine residents and the committee made it very clear that was not what they were hiring him for. They agreed to disagree and moved on to talking about other things. However, his panel size was not large and once the residents and attendings got to know him, some sections (for which rounding with residents was particularly challenging such as GI, Cardiology and GIM) agreed to let him be the attending for their patients on the residency service. In this way they would not have to come in and round on the weekends and would not have to leave their clinic during the day. The primary attitude before this transition, especially from GI, was that there was "no way anyone was going to take over for me as attending." However, shortly after seeing how well the hospitalist model worked, the prevailing attitude changed to "please be the attending for my patients" and from that to "there is no way I'm going to work in clinic and also take care of patients in the hospital." Having Barry as the attending for the residents was seen as a win for the residents too, since he was available throughout the day as opposed to the clinic doctors who were not.

At that time (1999 - 2001), the electronic medical record (EMR) was only a monitoring screen where providers could look up lab results and dictated clinic notes as well as hospital discharge summaries. There were old personal computers at nursing stations - some were on big carts in hallways that took 5 minutes to boot up. The nurses, well trained in saving energy by turning off lights when leaving rooms, dutifully applied that principle to the computers and promptly turned them off as soon as they retrieved what they needed. It took what seemed like forever to train them to leave the computers on so that providers could look up laboratory results as they made rounds.

During that first year there were still some attendings who were concerned that the hospitalist movement was not a good idea - they felt they would be abandoning their patients if they were not the attending and patients would not tolerate it. Barry vividly recalls the great interference Bob Mecklenburg, MD, ran with these attendings (Barry reported to him as he had become Chief of Medicine), so that he could focus on taking care of the patients instead of dealing with the politics. It was due to Bob Mecklenburg's astuteness and interpersonal skills that he was able to successfully expand the service. As it turned out, many patients were being admitted from outside the organization and so did not mind that they had a hospitalist attending because they knew no difference. Many came to know the hospitalists, appreciate their knowledge and skill and came to trust them as well as their regular attendings. This was not universal however, and it would take time to gain their full trust.

Since Barry was the only hospitalist, the hospital was still relying heavily on the NHAS to cover nights, weekends, and his time off, so others were promptly recruited to join him. Barry started Jan. 24, 1999. **Rick Kadera, MD**, who had completed the first hospitalist track residency at Oregon Health Sciences University (OHSU), joined him in May. **Kirk Chang, MD**, joined them when he finished his Chief year in July 1999. **Rich Davis, MD**, joined them in August or September of 2000 after finishing his internal medicine (IM) residency at Virginia Mason. As their capacity grew, so did the demand for their services, leading to the hiring of **Phil Royal, MD** (2000); **Jose Gude, MD** (2001 – 2006) from a hospitalist practice in New Orleans; Jose's friend **Mark Kohmetsher, MD** (2002) from the Franciscans in Tacoma; and **Ed Gacek, MD** (2000 – 2004), who didn't last long because he tried commuting from Port Townsend. Not long after, Barry was very pleased when Dan Hanson came over from the GIM clinic. They had bonded because they had a son born the same day, and had finished residency the same year. Dan saw what they were doing and noticed that they were actually doing more teaching than he was even though he was one of the residency associate program directors at the time. He left GIM and started as a hospitalist in January 2001. Barry also worked hard to get **Mike Ingraham, MD**, to join them from GIM (hired in 1998) because he would often see him rounding on his patients in the hospital, and was very glad when he finally did join later that year.

The first office for the hospitalists was in the Endocrine Section, which was in Lindeman Pavilion on level 2. Once they outgrew that space they were moved to Central Pavilion 11, directly across from the RN station. Once they outgrew that, the patient waiting area on Level 8 was enclosed and converted to an office where they are currently.

In late 2002, **A. James Bender, MD**, was named Medical Director of Hospital Services, which was a loose group including Critical Care, Emer-

413

gency Medicine, the Hospitalist Service and initially, Infectious Disease. As a result, Barry, who was serving as Section Head, began reporting to him instead of Dr. Mecklenburg. The first manager was **Sarah Blackwood**. After she retired to roam the country in her RV, **Val Ferris, RN,** took over.

During Barry's tenure, he started the Pacific Northwest chapter of the Society of Hospital Medicine (SHM) along with Kim Bell, MD, from Providence. They had monthly meetings in the Columbia Tower. During that time, he also gave the annual lecture at SHM on the topic of hand-held computers in medicine. There were not many options at that time (palm pilots, Psion, eventually pocket PC). He was also in the first cohort of SHM Fellows in Hospital Medicine and then in the first cohort of Senior Fellows in Hospital Medicine.

The hospitalists were the first to use Cerner for documentation. This was before computerized physician order entry (CPOE). They still had to print out the notes and put them in the chart, but at least they were legible and carried over important information from prior hospital days.

As Section Head, he continued to pursue his vision of making the hospitalist service a teaching service. During those first years, the residents had attending teaching rounds in the morning a few times per week. These were traditionally led by subspecialists. However, the hospitalists quickly got their nose under that tent too and before long were doing many of those sessions. They then realized that since it was their own teams that they were teaching, and that those same team members were with them all day, they could stop cutting into critical morning rounding time and work towards incorporating teaching into the rounding process. Rick started to work on a curriculum for the residents and **Jen Ashley, MD**, took that over once Rick left in 2006.

As soon as Rick joined Barry, they set the schedule as a one-week-on and one-week-off schedule. This has not changed since 1999. However, the total number of required weeks of work per year has decreased from 25 to 23. As they grew, they replaced locums at night with full-time hospitalists. They still needed locums in the afternoons to work the swing shift and help with admits. Ironically, since about 2002, they have started to look forward to the day, which they thought would come very soon, where staffing needs would be stable and matched to patient care needs. As of 2017, they were still growing and having that same conversation.

Barry remained Section Head until September 2003 when, during a day sail on Jim's boat with Val, he told them that he and his wife had decided to move to Italy for a year. Dan Hanson was chosen as his replacement and Barry was happy to know that the service he had grown from scratch would be in his very capable hands.

After Dan became section head in 2003, **Tom Gunby, MD** (hired at VM in 1985), starting asking questions about transferring over from GIM; Roger Bush, MD (1984 - 2013) made the move in about 2005 and both were stellar additions to the program as Tom was an Associate Program Director for IM and Roger was the IM Program Director. This helped balance the focus of the IM residency program to support teaching in the hospital, which has always been the largest portion of IM training. Other early additions to the team included **Alvin Calderon, MD, PhD** (2003 to present); **Mia Lee, MD** (2003 – 2015); and **Kathryn Kovacs, MD** (2005 to present). **Donna Smith, MD**, was promoted from ED Section Head to Hospital Medical Director in 2007. Though VM had completely implemented Cerner systems as its electronic medical record system (EMR) around 2002, it did not have computer physician order entry (CPOE) until 2005. This was very challenging to implement as Virginia Mason was one of the earliest adopters of CPOE, unlike other medical centers that delayed or abandoned CPOE. However, Virginia Mason successfully persevered due to its focus on safety and quality as an overriding value, and made the adjustments necessary for full implementation. The hospitalists were eager participants who were deeply involved in implementation and without whom, especially Barry Aaronson, it would not have happened.

As time went on and the popularity of the service grew, increasingly specialists, house staff and Graduate Medical Education saw the opportunity to have hospitalists be the attending-of-record and round with the house staff as part of the team. The hospitalists supported this enthusiastically as they saw it as a validation of their expertise in inpatient medicine and valued the teaching role. When they took over in 2003-04, however, it was immediately clear that they had bitten off more than they could comfortably manage, as they were challenged with the work volume. They were so enthusiastic to teach that rounding went on way too long. At one point, they had to ask specialists to take over care of some of their patients, which ironically created stresses for the specialists who had adjusted their work schedules to focus on outpatient care and were heavily dependent on the hospitalist service. This led, eventually, to growing the team. Between 2003 - 2008, more than 20 hospitalists were hired and the team grew to 16 after some natural attrition. Patients became accustomed to having hospitalists involved in their care and came to appreciate their expertise, even as the transitions in and out of the hospital became more challenging as PCPs were no longer coming into the hospital.

As the first five to seven years progressed, the hospitalist service was clearly transitioning from a provider group that was born out of necessity, struggling to maintain adequate staffing and self-identity, to one that was integral to operations, valued as teachers and necessary for improving quality and safety in the hospital. The team was maturing as clinicians, and just as other hospitalist programs nationwide, was developing their own sense of professionalism.

Michael Ingraham, MD, served as section head from 2008 - 2013, and during this time the Nocturnist program was developed. **Alvin Calderon, MD**, became Director of the internal medicine residency in 2008 and **Val Ferris, RN** served as the manager of hospital medicine from 2005 - 2007. **Cindy Davis, RN** was manager after her, followed by **Sharlene Hanlon** from 2010 - 2016. During Michael's tenure, efforts were made to implement physician extenders, such as Advanced Registered Nurse Practitioners (ARNPs). This was challenging though, as there were very few graduate nurses with hospital experience and no training programs. The section was not prepared to train physician extenders at that time, so early efforts came in fits and starts. It was a good experience to help understand, eventually, that a training program was necessary.

Evan Coates, MD (hired in 2006), became Section Head in 2013, just shortly after **Joyce Lammert, MD, PhD**, became Executive Medicine Director of the Hospital. Many big changes were implemented including moving to a daily admission process for the house staff teams, development of a new section of Hospital Medicine mission statement - "We make the Hospital Work for the Patient." The program moved forward on full implementation of geographic teams and instituted flow coordinators in 2014. These coordinators are instrumental in managing the flow of admissions and minimizing disruptions during the day. The first flow coordinator was **Aimee Vo** (2014 - 2018), followed by **Brooks Gatzemeier** (2015 - present) and **Sukhmani Gill** (2018 - present).

In 2019, as noted in the overview of Hospital Services (see chapter 27 in this volume), the decision was made to form a new department, the Department of Hospital Care Services, to improves care coordination and communication and help establish a common direction for the teams. Dr. Coates was chosen as the new Chief of Hospital Services, and Dr. Lammert stepped back to concentrate on her role as Medical Director of Physician and APP Recruitment, Development and Services.

With regards to teaching, members have been residency Program Directors, Associate Program Directors (Roger Bush, Alvin Calderon**, Brandee Grooms**), IM Teachers of the year and University of Washington School of Medicine liaisons. Many physicians in the section have led important organizational clinical quality improvement initiatives that have been recognized nationally, including sepsis (Evan Coates), heart failure, venous thrombosis prophylaxis (Rich Davis, Barry Aaronson), anticoagulation and diabetes (**Therese Franco, MD**). Several have also served as Kaizen Fellows and become Kaizen-Certified Leaders as the Virginia Mason Production System was embraced in their daily work. Barry Aaronson remains as a staff hospitalist in addition to his duties as Chief Medical Informatics Officer.

Through these efforts, the section has become key to the consistent recognition of the hospital, by many measures, as one of the best in the nation.

Stephanie Perry, MA, SFHM, became Director of Hospital Medicine Services in 2016 and is serving in that role at present (as of March

2019). She was hired as a conduit for all hospital-based services (critical care, hospitalists, neuro-hospitalists and psychiatry) and helped grow the team from 27 clinicians to 48 in a 2-year time frame (a 77% increase). **Patricia Vinson, MHA,** was hired in 2018 as Supervisor of Hospital Medicine to help manage this rapidly growing section.

In 2016, the section launched an Advanced Practice Provider Fellowship in Hospital Medicine. Therese Franco, MD, was tapped as the first director. This is one of only 8 programs in the country and has now produced 3 successful graduating classes, with a fourth that will finish in June 2019. This is the only such fellowship in the Pacific Northwest, and is run in partnership with Seattle University (the Nurse Practitioner program) and the UW (Certified Physician Assistant - PA-C program).

Another important member of the team is the administrative assistant. This role was filled by **Joanna Cornelius** from 2014 - 2016, **Anna Hazen** from 2016 - 2017 and **Monica Arreola** from 2017 - present.

Currently (as of March 2019), there are 43 physician hospitalists on staff, as well as 4 ARNP's and one PA-C. In addition to Drs. Aaronson, Hanson, Ingraham, Davis, Gunby, Calderon, Lee, Kovacs and Coates, they include the following individuals with the year of their arrival at VM:

Katherine J. Adler, MD	2008
Jordan D. Becerril, MD	2018
John P. Biebelhausen, MD, MBA	2014
Kelsey A. Brauer, DNP, ARNP	2018
Tina A. Chang, MD	2011
T.J. Cuff, MD	2017
Sandra M. Demars, MD,	2019
Jaspreet Dhami, MD	2017
Hannah J. Doss, DNP, ARNP	2018
Geetha Easwaran, MD	2009
Kevin D. Finch, MD	2017
Matthew Fitzpatrick, MD	2016
Therese Franco, MD, SFHM	2009
Marta Gorczyca, MD	2016

Brandee Grooms, MD	2007
Tonya M. Henninger, MD	2008
Sarah A. Hutchens, ARNP	2017
Angela Johnston, ARNP	2016
Shivani Kalu, MD	2017
Suheir Khajuria, MD, MPH	2016
Sara W. Kilkenny, DNP, ARNP	2017
Courtney D. Kraseski, MD	2019
Richard R. Kronfol, MD	2018
Timothy J. Lee, MD	2011
Ashleigh Leonard, MD	2017
Stephen A. Lopez, MD	2011
Christopher L. Lucas, MD	2018
Carly R. Magnusson, MD	2018
Joseph H. Parker, DO	2010
Ritu Piplani, MD	2017
Matthew S. Powell, MD	2015
Matthew M. Query, MD	2012
Elaine F. Sachter, MD	(1989 in GIM)
Jennifer Thompson, MD	2009
Richard Torres Jr., PharmD, PA-C	2017
Ashok Venugopal, MD	2017
Dennis Whang, MD	2017
Jamie Wong, MD	2014
Manu Yadav, MD	2018

In addition, there are 4 critical care physicians: Phil Royal, MD (2000); **Aneal S. Gadgil, MD** (2008); **Hashim Mehter, MD** (2014); and **Blake Mann, MD** (2012) along with anesthesiologist and Critical Care Section Head, **Eliot Fagley, MD** (2013 - present; Section Head 2018 - present); and 2 inpatient psychiatrists: **Scott Hansen, MD** (2012), and **Jay Owens, MD** (2019); **Karina Uldall, MD, MPH** (2011-2019) was important in developing some of this inpatient psychiatric work during her tenure aas well. Over the years, there have been many others who have served for varying periods of time as hospitalists, including physicians hired by Group Health and Pacific Medical Center. Some notable hospitalists include:

Erica S. Pascarelli, MD: Erica was a top-notch Virginia Mason residency graduate who joined the hospitalist team but left a few years later to be at home with her growing family.

Joshua T. Calvert, MD: Josh did his residency at Virginia Mason and worked as a hospitalist for one year before moving back to Oklahoma.

Janet C. King, MD: Janet did her training at UW before joining the hospitalist team. She went back to UW after a year at Virginia Mason to do a GI fellowship.

Alexandra M. Morrison, MD: Randy came to Virginia Mason in September 2004, and worked as a hospitalist for many years before moving to Harborview Medical Center in August 2015.

Amal L. Puswella, MD: Amal also graduated from the Virginia Mason residency program and worked as a hospitalist for almost 2 years before returning to California.

Mark G. Ochenrider, MD: Mark was a Virginia Mason residency graduate who worked nights in the CCU part-time for a few years while growing a primary care practice on the Eastside.

Wayne Strauss, MD: Wayne was another top-notch graduate of the Virginia Mason residency program, who left after one year to pursue a critical care fellowship.

Jennifer Ashley, MD: Jennifer did an excellent job in her residency at Virginia Mason and then joined the hospitalist team before moving first to Swedish Medical Center and then Bend, OR.

Megan McGilvray, ARNP: Megan was the first Nurse Practitioner on the hospitalist team. She was instrumental in helping us start to look at the success of geographic-based teams with her work on the observation unit. She moved closer to family in Maryland in 2017.

Janet Nagaminee, MD: Janet did her residency at Virginia Mason and left for a leadership position at Kaiser in California.

420

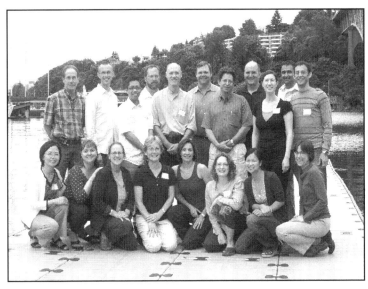

Freemont Rowing Center, Hospitalist Retreat, 2005
Back, L to R: Tom Gunby, Evan Coates, Alvin Caldaron, Roger Bush, Richard Davis, Michael Ingraham, Barry Aaronson, Dan Hanson, Brandee Grooms, Parag Nene, Seth Krevat
Front row, L to R: Mia Lee, Diane our manager, Kate Kovacs, Donna Smith, Randi Morrison, Katherine Alder, Theresa Tran, Tonya Henninger

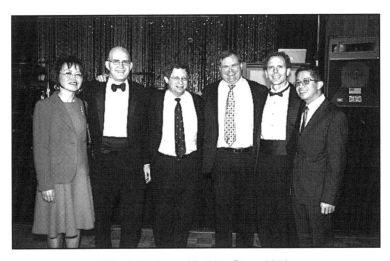

Virginia Mason Holiday Party 2012
L to R: Mia Lee, Dan Hanson, Barry Aaronson, Michael Ingraham, Tim Lee, Alvin Calderon

29

Emergency Medicine

by G. Ted Johnson, MD,
with contributions from Julianna Yu, MD

The practice of Emergency Medicine is all about the space in which it happens, and the history of Emergency Services at VM is inextricably tied to the 3 configurations that it has occupied over the past 40 years. For that reason, I will be spending a lot of time describing floor plans. I apologize in advance for any resulting boredom. I wish I could have included computerized diagrams, but my skills are not that advanced. At 65, I qualify as an old guy, vis–à–vis computers.

Everything I know about the Emergency Room (ER) at VM before 1975 is hearsay, because that's when I came to VM as a first year resident –in the parlance of the day, a flexible intern. (Ironically, I was anything but flexible.) At that time, the ER space was new and located in what is now the Central Pavilion, but was then called the East Wing. Its entrance was on the south side of the building, 2nd floor, at the intersection of Spring St. and Terry Avenue. It was the result of an addition to the East Wing, completed the year before, that interrupted Terry between Spring and Seneca. (Previously the East Wing had spanned Terry Avenue.) Opposing it on the north side of the building was the new hospital lobby, still present today.

Just prior to that, the ER had been located next to Radiology in the original clinic building (at that time called the Main Building), and before

423

that, the first ER had also been in the Main Building. It was entered from the outside by a door on the east side of the building near the corner of Spring and Terry. It consisted of two rooms and was staffed solely by nurses who, depending on the patients presenting, called for help from the residents and clinic staff physicians.

When I arrived in June 1975, the new ER was staffed by two attending physicians: **Scott Linscott, MD,** Section Head, and **Bruce Stevenson, MD**, both internists. Both were relative newcomers to VM, with Dr. Linscott hired in 1974 and Dr. Stevenson in 1975. (Emergency Medicine did not exist as a specialty at that time. Major trauma had already been centralized to Harborview and most of the critical patients presenting to the VM ER were medical, not surgical – thus, the hiring of internists.) One of these attendings was present for about 15 hours of each day–from 7 a.m. to 10 p.m., 9 a.m. to midnight, or some other variation of their choosing. Two interns were assigned to the ER for a four–week rotation and each did alternating 24–hour shifts. For 15 hours of the shift, they were supervised and taught by Dr. Linscott or Dr. Stevenson. For the 9 hours of the night, interns were there alone to deliver care independently. They were required to call the Medicine R2 for any chest pain and the Surgery R2 for any belly pain, but other than that, they had to do what they thought best, calling for specialty attending help – ENT, Neurology, Ortho, GYN, etc. – as needed. I remember it as being terrifying.

Patients entered at Spring and Terry. Immediately in front of them was the check–in desk. During windy weather, leaves blown in through the doors would accumulate at the foot of the counter. The secretary took the information while also fielding questions from hospital and clinic visitors entering though the same doors. Sometimes the patient needed to shout their complaint to be heard over the din. Confidentiality was not an option. (This was in the days before HIPPA.)

This check–in area was also the ambulance entrance to the ED. Generally patients who arrived by ambulance were directed to Room 7, which held 3 beds labeled A, B and C, separated by curtains. This was our "Trauma Bay" and critical care area, but in truth, Bed C was up against a wall and not conducive to any procedure involving more than one thin caregiver. If we could predict a catastrophic event, Room 7 is where we conducted Codes. As one might guess, there were six other rooms. Rooms 1, 2, and 3 were small and had standard doctors' office tables with two drawers on the end holding supplies and a third "drawer" at the bottom that pulled out to be a step patients used for mounting the table. There was also an extension that could be used to support the feet once the patient was lying down and foldaway stirrups for use during pelvic exams. These tables were practical for short visits, but quickly grew uncomfortable for longer stays involving IV fluids or surgical evaluations. They also lacked side rails to prevent the falls that occasionally occurred. Room 4 was the procedure room, used primarily for repairing lacerations, incising abscesses and stopping nosebleeds. For these purposes, it was large enough to accommodate a stretcher and had an overhead procedure lamp. All suture supplies lived in that room. Room 5 was a general treatment room with a stretcher – at least it was until a suicidal patient in Room 6 strangled herself with oxygen tubing that she found there. Subsequently, Room 5 was remodeled to be the "Psych Room", outfitted with a video monitor, locks on the cabinets and drawers, and a retractable garage door to cover the wall that contained gases, suction and monitoring equipment. Room 6 was smaller than Room 5 and designated as the "Orthopaedic Room". All casting supplies and the cast cutter were stored there, and, until fiberglass cast material was developed, the floor frequently showed streaks of plaster dust. In the corner between Rooms 6 and 7 there was an X–ray suite into which patients with traumatic hip pain were delivered directly by the ambulance crew. In 1975, CT scans were sort of new (VM had the first CT scanner in the Northwest, an EMI head scanner installed in 1974) and certainly were not a routine tool in the evaluation of the emergently ill. If one managed to arrange a CT scan for an ER patient, it had to be done downstairs in the Radiology Department.

The seven rooms and X–ray were arranged on a wide U–shaped hallway, with large double doors at either end to discourage but not prevent the public from entering the treatment areas. The reception desk facing

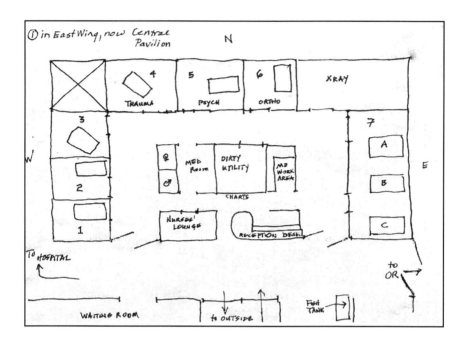

The Emergency Department at Virginia Mason 1975 - 1996

the doors to the outside closed the U. Contained in the center of the U were two tiny bathrooms, a med room, a dirty utility room, and a minute workspace for the docs. This tiny space accommodated two seated people at a counter, two phones, several rows of overhead shelves lined with reference books and four light boxes for X–ray interpretation with slots for film folder storage below them. There were, of course, no computers to clutter the counters, which were instead usually piled high with thick patient clinic charts in tattered manila folders that came from offsite storage facilities several hours after they were requested. (One pulmonologist, Gene Pardee, MD, was famous for marking important notes in the chart with a wooden tongue depressor–like a bookmark. Sometimes there were 10 or more of them.) There was a miniature nurses' lounge, approximately 5x7 feet, which sat three people in straight back chairs, but often accommodated several more standing or sitting on laps. That's where nurses lived when they were not in patient rooms. The coffee pot was perpetually "on" there and attracted one orthopaedic hand surgeon, Bob Stack, MD, who regu-

426

larly spent 30 minutes every morning drinking our very bad coffee, and talking with the nurses. On the wall behind reception, which also was the connecting hallway between the docs' area and the nurses' lounge, there were hooks for nine clipboard charts: Rooms 1–6 and 7A, B, and C. There was a slot for new charts and that's how we kept track of patient flow. A chart on the desk at one end of reception meant there were new orders. When the chart wasn't in play, it was hung back on the wall. All charting was done on paper, lab results were received by phone, and formal radiology interpretations were done the next day.

To the left, after entering the building and on the other side of the hall from the reception desk, there was a carpeted waiting room with upholstered chairs in several seating areas, and a window to the outside. Families passed the time there ordering take-out food and watching TV. Ironically, when the show "ER" was new in the early 90s, on several occasions I had trouble capturing the attention of a patient's family away from the show so that they could participate in their own "ER" drama. (When asked, "Which doctor on the show are you?" I replied, "The one who *doesn't* have sex with his coworkers.") There were no bathrooms for the waiting families or the public, but most of them quickly learned to push on through the double doors into the treatment area and compete with open–gowned patients holding rolling IV poles, and harried doctors and nurses, for the two toilets across from Rooms 1, 2, and 3.

In 1977, a third attending, **John Verrilli, MD**, was hired and attending physician coverage of the ED was extended to 17 hours/day. Nights remained staffed by the intern/resident team. Sometime before I finished my residency in 1979, John decided to leave the ER for an internal medicine office practice and I was offered the position. Unsure of what I wanted to do, I promised them two years. Scott Linscott left soon after I started and **Jacob Heller, MD** (1980) filled his spot. Bruce Stevenson became Section Head and remained so for many years. Soon we added another position. Physicians from those years included: **Carter Hill, MD** (1981– he trained in internal medicine with me at VM), **Bernard (Biff) Fouke, MD, Kevin O'Keefe, MD,** and eventually **David Frank, MD** (1988), another VM internal medicine graduate. It was around this time that the ED night shifts were identified as a major stressor for the young, inexperienced R1 residents who covered the ED as well as their other duties. As a result, we added yet another staff member to work overnight shifts. **Karen Early, MD (Karen Tom** after she married) had the longest tenure in that position.

This physical arrangement served more or less for about 20 years. When the hospital banned smoking inside, patients and staff (including a cardiovascular surgeon) used the ER doors to exit the building and smoke while standing on the sidewalks off the ambulance bay. We added locks to the two double doors leading to the clinical space, preventing people from wandering into treatment rooms and also limiting access to the bathrooms to just patients and staff. We created a small office for the new position of ER administrative director, which was in an unused corner just to the right as one entered from the outside. Later, the director moved to an office in the lower level of the Inn and that corner held a fish tank and a small play area for children. Otherwise, there weren't many changes until …

In the mid 90s, VM and Group Health (GH) formed an Alliance. As a result, GH closed their Capitol Hill hospital and Emergency Department, and all those patients came to our ER for their health crises. If Group Health patients needed hospitalization, they were hospitalized at VM. Prior to that event, plans had been underway for a completely new ED, which would have been expansive and most likely would have occupied the space now housing Hyperbaric Medicine. Architectural plans were underway and many of the ED personnel were intimately involved. However, in September of 1996, the timeline for the Alliance was moved up to December of that year, and the "new" ED plans were abandoned – it wouldn't be until 2011 that the badly needed upgrade would be finally completed.

The scramble to accommodate the increased number of patients and physicians coming to the ED as a result of the Alliance led to the use of ICU South in combination with the "old" ED, which was relabeled ED East. Previously, ICU South had been the southern half of 2 Main. It was in the original VM building. During my residency, it had been the Urology floor, housing lots of older men with catheters in four bed wards. (During my internship, I remember kneeling next to a bed in such a ward, watching the sun rise and crying in frustration because I was repeatedly unsuccessful in obtaining an arterial blood gas sample from a demented octogenarian who continuously yelled, "Help me, Jesus" through all of my attempts.) When 2 Main was converted to an ICU, cardiac monitoring was added in all the rooms and video monitoring was installed in the rooms not directly visible from the nursing station.

The space was a very long hallway running roughly north/south and entered from the outside through double doors approximately midpoint on the east side of the hall. There was an ambulance bay large enough for one stretcher just outside those doors and from there, another set of doors to the outside. We still accumulated leaves and other debris from the outside when the wind was blowing and any patient boarded in that part of the hallway got an icy blast of wind whenever the doors opened in the winter. At the center of the north end of the hall was another set of double doors that led into the hospital, just outside the surgical suites and across the hall from one of the newly configured ICUs.

For our needs, the nursing station at the northeast end of the space was modified to just barely allow 2 providers, a resident, several nurses and a Health Unit Coordinator (a.k.a. HUC or secretary). A small adjacent room on one side of the work area was initially intended for consultants or visiting surgical teams but when X–rays were first digitized, the space was needed for X–ray viewing. On the other side of the workspace, moving south, there was a tiny bathroom, then the med room and dirty utility room. Next to that was the "nurses' lounge", which also had a door opening onto another hallway that led to the ambulance bay and to the previous ED space and waiting room. The lounge contained a refrigerator–always full of decaying sack lunches–and later a microwave that was frequently broken and always densely encrusted with food spills. Still moving south, the entrance hall to the ED was next and then another patient room, which was designated "GYN". (I once delivered a baby there, or more correctly, the mother delivered the baby and I caught it.) Then there

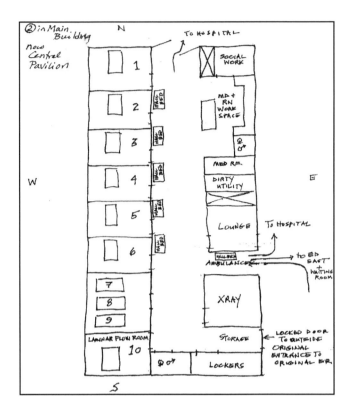

The Emergency Department at Virginia Mason 1996 - 2011

was a small workspace, which rapidly became cluttered with rolling IV poles, wheelchairs and both current and outdated equipment. Next to that was an emergency exit to the outside. Ironically, I believe it had originally been the entrance to the first Emergency Room when the building opened in 1920. Finally, at the southernmost end of the east side of the main hall, there a very small locker/coat room where staff hurriedly changed into scrubs, hoping not to be seen through the window in the door, or be interrupted by another staff member entering what was essentially a large closet. (At change of shift, when several staff were pressed for time, 2 or more people would be changing simultaneously, which could have its awkward moments.) At the south end of the actual hallway, facing the double doors to the hospital at the north end was our other bathroom. Neither of the bathrooms were wheelchair–accessible.

On the west side of the hall we had 6 single rooms starting with Room 1 at the north end. The very long hallway configuration dictated that the most acutely ill and unstable patients be placed in rooms 1, 2, or 3, closest to and across from the work station. When someone in one of the more distant rooms became sicker, patients had to be shifted. (One advantage of the very long hall was that, on *very* quiet night shifts, it allowed us to bowl using empty urinals as pins.) The seventh room housed beds 7, 8, and 9 in close proximity and separated by curtains. Yelling questions about bowel movements to the elderly hearing-impaired insured that everyone in the room was privy to the interview. Questions about sexual history and STDs were routinely whispered. Room 10 at the far south end of the hall was an isolation room with laminar flow.

Initially, patients needing X–rays were taken through several doors to the X–ray suite in the previous emergency space now referred to as ED East. That area had been repurposed as an Urgent Care facility also staffed by the ED team, initially by physician assistants and later, as the acuity of the patient population grew, by an MD/DO. With growing volumes, it became too time consuming to transport all those patients to X–ray and the GYN room on ED West was sacrificed for an additional X–ray suite. Patients could be taken to either of the 2 suites, making it challenging at times to know where your patient actually was. CT scans were still done one floor down in Main Radiology. (VM's first MRI was in a small building across the street from the hospital. On the rare occasions in those days that we ordered an MRI on an ED patient, we would need to call an ambulance to transport them there and back.)

Among the GH physicians who joined us at the onset were: **Neil Waddington, MD; Dorothy Lennard, MD; Roy Farrell, MD; Eli Dayton, MD; John Walters, MD; Keith Leyden, MD**, and **Tom Kinane, MD**. Coming later were **Julie McCormick, MD; Doug Migden, MD; Paul Dutky, MD; Tom Bohannen, MD; Patti Purpura, MD**, and **Joel Wasserman, MD**.

Initially, the vision was that VM ED docs would take care of VM patients and GH ED docs would do the same for their patient population. From 7 a.m. to midnight, there were 2 providers – one from GH and one from VM. Very quickly, however, it became apparent that we couldn't divide the patients along institutional lines. Patients didn't present in a balanced fashion so that sometimes the GH provider was slammed while the VM provider was underutilized and vice versa. Plus, the lower patient volume at night justified only one doctor, either GH or VM. So the standard practice changed to alternating an even distribution of patients as they presented. Difficulties arose as GH continued to demand that the ED provider write admitting orders and a history and physical on their admitted patients. That had been the standard at GH, but was not the standard at VM. The VM ED providers balked at writing orders that were supposed to cover the first 24 hours of a hospital stay, citing their professional organization's opinion that doing so was both a safety and liability risk. Compromises were made and the concept of bare bones admission orders emerged. They were, and still are called transition orders. Other differences in practice were encountered and negotiated. While in the ED, GH and VM patients were cared for in similar fashions though we called different consultants for their specialty problems and consultations. Somewhere along the line, Pacific Medical Center closed their hospital on Beacon Hill (the old Public Health Hospital) and brought their patients to us. Pac Med hospitalists joined the teams in the hospital, but no Pac Med ED docs joined us in the ED.

At the beginning of GH's second ten-year contract, VM stipulated that it wanted to employ all of the ED providers and GH acquiesced. I think they had gradually gained confidence that they could get what they expected from VM ED providers and didn't need to have control over their own ED staff. All of the current GH providers were offered positions, but many declined. New providers were hired to fill the empty spots. Staffing levels remained the same. Among the providers during this time were: **Al Johnson, MD** (1996); **Susan Egaas, MD; Ernie Franz, MD; Eric Mailman, MD; Sarah Dick, MD; Joanna Garritano, MD; Sydney Schneidman, MD; Janda Stevens, MD; Zao Nguyen, MD; Melissa Gagrica, MD; Lori Starke, MD; Julianna Yu, MD** (2008) and briefly,

Angela Heithaus, MD. Later **Chris Moore, MD** (2000); **Jay Bohonos, MD**, and **Josh Michael, MD**, covered nights in a rotating schedule. PAs were added to staff Urgent Care and to work nights alongside one physician. They included: **Susan Weissman, PA–C; Tom Catalina, PA–C; Ross Klein, PA–C; Laurie Merlino, PA–C; Megan Stroud, PA–C; Catherine Del Secco, PA–C; Valerie Quest, PA–C; Marilyn Wyse, PA–C; Mahmood Kakar, PA–C,** and **Christy Moore, PA–C**. In addition, most of our current staff physicians were hired during our tenure in ED West.

Patient volume continued to gradually grow, along with an increase in patient complexity. Hospital beds were often full and admitted patients had to board in the ED, taking spaces needed for incoming patients from outside. It became routine to fill all of our rooms on both the East and West sides, as well as 6 beds in the long hall of ED West and still have a full waiting room and ambulances lined up hoping to offload patients. In times of extreme volume surge, VM, as well as other EDs in the city, began to occasionally divert ambulances. This practice became increasingly common and began to represent a crisis in access. There were many times when all area hospitals were on "divert" (at which time medics would declare that nobody was on divert). Eventually, King County proposed a "No Divert Policy" and VM signed on and agreed to follow this county-wide agreement. Crowding in the ED only became worse as the numbers of homeless and drug–addicted patients increased. We added social work (MSW) coverage to better address the mental health and social needs of these patients, but only during business hours Monday through Friday, which were generally not the hours in which the homeless, psychotic and intoxicated presented for care. The MSW took over the X–ray read room since X–rays were now on the computers that, by this time, crowded our desks. Those same computers eventually, with the advent of the electronic medical record, made paper clinic charts obsolete, allowed us to access GH and Pac Med computerized records, and dragged us into CPOE–computerized physician order entry. Initially, it was a huge headache and slowed us down, but now, if the computer system crashes, writing an order on paper and handing it to the secretary feels like a return to the Stone Age. Gradually, we shifted our documentation to dictation, though how the transcriptionists could hear us over the general din at the overcrowded workstation, I'll never understand.

Meanwhile, a new building to the east of the main hospital was being planned on the site of 2 apartment buildings long owned by VM and scheduled for demolition. A new ED facility was to be included. Its design was based on a model of practicing Emergency Medicine that was controversial within the section but supported by administration.

The plan was called SORT and was built on the idea that about 30% of patients presenting to the ED could quickly be identified as needing admission to the hospital. If those patients were stable, it followed that they could be sent directly to a hospital bed. Once there, they were to be immediately greeted by a hospitalist, who would then proceed with evaluation and treatment in a rapid fashion. The midday provider in the ED was labeled the "SORT doctor" and was responsible for identifying those patients – sorting them – and also caring for ambulatory or "fast track" cases. A small portion of the waiting room was carved out for 2 Triage Rooms where ambulatory patients were interviewed and very quick, simple cases were treated. This location also provided rapid access to the patients coming in by ambulance. The SORT doc would see the patient on the ambulance stretcher and then either send them directly upstairs to a hospital bed or into an ED room for further evaluation, stabilization and treatment. The theoretical benefits of this model included shorter ED stays, decreased ED crowding and improved patient satisfaction. In trials however, this plan didn't prove feasible for reasons including hospital bed availability, hospitalist staffing and practice patterns, and an overestimation of the actual number of patients who were stable enough to be in this category. But by the time this was realized and in anticipation of achieving the theoretical benefits of the plan, construction of the new ED was underway and thus the current ED has fewer beds overall, a smaller waiting room, and a separate four bed area originally designated for SORT, but never used for that purpose. It opened in October of 2011, in the new

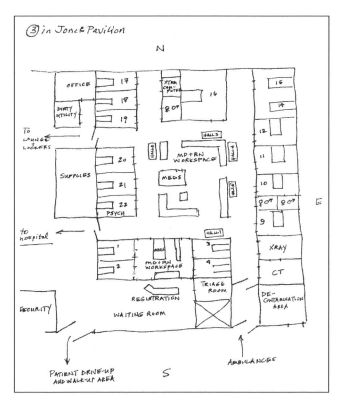

The Emergency Department at Virginia Mason 2011 - present

Jones Pavilion along Boren Avenue between Spring Street and Seneca.

The current ED in the Jones Pavilion is vast. Sometimes I think it has its own weather patterns. It occupies the entire Level 7 of that building. A few words at this point about floor numbering: Since the medical center is built on a hill which falls away in two directions from its high point at the corner of Boren and Spring and is composed of several buildings, labeling the levels so that they are consistent has been a challenge. Level 1 is on the 9th Street side of the campus. Everything flows uphill from there, skipping the occasional number in order to make it work out. (For example, there is no Level 4 in the Lindeman Pavilion.) Hence ground level entry to the ED is Level 7 of the Jones Pavilion. There is a large ambulance/car drive–through area in the southeast corner. It must be entered from Spring Street. Ambulances exit onto Boren and cars exit back onto Spring Street.

Through a vestibule, in which the ambulance crew can find coffee and some counter space for their charting, a long hall leads north past X–ray and CT on the right, to the charge nurse stationed in the southeast corner of the big room. (This hallway is so long that we no longer see any leaves blown in from the outside.) Admitting staff who do registration sit adjacent to the charge nurse. From there, crews are directed to a specific room, or, for direct admits, to the left (west) through electronic doors that give onto banks of elevators for the Jones Pavilion above us, or to the Central Pavilion, level 7. Our connections to the Central Pavilion (previously the East Wing of the hospital) are several and not necessarily intuitive. Two of the quickest routes to the cafeteria and coffee bar involve going outside.

The waiting room is entered from the ambulance bay as well. It is narrow and has no windows. There is a small desk for triage and another for registration. A small "consult room" opens off the back corner and, in times of high volume, is used for drawing blood and starting evaluations on patients in the waiting area who cannot as yet be roomed. From the waiting room, double doors open to what was originally intended to be the "Fast track/SORT" area. It is a rectangle, commonly called the Blue Zone, with Rooms 1–4, two at either end, and a workstation and medication station in the center. The three daytime providers are labeled Red, Yellow and Blue. For a while after the SORT plan didn't work, we experimented with the Blue doc being confined to Rooms 1–4 and only seeing low acuity patients. The goal was to reduce those patients' wait times. The volume of that type of patient, however, was never great enough to fully utilize one provider and the other two providers were frequently overwhelmed with more acute patients causing them to have longer waits and stays. As a result, we returned to a system in which patients are assigned to the providers in rotation with no consideration of the acuity of their illness. Now any of the providers can have a patient in Rooms 1–4, but the name "Blue Zone" stuck.

Through another set of double doors off the Blue Zone, one enters the main clinical area of the ED. It is a large rectangle with rooms arranged around the outer rim and the work area in the middle. Starting in the southeast corner where the ambulances enter, the rooms are labeled 9 through 12. In the northeast corner is the only double room, containing Beds 14 and 15. (The missing numbers 5–8 are X–ray suites, which apparently are required to have numbers. The absence of Room 13 is an obvious nod to superstition, which seems consistent throughout the Medical Center. In no building is there a level 13.) Room 16 occupies the north end of the ED, along with bench seats at the ends of the two north–south hallways. In the northwest corner is Room 17 and continuing south from there, Rooms 18–22. Room 22 was designed as a psychiatric room and it's always the first room used for that purpose, but we frequently have to rapidly configure up to three to four additional rooms for psychiatric safety. Between Rooms 19 and 20, double doors lead to a hallway off of which are situated a small cluster of administrative offices, a dirty utility room, a wall of mail slots for the providers, a large supply room, a bathroom, a stairway to the sidewalk on Seneca or to the Level 5 skyway from Jones to the Central Pavilion, a doorway to the elevators and a secure door to the staff lounge. The lounge contains lockers, a small kitchen with dishwasher and two microwaves, several computers, a bathroom with shower, a large table, a TV and the only transparent glass windows in the ED through which one can appreciate a panoramic view of downtown and also get some idea of the prevailing weather, which in turn may affect the route you choose to the cafeteria or the coffee bar. Everyone now changes clothes in one of the bathrooms rather than in semi–public areas. The bathroom doors do not have windows.

The large rectangular configuration of the main area was intended to provide a view of what's going on in any of the rooms, but for reasons of confidentiality, the curtains are always drawn over the glass doors, so there is, in fact, no visibility. Moreover, even with the drapes open, visual access to the rooms would be incomplete. Presumably for easy access, the medication room was positioned in the center of the otherwise open work area and it effectively obstructs visual sight lines to patient rooms and among various workstations. The secretary sits in the southwest corner of the space and the charge nurse in the southeast corner where ambulances first encounter someone upon entering. Initially, the plan was that there would be a provider with nurses at either end of the central rectangle and a provider in the SORT area, seeing people in Rooms 1–4. But for various reasons, it has evolved that all the providers are clustered next to the secretary and across from Room 22 (ensuring that the providers are hyper–aware of any verbal abuse and threats being dished out by restrained psychotic or intoxicated patients). Most of the nurses have stations in the north half of the workspace–except for one who is situated in the Blue Zone. Locating the nurse who is caring for your patient remains a challenge for providers but also helps to maintain aerobic fitness. In short, it is not a perfect space, but it does have some advantages over our previous space, ED West and East.

The hospital ward on Level 7 of the Central Pavilion was initially viewed as a potential overflow area for ED patients but it was quickly realized that it was too far away for the ED providers to efficiently manage patients placed there. It became Patient Accelerated Care or PACE and has recently been re–named Observation. ED patients requiring longer stays, but not necessarily admission to the hospital, are placed there on Observation Status under the care of hospitalists.

As volumes continue to fluctuate and surge erratically, we often experience a shortage of ED beds as well as waiting space and have had to resort once again to placing patients on stretchers against walls in the open aisles. The waiting room is often filled beyond capacity. We have a larger space for arriving ambulance crews than in our previous quarters, but, too frequently, there are several of them waiting there with their patients for a space to open up in the ED. This situation has a negative impact on patient safety as well as on patient and staff satisfaction.

As of January 2016, GH has changed their affiliation to the Swedish/Providence system of hospitals, which has raised concerns about impact on the VM ED and hospital revenue going forward. With the departure of GH patients, however, the ED providers hope that our frequent overcrowding will be eased temporarily.

Section Heads have all been physicians. As mentioned above, the first section head was **Scott Linscott**, followed by **Bruce Stevenson** from

1979–1997. He was followed by **David Frank**, who was trained as an internist at Virginia Mason and served as section head until 1999. In August of that year, he was followed by **David Dabell** who was specifically recruited for the position of section head. He served until spring of 2004 and was succeeded by **Chris Moore**. In spring of 2006, **Donna Smith, MD**, a pediatrician, took over the position until 2008 when **Julianna Yu, MD**, stepped in. Julianna served as section head until the fall of 2017. **Scott Osborn, MD**, took over as section head until the spring of 2019. The current section head is **Joshua Zwart, MD.** When first formed, we were a section in the Department of Medicine. As Emergency Medicine grew as a specialty, many in the section felt we should be a separate department, but the institution disagreed. We are now a section in the Department of Hospital Care along with Hospital Medicine, Critical Care, and Neurohospitalists. For national consistency, however, we refer to ourselves as the ED – Emergency Department.

As of 2016, the staff coverage is two AM providers, two PM providers and a third provider bridging those shifts from 11 a.m. to 9 p.m. Nights are staffed by one MD, and one PA. Total medical staff now numbers 15 MD/DOs and three PAs. The physicians include **Drs. Bohonos, Michael, Moore, Dabell, Frank, Heller,** and **Yu**, as well as **John Lacambra, MD; Carly Maak, MD; Maria Vasilyadis, MD; Krista Caldwell, MD; Jonathan Hall, MD; Lisa Wilson, MD; Scott Osborn, MD; myself, Ted Johnson, MD,** and until recently **Thomas Wu, MD.** The PAs are **Susan Weissman, PA–C; Robin Moore**, **PA–C,** and **Jason Montemayor, PA–C.** There is currently 24-hour coverage by an MSW as well to help meet the needs of the mental health/substance abuse/homeless populations, which continue to grow.

Residents continue to rotate through the ED, but residency has changed greatly over the years. There are restrictions on how many hours a resident may work consecutively, so there are no more 24-hour ED shifts. Instead, a resident is assigned to a specific provider and works that person's shifts along with them. It has been many years since they have cared for patients in the ED without direct supervision by an ED doc.

The practice of Emergency Medicine has obviously evolved along with the spaces we've occupied. Universal precautions have become standard practice and second nature. Pulse oximetry and pain scale ratings have become vital signs along with blood pressure, heart rate and temperature. MRI has become another valued imaging tool, CT scanning has become as common as plain films and they are all viewed on the computer. (I don't believe we have any light boxes in the current ED.) And speaking of computers, they are vital to our work. No reference books line any shelves. No fat, tattered patient charts litter our desks. We order on–line, receive results on–line, read patient histories on–line and document by dictation, voice recognition software or real–time data entry. Who knew that typing skills would be so crucial?

We now have very specific treatments for strokes, myocardial infarctions and sepsis, and strict pathways and a sense of urgency guide our care. The increasingly frequent presentation of agitated and violently psychotic and intoxicated patients has mandated that we develop detailed plans for evaluating those individuals while simultaneously guarding their safety and that of staff. Previously, patients were admitted to the hospital under the care of their primary provider or a specialist service, which meant that the ED provider needed to communicate by phone with many other providers and got to know them by voice at least. With the development of the hospitalist and intensivist services, ED providers now only speak with outpatient providers when specific specialty care is needed in the ED or questions of follow–up need to be addressed. This means that while we know the hospitalists and intensivists well and often see them face–to–face, there are many outpatient providers whom we only recognize by name, if that.

As the way we practice has changed, so has the way we dress. When I started in the ED, the doctors (all men) wore dress shirts, ties and long white coats. This was the dress code of the clinic (also all men) and was transferred intact to the ED. It looked very business–like but turned out to be inappropriate for what is a practice with frequent and unpredictable moments of physical involvement – joint relocations, blood spurting from wounds, lumbar punctures, CPR. It can be very strenuous and messy.

Over the years, dress shirts and ties have been abandoned in favor of more casual shirts and currently, most providers wear scrubs with or without a white coat for additional protection. It allows for freer movement, is easily replaceable in the event a patient vomits on you and tends to make the team look far less hierarchical.

Our current major challenge is to adapt to the departure of Group Health. In theory, our census will fall and may require new staffing patterns in order to maintain financial viability. The next few months will give more information with which to make decisions. In the meantime, I am retiring as of 2/29/16 – just days away. Our current workspace with its advantages, idiosyncrasies and shortcomings will be my last workspace … and likely the one I will remember best, since it's most recent. I will miss the energy and banter generated by a team of skilled, smart, empathetic and motivated people. I will miss being part of the drama … and farce … that is the practice of Emergency Medicine. It's been a stimulating and satisfying 36–year career and I'm grateful to Virginia Mason for having me. I wish our section and the institution well – for many reasons, but not least among them the fact that I intend to continue to get my own health care here, and that they're paying me a pension. I will follow their progress with interest.

July 2019 Update by Julianna Yu, MD

As of July 2019, we have an outstanding staff of board–certified emergency physicians and an experienced physician assistant team. The Virginia Mason Emergency Department has an excellent reputation locally and regionally, and each year we are approached by new residency graduates from top Emergency Medicine programs across the country hoping for a position with our team. As we have had very low turnover in the past several years, it may take years until full–time positions open up. We are fortunate to have several locums physicians as a result of the high desirability of our practice.

Our current challenges moving forward into 2020 include ensuring we are well–staffed to care for an increasingly aging and medically complex patient population in a growing city that brings in many new residents for high tech jobs every year, while also struggling with homelessness, a mental health crisis, and the opioid epidemic. We are preparing to support new labor and delivery services, and will need to ramp up our obstetrics and pediatrics training and equipment to deal with obstetrical emergencies. The ED is now not only the social and medical safety net for many, but we are also critical in ensuring appropriate resource utilization of health care services in the medical center. Increasingly, emergency physicians are poised to discharge and manage many conditions as outpatients, which in the past used to result in automatic admission to the hospital, such as transient ischemia attacks (TIAs), chest pain, GI bleeds, etc.

Current physicians include **Drs. Caldwell, Dabell, Frank, Lacambra, Maak, Michael, Osborn, Vasilyadis, Wilson, Yu,** and **Helen Y. Chiu, MD; Travis Omura, MD; Reed W. Simons, MD; Amanda J. Trau, DO,** and **Joshua M. Zwart, MD,** who serves as current Section Head. Current PA–Cs include **Robin Moore, MS, PA–C; Chelsea C. Walter, PA–C,** and **Shawn McLane, PA–C.**

We are fortunate to be the "Front Door' of Virginia Mason and look forward to being here for another 100 years.

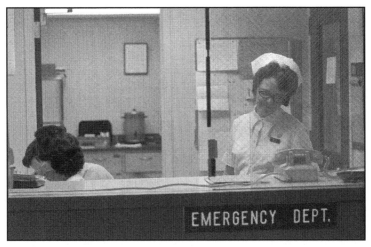

The Emergency Department Entrance in the 1960s (PH 8217, VMHA)

30

Critical Care Medicine

by Tony Gerbino, MD

The Origins of Critical Care

The evolution of critical care at Virginia Mason mirrors changes in the field over the last century. Virginia Mason's critical care experience began in the mid-1960s with creation of the Special Care Unit (SCU), an 8-bed unit that grouped patients with higher acuity of illness. This practice began in the mid-nineteenth century when the British nurse Florence Nightingale began cohorting seriously ill soldiers in the Crimean War so that sicker patients could receive more attention. Patient cohorting was resurrected during WWII with creation of "shock wards" for military casualties.

Special units for the severely ill were adopted on a widespread basis in the 1960s as technology developed to monitor and treat organ failure. For example, the development of hemodialysis was accelerated when the epidemic of hemorrhagic fever in the Korean War led to acute renal failure in military personnel. In the 1950s, the polio epidemic resulted in large numbers of patients with respiratory failure who required mechanical ventilation with the "iron lung," accelerating development of positive pressure ventilators. Cardiac monitors and defibrillators began seeing widespread use in the 1960s, and the explosion in increasingly sophisticated forms of life support over the next two decades led to a dramatic increase in critical care beds. Virginia Mason's SCU was formed to accommodate the expertise needed for these new technologies.

The Special Care Unit at Virginia Mason

The SCU included two private monitored beds for cardiac patients with myocardial infarction and those recovering from cardiac surgery. Cardiac monitors allowed detection of arrhythmias that for the first time could be treated with defibrillators and transvenous pacemakers. **Becky Walsh, RN,** who would remain involved in the critical care program until her retirement in 2014, recalls her first days in the SCU in 1969: "Back then the patients infarcted, then we dealt with ventricular arrhythmias and heart block" with our new technologies. Nurse training for the SCU included classes in electrocardiogram interpretation, "code" management in case of cardiac arrest, and care of the ventilator patient.

Six additional SCU beds were housed in a single room separated by curtains and primarily used for post-operative patients and those undergoing special procedures. The first hemodialysis at VM was performed in the SCU under the care of **Burton Orme, MD**, and Becky Walsh, RN on a young woman with hemolytic uremic syndrome (the first SCU medical director was a nephrologist, **Richard Paton, MD**). The SCU also witnessed VM's first kidney transplant in 1972. The donor was a brain-dead head injury patient from Alaska and the recipient was a renal failure patient from Port Angeles. "Both were in our SCU," said Ms. Walsh. "The two wives met together in the waiting room and supported one another."

The Growth of Critical Care Services: Coronary and Intensive Care Units

The Coronary Care Unit opened in 1970 on the 8th floor of the Main Hospital and the SCU evolved into the Intensive Care Unit (ICU) in the mid 1970s. The need for more critical care beds led to the opening of a new unit on the north end of level 6 in 1976. Later, an adjacent unit was built to the south for a total of 24 beds and renamed the Intensive Care Unit (ICU). Although monitoring equipment became increasingly sophis-

444

ticated, newly minted nurse **Susan Dunn, RN** recalls that in 1984 "cardiac monitors were like oscilloscopes that we adjusted with a screwdriver." **Neely Pardee, MD,** a pulmonary section member, became the medical director in 1976, and that job was later assumed by **William Horton, MD,** an anesthesiologist. **Johanna Viking, RN,** was the first ICU Nurse Manager.

In the 1980s, house staff teams followed their patients in and out of the intensive and coronary care units. The ward attending, or "primary managing physician," provided guidance and teaching. If patients were mechanically ventilated there was a mandatory "ventilator consult" from one of the pulmonologists. **Neil Hampson, MD,** joined VM in 1988 and suggested a new model of ICU staffing based on his pulmonary/critical care fellowship training at Duke University. A designated ICU house staff team for internal medicine patients was formed and Hampson began thrice weekly critical care teaching rounds, a practice that won him Teacher of the Year in 1991. Soon after, non-surgical patients who transferred to the ICU or coronary care unit (which had been incorporated into the ICU in 1992) were assigned a new attending with expertise in critical care medicine. "This change was met with some resistance, but succeeded," noted Dr. Hampson. Never has the process of change in medicine been more simply or aptly stated.

As patients became sicker and the unit became busier, the role of "Teacher-Manager" was created in 1996. Internal medicine attendings with expertise in critical care spent one month at a time rounding in the ICU with house staff and being available to assist with management. Around the same time, the increased census due to Group Health patients led to an expanded 20 bed ICU on the 7th floor of the Main Hospital (20 beds) while the 12-bed 6-North unit remained open and was preferred for post-surgical patients. **Ted Gibbons, MD**, of cardiology, and pulmonary section member **Steve Kirtland, MD,** were co-directors of critical care during this time, with Dr. Kirtland continuing alone in this role until the early 2000s. It was Dr. Gibbons who christened this new combined unit the "Critical Care Unit," or CCU as it is known to this day.

Critical Care Certification

Board certification for critical care medicine became available in 1989 and was achieved first at Virginia Mason by Neil Hampson, MD, and **David Dreis, MD.** Both were pulmonary section members throughout their career, with Dr. Hampson also responsible for development of VM's hyperbaric program until his retirement in 2010, and Dr. Dreis serving as Chief of Medicine from 1991 to 1999. Ted Gibbons, MD, a member of the cardiology section, and **Brian Owens, MD**, an anesthesiologist, obtained board certification shortly thereafter. By 2001, all CCU attendings had critical care board certification.

The first professional organization for critical care nurses was formed in 1971. The American Association of Cardiovascular Nurses became the American Association of Critical Care Nurses (AACN) in 1976 and began offering professional certification as a critical care registered nurse (CCRN) at that time. The ICU/CCU orientation and nurse residency programs were developed in the 1980s in collaboration with the first critical care nurse specialists. **Susan Osguthorpe, RN, MN** became the Nurse Director of the ICU in 1984. **Charleen Tachibana, RN, DNP,** current Senior Vice President and Chief Nursing Officer, was involved with the critical care program starting as a bedside nurse in 1977 and in various administrative roles until 2015. Both of these individuals were instrumental in supporting the professional development of Virginia Mason's critical care nurses, including CCRN certification, advanced degrees, and funding to attend national conferences. In 1996, VM began participating in the newly formed Puget Sound Critical Care Consortium. This organization included clinical specialists and critical care educators who provided didactic classes to CCU nurses from all area hospitals.

The New Critical Care Section Takes Shape

Critical care staffing around the country in the early 2000s was influenced by the Leapfrog Group, a national consortium of large businesses formed in 1999 with the goal of improving the quality of health care. One quality benchmark identified by the Leapfrog Group was the presence of a

446

dedicated, on-site intensivist available during daylight hours. This recommendation led to creation of the critical care program in 2002, with newly hired but seasoned **Mike Westley, MD**, as its Head.

Dr. Westley completed training in pulmonary/critical care medicine at the University of Washington in 1981 and had been practicing pulmonary medicine in Anchorage, where he also served as Chief Medical Officer and Director of Quality Resources. In the late 1990s, Dr. Westley (who was an avid sailor) left his job in Alaska and with his grown sons sailed around the world for two years. Upon return from this sojourn, he began looking for work, including an interview with the Virginia Mason pulmonary section for a locum tenens position. Mike did not get that job, but so impressed newly appointed Medical Director of Hospital Services **Jim Bender, MD,** that he became the first Medical Director of the Critical Care program in late 2002.

Dr. Westley brought a passion for patient-centered care and safety that borrowed from the airline industry and was an excellent match for the ascendant Virginia Mason Production System. In addition to Dr. Westley, the CCU was staffed by all members of the pulmonary section (Drs. Hampson, Kirtland, **Gerbino, Horan, Mahoney** and **Kregenow**), all of whom were boarded in critical care medicine. The CCU attending rounded, admitted, and supervised all care for patients admitted to the CCU internal medicine house staff team.

While the new hospitalist service provided in-house overnight attending coverage for patients who were not in the CCU, the CCU had no in-house nighttime attending. "Mike thought it was crazy that hospitalized patients outside of the CCU had 24 hour in-house attending coverage courtesy of the new hospitalist program, whereas CCU patients - the sickest in the hospital – did not," recalls **Phil Royal, MD.** Dr. Royal joined VM as a hospitalist in 2000, and became the first CCU "nocturnist" in 2004. Also notable for "nocturnal" contributions is **Vamshi Thandra, MD** (2011 - present). Dr. Thandra completed his internal medicine residency at Virginia Mason in 2009 and joined the critical care program in 2011. While night coverage is often a CCU staffing challenge, the skill and compassion these two individuals continue to provide have contributed greatly to the quality and stability of CCU care over the years.

The last two decades of critical care medicine have been characterized by changes in the organization and processes by which critical care services are provided. There has been increased focus on patient-centered care, a multidisciplinary approach, and quality improvement and safety. In 2003, Westley and CCU nursing leadership began a series of initiatives that reflected these new emphases and anticipated what would become standard care in CCUs across the country.

Quality Improvement and Safety

Quality improvement efforts during this time began with participation in the Institute for Healthcare Improvement's Critical Care Collaborative. The goal of this collaborative was "for teams from a variety of organizations to work with each other to rapidly test and implement changes that lead to lasting improvement." These changes included a "ventilator bundle" in 2003 that included best practices for mechanically ventilated patients, and standardized ventilator protocols for ARDS and weaning. Manager of respiratory therapy **Joe Streiff, RRT,** was instrumental in implementing these RT-driven protocols. "Code" drills started in 2004 to improve resuscitation of those with cardiac arrest. The medical emergency response team, or MET, was also started in 2004 and was the forerunner of today's rapid response team. In 2005, a "central line bundle" was implemented to establish standard work (including the first use of ultrasound in the CCU) and a safety checklist. Mike also made untiring efforts to "encourage" hand washing, including frequent safety inspections and enlistment of patient families in this effort. Assistant Nurse Manager **Shirley Sherman RN, MN,** Mike, and the CCU charge nurse began bedside "safety rounds" in 2006, a practice that occurred both day and night.

A Multi-Disciplinary Approach

By the early 2000s clinical research had emerged indicating that multi-disciplinary CCU teams delivered care more effectively than lone practitioners.

In keeping with this new understanding and the increasing complexity of care, nurses and respiratory therapists began presenting to the CCU team and family on morning rounds. Shortly after, a pharmacist with critical care expertise began accompanying the multidisciplinary rounding team. **Lisa Chamberlain, PharmD**, was the first to regularly participate in CCU rounds and continues to lead pharmacy contributions to the CCU. These contributions include evidence-based use of medications, appropriate medication dosing, antibiotic stewardship, continuity of care, and numerous other tangible and intangible benefits. In the last few years, daily on-site radiology review between the CCU team and a radiology attending began. In addition, a daily multidisciplinary morning huddle is now held that includes physical, occupational, and speech/language therapists, medical social workers, registered dieticians, palliative care providers, and nursing.

An Open, Family-Friendly CCU

Another major change during this time was to make the CCU more family friendly. The first step was to eliminate "visiting hours" so that family members were welcome at all times of day (2005). Families were invited to join in morning work rounds and nursing sign-out at shift change, and formal family meetings became routine. This work engendered trust and made patients' goals, values, and prognoses more transparent. This created a natural opportunity to introduce palliative care to the CCU, an effort led by Drs. Westley and Kregenow who both became certified in palliative care medicine. Mike stepped down from the medical director position in 2011, but change continued in the CCU under new director **Ian Smith, MD** (2011 – 2014).

Dr. Smith joined Virginia Mason in 2006 as the second full-time hire for the critical care section after completing a pulmonary/critical care fellowship at the University of Washington. Dr. Smith shared CCU leadership with Shirley Sherman, RN, MN (1983 - 2018). Shirley had worked many years as a VM critical care nurse, became CCU Assistant Nurse Manager in 2006 and Nurse manager in 2011. Under Ian and Shirley's guidance,

CCU care continued to advance. Following the pioneering work of Johns Hopkins University intensivist and quality improvement guru Paul Pronovost, MD (later popularized by physician-author Atul Gawande), rounding checklists were introduced that included daily goals of care and safety measures. Based on emerging evidence, respiratory therapy-driven protocols that speeded liberation from mechanical ventilation were introduced, and nurse-initiated protocols were begun to titrate sedation, including daily pauses in sedative medications. Dr. Smith also developed the first "Code Sepsis" protocols, wherein sepsis was identified before transfer to the CCU, permitting early treatment that improved outcomes.

The New Jones-9 CCU Arrives

A new CCU on the ninth floor of the Jones Pavilion opened in 2014 and along with it came a new critical care medical director, **Aneal Gadgil, MD**. Dr. Gadgil joined Virginia Mason's critical care section in 2008 and served as CCU medical director from 2014 - 2018. He continues to provide critical care services in addition to an expanded administrative role as Medical Director of Utilization Review and Clinical Documentation, and Associate Medical Director of Business Services. The Jones-9 CCU includes dedicated space for multidisciplinary meetings, teaching, the CCU pharmacist, and an adjacent imaging suite and radiology reading room. The physical plant also provides adequate space for family in both patient and respite rooms.

During this time, VM was one of 68 hospitals (and one of two in Washington state) to participate in the Society of Critical Care Medicine's ICU Liberation Collaborative that studied the "ABCDEF" bundle. This study proved for the first time that implementation of the bundle – adequately treating pain, spontaneous breathing trials, limiting sedation, assessing delirium, early mobility, and inclusion of family - improved outcomes for critically ill patients. This study also reflects the culmination of many individual improvements made in CCU care over the prior fifteen years.

Two relatively new Virginia Mason programs became more visible with the move to the Jones-9 CCU. With the growth of VM's palliative care program, palliative care consultation is now commonplace in our CCU. In addition, the growth of the neuroscience program has led to an increase in CCU patients with primary neurologic diagnoses. These patients include those recovering from neurosurgery as well as those with diagnoses of subarachnoid hemorrhage, stroke treated with thrombolysis or catheter-based thrombectomy, and status epilepticus.

A "Surgical CCU" and Anesthesia-Critical Care

Current medical director **Eliot Fagley, MD**, has been at the helm of the critical care service for less than two years, but the pace of change has continued. Dr. Fagley came to Virginia Mason in 2013 having served as anesthesiology and critical care faculty first at Washington University and then at the University of Washington. Dr. Fagley began attending in the CCU shortly after his arrival, but he was not the first anesthesiologist at VM to do this.

Robert Hsiung, MD, completed a preliminary internship at VM in 2002 and then an anesthesiology residency and critical care fellowship at Stanford. Dr. Hsiung's addition to the CCU in 2008 was motivated by the different skill set an anesthesiologist would bring to the CCU. Dr. Hsiung continues to serve as both critical care and anesthesiology attending.

In addition to continuing the work pioneered by Drs. Pardee, Horton, Hampson, Kirtland, Westley, Smith, and Gadgil, Dr. Fagley has brought a focus on post-surgical care. This focus has led to the addition of a second CCU team focused on the post-operative patient. The goal is to make CCU care an extension of intraoperative management, improving care in both arenas. This second CCU team, currently consisting of a surgery intern and CCU attending, is present throughout the day and able to attend immediately to changes in patient status. As a result of its peri-operative focus, this newly created CCU service has been staffed primarily by anesthesiologists. In addition to Drs. Fagley and Hsiung, Stanford-trained **Sarah Bain, MD** (2013 -present) and **Sara Nikravan, MD** (2017- 2019) have provided both anesthesiology and CCU services, as does **Brooks Ohlson, MD** (2018 - present). Additional critical care faculty during this period have included **Rebecca Gooch, MD** (2017 - 2020) and **Hina Sahi, MD** (2016 - present).

One of the biggest changes in CCU organization related to the "surgical" CCU team is the transition to a "closed collaborative" CCU. Previously, surgical teams would often have primary care of patients residing in the CCU, while hospitalist teams occasionally provided short-term care for patients whose acuity straddled the critical care and intermediate care units. In the new model, all patients physically located in the CCU are assigned to one of the two CCU teams with other disciplines serving as consultants. The transition to a unit-based model has occurred simultaneously with similar changes in the hospitalist group, and preliminary metrics suggest this reorganization has led to shorter CCU stays, shorter hospital stays, and fewer readmissions after discharge.

Past is Prologue

Though the trajectory of care is inexorably forward, sometimes past is prologue. The 1980s and 1990s saw several VM house staff graduate, receive pulmonary/critical care fellowship training, and then return to practice at Virginia Mason. These include former Chief of Medicine **David Dreis, MD** (1983 - 2014), **Bill DePaso, MD** (2001 - 2015), and current Chief of Staff Steve Kirtland, MD (1995 - present), who was in part mentored by Dr. Dreis. These faculty have mentored more recent Virginia Mason house staff who, after fellowship training elsewhere, have returned to become mainstays of VM's critical care section.

Dr. Kirtland provided mentorship to Virginia Mason internal medicine resident **Hashim Mehter, MD**, who completed residency in 2010, and was hired in 2014 as Virginia Mason's first home-grown, full-time intensivist. Subsequently, **Blake Mann, MD,** has charted a similar path (VM internal medicine '13), joining VM as a full-time critical care physician in 2017. As previously mentioned, Vamshi Thandra, MD, completed a VM internal medicine residency in 2009, and Brooks Ohlson, MD, completed a VM anesthesiology residency in 2016 before returning to VM in 2018 to provide anesthesiology and critical care services.

Among the many changes in the critical care program over the decades, the one constant may be this cycle of renewal, wherein our trainees return to VM to join the next generation of leaders. This fact not only leaves us enthusiastic about the future of Virginia Mason's critical care program, but also for the daily opportunity to teach and mentor our current house staff in the critical care unit.

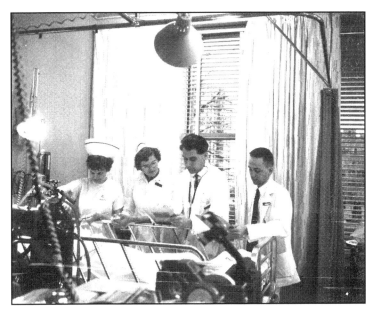

Early Days in the ICU - 1960
Natalie Goemaere RN, an unidentified nurse, and two unidentified physicians stand at the bedside of a patient in the intensive care unit (PH 0937, VMHA)

31

Graduate Medical Education

by Brian D. Owens, MD,
with contributions from Gillian Abshire, RN, MSN

Virginia Mason (VM) has recorded many "firsts" in the 100 years since its founding. One not widely recognized is the Graduate Medical Education (GME) program, said to be among the first, if not the first in the Pacific Northwest. It began when two interns, **A. Stephens Graham, MD**, and **Julian Coleman, MD**, joined a recently founded Mason Clinic for the 1925–26 academic year. Since then GME has been a critical piece in VM's successful journey as a learning institution. This history is dedicated to the residents and faculty who have served the institution so well over all those years.

In an academic medical center, most clinical care on teaching services is directed by residents and supervised by faculty attending physicians. VM training programs are highly sought after and attract excellent medical students from outstanding medical schools nationwide. They come seeking training in their chosen fields and bring with them "outside eyes" – diverse perspectives and broad experience that can and have provided the impetus for productive change not only in GME but throughout the organization.

To begin this history one must acknowledge **Donna Hegstrom**. In 1964, Donna became the first secretary in Virginia Mason's newly created Medical Education Office. She worked in the department for 28 years and retired as the Administrative Manager of the Office of House Staff Affairs in 1992. During that year, she wrote an essay about GME at Virginia Mason, which is the most accurate history of the department available between 1925 and 1992, and referenced often for the writing of this chapter. [1] Donna's career spanned a time of unprecedented change. GME progressed from a cottage industry in which physician medical educators imparted skills and knowledge to residents in accordance with institutional tradition, to a significantly more organized structure under national oversight, first by the Liaison Committee on Graduate Medical Education (1972–81) and then by the Accreditation Council for Graduate Medical Education (ACGME). Today ACGME provides infrastructure and policy to standardize requirements for sponsoring institutions, programs and curricula; to evaluate compliance; and, when necessary, to assist in meeting required standards and avoiding loss of accreditation. Donna was the only person at VM to experience all that change firsthand. As an interesting aside: In the 1980s, Mrs. Hegstrom received a letter from Dr. Graham, one of the interns who came to VM in 1925, describing his experience. [2] Portions of this letter are quoted below and highlight the fact that Team Medicine and humanism are continuous threads through decades of care and education at Virginia Mason.

Dr. Graham remembers: "My most cherished honor was the appointment ... along with Julian Coleman, as the first interns of the Virginia Mason Hospital. Actually, however, acceptance was somewhat of a gamble." Dr. Graham had been accepted to a few other programs back East, including the prestigious St. Luke's Hospital and Johns Hopkins, but they weren't exactly what he wanted. As he noted, "While still bewildered and uncertain, I received a call from my classmate, John Blackford's brother, urging me to accept the appointment in Seattle. In my frustrated state I accepted and have never regretted it.

"From the very beginning ... we realized how fortunate we had been in accepting appointments. In addition to **Dr. Mason, Sr.**, who on the first day insisted we address him as "Tate" – not even 'Dr. Tate'– and became my immediate idol, we were tremendously impressed with **John**

Blackford, Minor Lile, the Dowlings, Lester Palmer, Pius Rohrer, John Dare, Sr. and **Miss Fraser.**" He cryptically describes his first days in Seattle: "Met at station on July 3 by Dr. Lile. Quick trip to Mason Clinic … thence around the lake to the summer home of Dr. Mason and distinguished friends, constituting one large open house for three glorious days. Became acquainted with the men of the Staff and their families, as well as leading citizens, including one well on his way to becoming the world's greatest producer of planes (Boeing) who continued to be friendly throughout our entire stay."

Dr. Graham describes the state of Seattle medicine at that time: "Incomprehensible in a city of 340,000, VM Hospital and the considerably larger Sister's (Providence) Hospital had never had an intern and the remaining three or four hospitals had extremely few for a city so large. The doctors of the staff were at a loss as to how to use us … We made certain suggestions and explained we were trained to perform, and could carry out nights and weekends, lab studies, including blood chemistry, Wassermans, … x-rays, give nitrous oxide and ether and perform spinals, give transfusions, undertake deliveries if labor was precipitate and (the) responsible physician was not available (how wonderful it proved during periods of dense fogs)" and be "avid performers of autopsies. Amazed, yet delighted, they could avoid the expense of technicians (on) nights and weekends … We alternated weeks for covering night calls. With Mr. Dare's blessings, the man 'off' could 'moonlight' on the Doctors' Exchange for house, apartment and hotel calls … In lieu of fees we received tickets to shows, games and premium distilled products from Canada."

He describes a different world medically that is hard to imagine now. They would do "itinerant surgery in distant small towns" with the interns "chauffeuring Tate and the OR crew in his huge Lincoln," and "dramatic life-saving emergencies (in) out of the way places in dense fog, as when I administered IV mercurochrome to a young girl near death from erysipelas and septicemia (with) the distinguishing features of (her) face obliterated." She apparently survived and they shared a "fabulous luncheon at La Blanc's arranged by Dr. Mason" six weeks later.

457

Perhaps the most dramatic story is that related to a "post-tonsillectomy hemorrhage (on) a dense foggy night that prevented the patient's MD, from reaching VM. (She was) a lovely 18-year-old girl, reputedly a heiress … Hours later when everyone descended upon her room they found both of us asleep, head to head, as I leaned over to compress (a) wad of cotton soaked in adrenalin with (my) index finger."

The number of interns increased to four by 1928. [3] The group included **Joel Baker, MD; Louis Edmunds, MD; John Wilkinson, MD,** and **Gordon James, MD.** [4] "In 1938 a new building was erected to the west of the Hospital, designed to house new interns' quarters, a library, a medical artists' studio, the Hospital laundry and a power plant … In addition to regular internship training, the Hospital made its first residency appointments in Surgery and Medicine in 1939." [3] The surgery residency program is the oldest in the Pacific Northwest, and the internal medicine residency program was one of only two in the state, with the other at the UW. [1]

Over the next 15 years, the hospital was able to recruit six to eight interns per year, which was barely adequate. In 1953, however, the nationwide Internship Matching Plan began, which was designed to prevent hospitals from contracting with prospective interns prior to their graduation from medical school. As a result, recruitment fell, and the hospital was only able to recruit for five of its 10 spaces in 1955. At that time, **Alan Nourse, MD**, was an intern and he describes it as very "hectic." [3]

By 1962, VM sponsored seven residency programs and more than 35 interns and residents, including five women. Sponsored programs included five that continue today: internal medicine, general surgery, anesthesiology, diagnostic radiology and a "rotating internship", which is now our transitional year program. In 1962, there were also training programs in pathology and obstetrics/gynecology, which were later discontinued. The number of applicants in 1964 was 29 for nine positions. In 1965, the "first straight medicine interns were appointed … and **Ted Rynearson, MD**, was one of the two." [1]

Although VM GME had decreased to five ACGME accredited programs by 1992, it had grown as a result of expansion in every program, so that there were 96 interns and residents at that point, with 42 women. The number of applicants was over 1,100 for 32 positions! [1] Over the next 25 years, GME at Virginia Mason had grown further to sponsor eight ACGME-accredited programs with 126 +/- interns, residents and fellows. The sponsored programs and number of trainees are as follows: internal medicine (35), general surgery (32), anesthesiology (27), radiology (12), urology (four when this newer program, accredited in 2013, fills its resident complement in the 2018–19 academic year), transitional year (12), pain medicine fellowship (two - accredited in 1994) and female pelvic medicine and reconstructive surgery fellowship (two - accredited in 2012). An anesthesiology-based regional anesthesia fellowship was accredited as well in September 2018.

A special note should be made of the evolution of the "Transitional Year Program." This program was accredited by ACGME on July 1, 1983, but is actually the program that has continued since the first arrival of interns in 1925. This program serves as a first year for many interns later entering either residencies at VM in radiology or anesthesiology, or transferring to other institutions for residencies in a wide variety of other disciplines.

GME has benefited from the efforts of numerous people over the years including physicians, executives and administrative staff. We have been fortunate to attract passionate team members who have served our programs and residents well.

Prior to 1962, GME oversight at VM was the responsibility of the Chair of the Intern–Resident Committee. The three physicians who held that position include **John Walker, MD** (radiology); **Thomas Carlile, MD** (radiology); and **Randy Pillow, MD** (internal medicine). Since 1962, there have been seven Directors of Graduate Medical Education (DGME). In 1998, an ACGME directive required that every institution sponsoring GME appoint a senior institutional leader to oversee the GME enterprise. As a result, the DGME is also the Designated Institutional Official (DIO).

Hugh Lawrence, MD (thoracic surgery), was the first DGME, between the years 1964–72, which preceded the formation of the Liaison Committee on GME (LCGME) that is largely responsible for creating the infrastructure and curricula to enable our programs to gain accreditation. He founded the Department of Medical Education, formed the teaching faculty, and established program director positions. Dr. Lawrence benefited greatly from the supportive leadership of VM's Clinic Chairmen, Joel Baker, MD (surgeon) and John Walker, MD (radiologist). He personally increased recruiting efforts to attract resident candidates from medical schools across the country.

Bob Hegstrom, MD (nephrologist) assumed the DGME duties for the next seven years. Does the name sound familiar? He and Donna were husband and wife. He also served as the internal medicine program director during the same period. Bob led VM through LCGME's first accreditation process and continued the significant curricular modifications the process mandated. He improved institutional support for residents, faculty and program leadership to improve program competitiveness.

After Dr. Hegstrom, **Paul Fredlund, MD** (endocrinologist) served as DGME for two years before **Jim Coatsworth, MD** (neurologist) took the reins for 10 years between 1981–91. Donna remembers Jim as an outstanding DGME with impeccable interpersonal skills, who never failed to act in the right way for the right reasons to ensure the best and kindest outcome for all concerned.

Between 1991 and 2003, **Jim Benson, MD** (endocrinologist), was the DGME and VM's first DIO. Fortunately for all, Jim was incredibly organized, a trait that helped prepare them for the next significant ACGME initiative. In 1998, ACGME began to transition GME from a process-based system to one that was outcome-based (to be discussed later). Most of the structural modifications to implement this change came after 2003; however, the cultural adjustment for residents, faculty and leadership began immediately. Just to make it interesting, the concept of national duty-hour regulations and fatigue mitigation became a reality in 2003. Jim worked with operational leadership to address the workflow and provider issues created by the new requirements at the end of his appointment.

Brian Owens, MD, joined Virginia Mason in 1988 and became the associate program director of the anesthesiology residency in 1990. He was the anesthesiology associate program director or program director (PD) for all but a brief period until 2003. In August 2003, **Dr. Gary Kaplan** appointed him to replace Dr. James Benson as the director of GME. He continued in that position until August 2016.

Several themes characterized his time as DGME: encouraging residents to engage in improving health care and helping them to be heard, both locally and nationally; aligning institutional educational and operational efforts; and directing GME outcomes toward societal expectations for physician providers. Big picture initiatives included implementation of the ACGME's outcomes initiative; integration of GME into VM's management or production system, VMPS, and vice versa; conversion of the Graduate Medical Education Committee (GMEC) from its mostly administrative function to a productive operational unit; improved integration of operational and educational leadership at program and institutional levels; initiation of national involvement in GME; and implementation of ... wait for it ... yet another ACGME accreditation system. Dr. Owens was an active participant and leader in the Alliance of Independent Academic Medical Centers (AIAMC), serving as a member of the Board of Directors from 2008 – 2014, as Chairperson of the Annual Meeting Program from 2009 – 2011, as a member of the Executive Committee from 2010 – 2014, and as President of the Board of Directors from 2012 – 2014. Dr. Owens has received many awards at the local and national level, including the AIAMC Innovation Award and their Weinberg Award, which he received in 2015. The Weinberg Award is given to individuals who demonstrate leadership in academic medicine, both locally and nationally; serve as an advocate for the independent academic medical center; and have articulated a vision for the future of academic medicine in the AIAMC.

Effective August 2016, **Joyce Lammert, MD, PhD,** became VM's DGME/DIO. The handoff was perfect — Joyce was Dr. Owens' direct supervisor for the previous four years. Joyce is a creative and outspoken proponent for residents, faculty and training programs, and, as a bonus, she is a graduate of VM's internal medicine residency. She was appointed to the Board of Directors of the AIAMC in March 2019, maintaining VM's prominence in GME nationally. In July 2019, Joyce transitioned from her role as DGME/DIO and Executive Medical Director of the Hospital, and **Ryan Pong, MD,** who has served as both Transitional Year Program Director and Deputy DIO will step into the DIO role. The good ship GME has a new captain to keep her on course for a better tomorrow.

For most if not all of Dr. Owens' 28 years at VM, the DGME has had an administrative partner. There have been three members of the executive leadership team who served in this role: **Joyce Jackson, Sarah Patterson** and **Lynne Chafetz,** although Dr. Owens never had an opportunity to work with Joyce. Sarah was the GME administrative partner between 2001 and 2004. When Dr. Owens became DGME/DIO, she guided his transition into executive leadership. She was a strong proponent for integration of VMPS into the GME curriculum. Her passion for the VM management system and her skill and knowledge in using and teaching those tools and processes laid the foundation on which the current work is built.

Lynne Chafetz was the GME executive administrative partner of Jim Benson between 1997 and 2001. In 2004, she returned to this role as Dr. Owens' partner. The degree to which Lynne's leadership changed the working relationship with the DGME/DIO cannot be overstated. Lynne has a passion for all aspects of GME. She is a resident advocate in the very best of ways and she sees the programs as a direct conduit to improving medical care in both the near and distant future. VM's success in aligning its operational and educational value streams; improving communications between their programs and residents, their sponsoring departments and the institution; seeking a national GME presence; and mobilizing the talents of residents, faculty and GME leaders to improve VM as an institution and the resident and program performance would not have been achieved without Lynne's leadership. Her work has been recognized both locally and nationally with several awards including receiving the VM Mary McClinton Award and the AIAMC award for Innovation in GME;

appointment to Women of Impact, a national group of executive-level women leaders from diverse sectors of the health care industry who seek, through collective impact, to advance change in our health care system; and service as a director and officer of AIAMC and as vice-chair of the AIAMC's *National Initiative VI: Stimulating a Culture of Well-Being in the Clinical Learning Environment*. She also recently received the 2019 Weinberg Award from the AIAMC.

Another position that is critical to the GME programs is Administrative Manager of GME/Director of GME Administration. Donna Hegstrom's service in this role from 1964 to 1992 was previously noted. When she retired, **Maureen Beaulieu**, a mainstay in the Department of Anesthesiology office replaced her. Maureen left in the mid-1990s to complete nursing studies. GME lost an outstanding advocate; patients gained a wonderful nurse. **Bonnie Plymire,** program coordinator for general surgery and anesthesiology, took over and was a valued resource for Jim Benson as they worked through ACGME's Outcomes Initiative and Duty Hour Standards. Bonnie had an unparalleled ability to connect with residents; it was a rare occasion when there were no residents discussing the programs and their experience in her office. Bonnie retired in 2004. **Steve Stahl** moved from HR to GME for about a year before returning to his original department. **Heather Seabott**, a "go to" internal expert in understanding and interpreting the ACGME requirements and standards, brought this detailed knowledge from her anesthesiology and general surgery program coordinator position to manage GME between 2005 and 2009. In 2009, Heather returned to her coordinator role and was instrumental in the work to gain accreditation for new fellowship programs in urology (female pelvic medicine and reconstructive surgery fellowship), and regional anesthesiology. All are grateful for her ongoing work in the two programs mentioned, and in general surgery.

Fariba Fuller then came to GME from KPO. She brought with her a wealth of VMPS knowledge and practical application skills. She created the framework for an elective to train residents in the implementation of VMPS principles and processes to health care.

Gillian Abshire accepted the offer to become the Director of GME Administration in 2011 and continues in that position today. She is a game-changer and a paragraph cannot adequately recognize her contributions. She changed GME administrative staff from a group of individuals to a team that uses standard work, allowing team members to share best practices to benefit all programs. Gillian created a system that encourages administrative staff to grow and job descriptions that provide transparent incentive for advancement. She aligned policies, procedures, support and benefits for residents with that of other VM staff and reduced the need for GME systems that duplicate those of the institution. Gillian is a Kaizen fellow; she took Fariba Fuller's framework for the systems-based practice elective and turned it into a reality. It is the most popular elective at VM. Her guidance has been instrumental in helping all program directors achieve VMPS for Leaders' certification, and, in fact, there is now a cohort of residents, alumni and program managers who have completed that course. As a result of her efforts, people in GME recognize opportunities for improvement and use their skills to address them. There are so many examples of excellent work bearing Gillian's signature. The bottom line is this: Gillian is all about the team and for her, the team includes any person or operational unit that touches GME.

Between 2004 and 2009 the leadership structure of GME included an Administrative Director, **Debra Madsen**. Debra is an attorney with experience as an assistant dean of a law school and she was one of VM's first Kaizen fellows. She was a resource for everyone in GME and a force for improvement. She was a driver in the work to more closely associate GME and its residents with support services in HR and finance that served all other VM departments. As a result, GME personnel and benefit policies were simplified and aligned with those of the institution. Debra's contributions were many. One remarkable effort was her work to make the Eastgate Resident Continuity Clinic a reality. This is an award-winning, public-private partnership with King County that provides VM internal medicine residents the opportunity to provide care to the underserved. It is a primary care gem!

As stated earlier, when accreditation began in the 1970s, individual program directors were required and somewhere along the timeline, program coordinators were added. The two form the physician/administrative dyad to provide direct leadership for sponsored programs. They keep the programs among the most competitive in the country. Certainly, attention to detail to ensure compliance with requirements is important; however, their dedication to resident well-being and professional development, and their longevity in their positions is much more important to create the environment in which residents recognize their worth and flourish.

The following is a list of program directors (with the most accurate inception date for each program in parentheses):

Anesthesiology (1959): Don Bridenbaugh, MD; Robert Balfour, MD (1970s); Manny Batra, MD; Mike Mulroy, MD (1980 – 1998!); Steve Rupp, MD; Brian Owens, MD; Joe Neal, MD; Spender Liu, MD; Julie Pollock, MD; Jim Helman, MD; Grete Porteous, MD.

Diagnostic Radiology (1972): Radiology designates two physicians as associate program directors and they share duties: Al Alzose, MD; Marie Lee, MD; Lucy Glenn, MD; Ingrid Peterson, MD; Felicia Cummings, MD; Larry Holder, MD; Wendy Hsu, MD; David Coy, MD; Jennifer Kohr, MD; Erin Cooke, MD.

General Surgery (1941): Phil Jolly, MD; John Ryan, MD; Rick Thirlby, MD (1992 – 2015!); Lily Chang, MD.

Internal Medicine (1979): Robert Hegstrom, MD; Jim Benson, MD; David Dreis, MD; Judy Bowen, MD; Roger Bush, MD; Alvin Calderon, MD; Brandee Grooms, MD.

Transitional Year (1983): Norm Rosenthal, MD; Jim Benson, MD; L. Keith Dipboye, MD; Ryan Pong, MD.

Urology (2013): Kathleen Kobashi, MD.

Pain Medicine (1994): Gale Thompson, MD; Hugh Allen, MD; Daniel Warren, MD; Kevin Vorenkamp, MD; Christine Oryhan, MD.

Female Pelvic Medicine and Reconstructive Surgery (2012): Kathleen Kobashi, MD; Alvaro Lucioni, MD.

In addition to program-specific staff, some GME staff serve all programs, and the GME program continues to evolve. The Medical Director of Simulation (with **Rob Hsiung, MD,** serving as the first appointee
to this position) and the Simulation and Training Coordinator have been
added in the past seven years as simulation efforts were expanded. These
programs are critical to education and patient safety and have improved
resident training immensely. The growth of simulation and innovation experiences for the residents has contributed to the creation of the Floyd
Jones Learning, Innovation and Simulation Center, supported by a $5 mil-
lion gift from Floyd Jones. Finally, there is the administrative assistant, a
"jack of all trades" to GME, the voice of GME to outside callers and the
face of GME to the numerous people who visit the department.

There have been many changes in GME over the past 25 years, with
some noteworthy highlights: ACGME, Virginia Mason Clinical Learning
Environment and National partnerships. The three are related.

For the first 17 years of its history ACGME's accreditation metrics
were process-based. ACGME personnel visited institutions and programs
to determine if they were in compliance with requirements, if residents'
learning experiences included prescribed numbers of weeks studying specific disciplines, and if they provided appropriate support to program leadership, support staff, faculty and physicians-in-training. That changed in
1998 with the Outcomes Initiative. ACGME sought to shift its focus from
processes to outcomes. Nineteen years later the work continues; accreditation and GME are remarkably changed.

ACGME's Outcomes Initiative began with a rigorous effort to identify
outcomes essential to a successful professional career. The six competencies
chosen continue to guide GME in 2017: patient care, medical knowledge,
practice-based learning and improvement, interpersonal and communication skills, professionalism and systems-based practice. Not surprisingly,
the competencies have spread beyond GME and are used by numerous
organizations in medicine, including the American Association of Medical

Colleges (AAMC), the Accreditation Council for Continuing Medical Education (ACCME) and the American Medical Association (AMA).

Virginia Mason welcomed the Outcomes Initiative and began implementation early in the new millennium. Competencies were incorporated into curricula, and evaluations were modified to collect competency-based information about resident performance.

The method chosen to address change is unique. In 2001, Virginia Mason adopted the Toyota Production System as its management system. The Virginia Mason Production System (VMPS) provided tools, processes and progressive instruction to enable staff to "work on their work." Using VMPS, various teams addressed all aspects of our teaching programs: recruitment processes, the on-boarding of new personnel, optimization of workflow for support staff, the evaluation system, workflow and teaching opportunities in both the hospital and clinic settings, patient care handoffs, faculty-resident feedback, disparity in health care and many more.

It became obvious to all that educational and operational units/functions had to be more closely aligned to prevent each from adversely affecting the other as they eliminated waste to make processes more efficient and effective. The work took many forms, required scheduled communication at all levels and relied on operational leadership for support and implementation. **Gary Kaplan, MD,** CEO; **Sarah Patterson,** COO; **Steve Rupp, MD**, Chief of Anesthesiology and Perioperative Services; **Lucy Glenn, MD**, Chief of Radiology; Joyce Lammert, MD, Chief of Internal Medicine; **Catherine Potts, MD,** Chief of Primary Care; and **Donna Smith, MD,** Chief of Clinics, were early operational leadership champions.

An interesting story from 2009 highlights work with ACGME. GME planned a one-week VMPS workshop to redesign the chaotic 60-to-90 day accreditation visit preparation. The goal was to create an environment of continuous preparedness for ACGME visits, one in which improvement was ongoing and driven by information from all sources available, including data collected by ACGME. The group asked ACGME if they had a representative interested in joining the team. To everyone's surprise, Ingrid

Philibert, Senior Vice President, Field Activities, the ACGME executive who oversaw accreditation visits, joined them for most of a very educational week. Although not known to the team at the time, the workshop aligned with ACGME efforts to update accreditation practices. Within four years, ACGME introduced the Next Accreditation System (NAS) emphasizing fewer accreditation visits, improved information flow between ACGME and programs and an emphasis on continuous improvement efforts rather than spot checks of compliance with requirements. Perhaps the workshop at VM contributed in some small way to the new system.

As efforts to address opportunities for improvement increased, GME needed more people involved in the activities. That realization led to the use of the Graduate Medical Education Committee (GMEC) to engage leaders, faculty and residents in improvement efforts and to having program directors complete VMPS for Leaders' training. The GMEC prioritized areas to address. **David Coy, MD,** and **Adnan Alseidi, MD,** led work to provide frequent, actionable resident feedback. The work built on an effort begun as a National Initiative project (see below). **Alvaro Lucioni, MD,** worked with Patient Safety to improve resident engagement with VM's Patient Safety Alert system. The work benefited all VM employees. **Jim Helman, MD,** and **Alvin Calderon, MD,** took on the challenge of improving faculty engagement, creating transparent expectations for faculty and identifying resources to assist them in achieving professional satisfaction as educators. **Ryan Pong, MD,** and **Jennifer Kohr, MD**, are leading efforts to improve opportunities for residents to complete scholarly activity during their time at VM.

The ACGME competencies combined with VMPS to stimulate significant interest in patient safety and quality improvement among residents, specifically in preparing themselves for a professional career where they would participate as members and leaders of teams to address opportunities to improve health care for individual patients, as well as for society. It was an opportunity for training beyond basic orientation to VMPS. Gillian Abshire, with the help of many others including **Alvin Calderon, MD, Craige Blackmore, MD** (Center for Health Care Improvement Science

- see chapter 36 in this volume), **Robert Mecklenburg, MD** (Center for Health Care Solutions), Patient Safety, and the Kaizen Promotion Office, created a systems-based elective that emphasized a multidisciplinary, team-based, patient-centered, value-driven approach to patient care that quickly became the most popular elective offered to VM residents.

GME's work in quality improvement, combined with VM's national reputation in the area, has changed the profile of people we recruit and opportunities for graduates. VM continues to attract residents looking for an outstanding educational experience in the subspecialty area of their choice. Increasingly, they attract residents who come with experience in systems design and engineering, quality improvement in medicine or other industries or advanced degrees in business, computer science, systems science, etc. Likewise, VM graduates are sought after for their clinical expertise and for their experience in patient safety and quality improvement that few other institutions can provide.

In 2005 VM's patient safety and quality improvement (PS/QI) efforts drew the attention of the Alliance of Independent Academic Medical Centers (AIAMC), who contacted GME to determine if there was an interest in joining their organization. AIAMC is a national organization of institutions very similar to VM. Member organizations are neither university nor medical-school based; they sponsor GME and many have research institutes in their organizational structure. When VM joined in 2006, AIAMC was searching to reenergize their membership. They chose PS/QI, an area where residents, for the most part, were invisible at the national level. To accomplish the goal of integrating PS/QI and GME, the organization developed National Initiatives - 18-month, national collaboratives that included formal education as well as experiential learning. National partners included ACGME and the Institute for Healthcare Improvement. Teams chose projects to benefit their programs and institutions. The goal was to integrate residents and faculty with multidisciplinary teams to learn about and use PS/QI principles. There have been six National Initiatives (NI) since 2007; VM has participated in all of them.

In NI 1, **Joe Panerio-Langer, MD,** an internal medicine resident, led a team of residents from internal medicine and general surgery to redesign the patient care handoff system from one that was paper-based and non-standardized to one embedded in the electronic medical record (EMR), templated for essential information and linked to information in the EMR progress note. **Rosemary Tempel, RN,** provided truly phenomenal project coordination. **Keith Dipboye, MD,** Transitional Year PD, directed programming to integrate the handoff into VM's EMR. **Bob Caplan, MD,** and **Cathie Furman,** executive leaders for quality, allocated $50,000 for programming costs. The handoff tool was made available to any caregiver at VM to communicate patient care information for coverage periods.

The NI 2 team worked with a multidisciplinary preoperative team to develop VM's Attestation Procedural Pause. GME team members were: general surgeons **Rich Kohler, MD** (faculty), and **Alison Porter, MD** (resident), and anesthesiologists **Mike Mulroy, MD** (faculty), and **Jon Narimasu, MD** (resident). Once again, Rosemary Tempel, RN, contributed her project management skills. Dr. Porter published the work in the *Joint Commission Journal of Quality and Safety* in January 2014; Dr. Narimasu presented the work at the Annual Meeting of the American Society of Anesthesiologists in 2010. The team won VM's Mary McClinton Award in 2012 and the Joint Commission noted that the procedural pause was the best they had ever witnessed.

NI 3 focused on feedback from resident contributors from all VM programs. Faculty leaders were **David Coy, MD; Ryan Pong, MD; Adnan Alseidi, MD**, and **Alexandra Morrison, MD**. The team developed a template for frequent, brief, resident-initiated feedback sessions. Work in improving feedback continues as one of VM's GMEC improvement tactics.

In 2013, the AIAMC chose health care disparities as the focus for NI 4. **Ananth Shenoy, MD,** and **Lauren Sullenberger, MD,** internal medicine, and **Justin Lieberman, MD**, anesthesiology, led VM's team to educate providers about health literacy. They produced short educational videos to highlight tactics and tools providers can use to improve patient comprehension of critical conversations.

470

NI 5 kicked off in 2015 and was completed in 2017. The team focused on improving VM's care for patients at risk for alcohol-related health concerns. The team consisted of primary care internal medicine residents: **Amy Thomson, MD** (team leader and chief resident); **Carly Magnusson, MD; Leighe Lincoln, MD; Michael Chu, MD,** and previous chief residents **Leah Geyer, MD,** and **Camille Johnson, MD.** Gillian Abshire provided operational leadership and faculty guidance came from **Karina Uldall, MD** (psychiatry); **Elly Bhatraju, MD** (primary care); **Norris Kamo, MD** (primary care); and **Mark Levy, MD** (primary care). Their work has improved screening for alcohol-related risk and created a resource guide that assists primary care providers with options for patients who desire treatment.

NI 6 ran from the fall of 2017 to the spring of 2019, focused on creating a culture of well-being in the clinical learning environment. A team of residents, program directors and GME leaders from across programs worked on eight projects in the three domains of "access to resources," "asking for help," and "creating connections."

VM plans to participate in the next National Initiative, which will focus on team-based, interprofessional collaborative care, and VM's team will be multidisciplinary, including GME, nursing, pharmacy and quality leadership, truly reflecting "team medicine".

VM's association with AIAMC has benefited many. Residents have an opportunity to work in national collaboratives and to see first-hand how other institutions work to address PS/QI. Along the way they have been exposed to national experts in education from ACGME and in PS/QI from the Institute for Healthcare Initiatives (IHI) and other organizations. Patient Safety and Quality at VM are improved by the tools and processes developed in team projects and VM's operational and educational missions benefit from a better understanding of each other's work.

This summary is far from complete and it is possible that others might choose different areas to highlight, such as the program's role in training physicians or leaders employed at VM and other institutions, or faculty and resident contributions to scholarly activity. However, the impetus for change has been driven by our national accrediting body; by Virginia Mason's culture and management system, VMPS; and by the decision to involve VM's GME Department in an organization committed to making GME and residents visible in the national movement to improve patient safety and quality improvement. As a result, Virginia Mason is on the right path to prepare the next generation of physician health care providers to address the challenges they will face as they create systems to improve care to individuals and populations at reduced cost.

Although this chapter has drawn attention to many people who have contributed to GME success, there are others that may have been missed. Truthfully, every resident and faculty member deserves to be named. They are the people who make the department one with a reputation for educating physicians who provide excellent care and who have proven over decades that they are leaders in their chosen professional endeavors.

References:

1. Hegstrom D. "Medical Education at Virginia Mason Hospital, 1962-1992." Virginia Mason Archives.

2. Letter from A. Stephen Graham, MD. "Reflections, Intern 1925-1926." Virginia Mason Archives.

3. Nourse AE. *VIRGINIA MASON MEDICAL CENTER: The First Fifty Years.* Seattle, WA: Frayn Printing and Publishing Co.; 1970:12.

4. Low, DE "From the Archives, Louis H. Edmunds, Orthopaedic Surgeon." *Bulletin*, v66(1); Spring 2012.

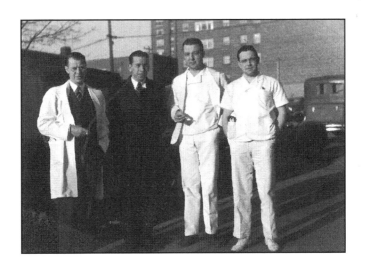

L to R: Surgeon Eugene Potter and internist John Wilkinson,
with interns William Cole and Larry White, circa 1937
(PH 6827, VMHA)

1954 - 1955 Housestaff
Back L to R: Randy Clements, Robert Schutt, Davis Lucas, Fred
Casserd, Doug Erickson, Ralph Nuzum, Wally Coburn, Charles Cobb, Ralph
Foster, Dave Bossler, Wally Nelson, Will Taylor, Lester Margetts, Vince Picconi,
Fred Blackhurst, Carl Lindstrom
Front, L to R: Clint Merrill, Tom Kerns, Ted Steffen, Maryonda Scher
(& daughter), Melvern Laidlaw, Nancy Elliott, Dave Witten,
Ralph Knopf (PH 1021, VMHA)

2014 - 2015 Housestaff
5th Row, L to R: Joshua Gulvin, Dion Booras, Bradley Hansen, Khalda Ibrahim,
G. Ryne Marshall, Kevin Finch
4th Row, L to R: Jeffrey Rouse, David Drimmer, Zachary Kane,
Carly Turgeon, Shanley Deal, Robert Henley
3rd Row, L to R: Nikolas Sirs, Ashleigh Leonard, Lauren Scovel, Alex Sheu,
Derek Khorsand, Kate Khorsand, Mahsa Karavan,
Julia Shlyankevich
2nd Row, L to R: Frank Kuo, Gregory Morris, Nathaniel Ott, Sana Jaffri, Jihoon
Lim, Crystal Kiewert, Caitlin Robinson, James Barlow
1st Row, L to R: Daniel Gealy, Jillian Warner, Justin Koo, Serena Frazee,
Sarah Lee, Lauren Powell, Monika Wells

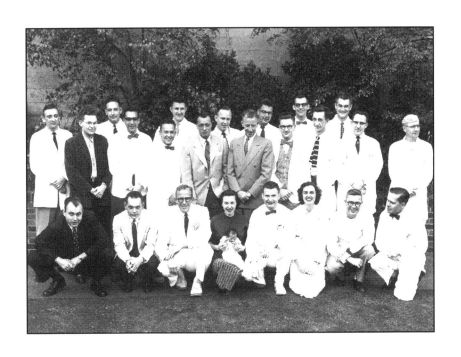

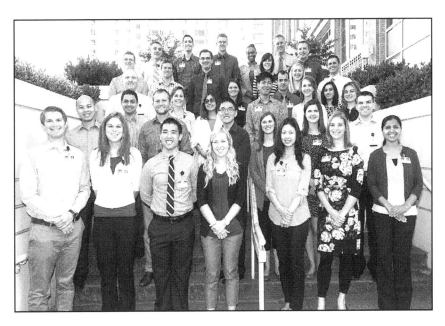

32

The History of Spiritual Care at Virginia Mason

by Cynthia Kirtland, M.Div.

In 1969, clinic physician **Robert L. King, MD,** formed a group called the Chaplain's Committee to explore the possibility of providing spiritual and emotional support to patients and family members at Virginia Mason. That committee, together with hospital administrator **Austin Ross,** recognized the fundamental importance of meeting the spiritual needs of patients during illness or at the end of life.

In 1971, the **Reverend George H. McCleave, DD**, a retired Presbyterian minister, approached the committee with the idea of establishing a volunteer chaplaincy at Virginia Mason through the Greater Seattle Council of Churches. Members of the Committee thought this would be a good opportunity to see if a resident chaplain would work in the hospital setting. McCleave and clergy from four faith communities in Seattle each spent one day a week at the hospital, caring for patients, their families and staff.

Rev. Richard Garlichs, an Episcopal priest, was the first chaplain to be hired at Virginia Mason; he began in January 1974 as a half-time resident chaplain. At the same time, Dr. King, chair of the Chaplain's Committee, began the process of securing funding from the community for a hospital chapel. It was opened and dedicated on June 1, 1975. The original chapel featured a stained glass window created by an art studio on Mercer Island and commissioned by a VM family in memory of their son.

In June of 1976, Rev. Garlichs received national accreditation to offer clinical pastoral education (CPE) at the hospital for seminary students and graduates. That program trained students to become certified as hospital chaplains while providing spiritual and emotional care.

Rev. Garlichs retired on January 31, 1985. That same year **Rev. David Wendleton** was hired as a full-time chaplain and CPE supervisor. He expanded the role of spiritual care to include participation with the Bioethics committee, the Institutional Review Board of the Research Center, and provide staff support, along with supervising CPE students year round. He worked at Virginia Mason for 13 years.

In February 1999, **Rev. Cynthia Kirtland** was hired; she is currently the supervisor of the Spiritual Care and Support department. Three chaplains plus volunteers provide patient and staff support throughout the organization, working closely with the palliative care and patient relations service lines. The department is currently building a peer-to-peer support program to care for colleagues in difficult situations. Spiritual care is now viewed as so essential to the care of patients that it is a Joint Commission requirement for hospital accreditation.

33

Fostering Relationships at Virginia Mason

by John Kirkpatrick, MD

The Doctors' Dining Room

In 1976, the doctors' dining room served as a gathering place for administrators and docs of all specialties. It sat between the cafeteria and the ophthalmology department, next to the Executive Conference Room, with round tables, a cafeteria line and good, subsidized food - all you could eat for $1.50. There was even a smokers' table saved for John Huff, Pat Ragen, Roy Correa, Dick Anderson and Wei Li, who were occasionally joined by pipe smokers Fritz Fenster and Lee Burnett. A clinic-wide initiative to make VM a non-smoking facility in the early 1980s put an end to that.

Doctors would gather to socialize, chat about interesting cases or listen to investment advice. One dermatologist was such a zealot for Howard Ruff doomsday economics that he sold his house and bought an apartment complex in Seattle and a farm 60 miles from the big city. There he grew crops to provide food for himself and his family when the grocery stores and supply chains went belly-up, and armed himself with guns to defend it. He later took a position in Saudi Arabia.

Friendly discussions around the tables were the norm. The clinic was like a family then, and internists, surgeons, radiologists, anesthesiologists, pathologists, gynecologists and administrators all came. Doctors saw just eight patients a day in those years, so there was time. The food wasn't gourmet but it wasn't bad. I recall there were two very tall, skinny guys, Bob Rudolph and Reilly Kidd, who took advantage of the pricing and completely filled their trays.

Interesting medical discussions ensued. One famous conversation involving Ken Wilske and Dick Kozarek led to methotrexate being used in the treatment of inflammatory bowel disease. Clinic politics were discussed. The debate was never-ending over who was responsible for the time delay between surgical cases – anesthesiologists or surgeons – and the obvious next question: why were freestanding ambulatory surgery centers so much more efficient? The dining room was an open forum for administrators and specialists of all types. Some came for ten minutes, just long enough to catch a bite to eat, while others had time to linger. It was a place where friendships were forged and enhanced as leisure activities, vacation sites and personal stories were exchanged. The number of bike-to-work advocates increased partially because of the enthusiasm they expressed at the lunch table, but we also learned there about a number of injuries they sustained on their way to work.

The Breakfast Club

Several physicians, administrators and hospital staff met regularly in the cafeteria in the morning.

According to "member" Janet Walthew: "I worked at VM from 1972 to 1997. The Breakfast Club was part of the VM culture long before I joined VM. It was a gathering place in the hospital cafeteria for early risers who enjoyed coffee, breakfast, a discussion of current events and fellowship before going our separate ways for the day.

"Fritz Fenster, MD (hepatologist) was considered the Chairman of the Breakfast Club. His birthday was Halloween and always a good excuse for a celebration. One year we had a plaque made and installed on the back of his chair that read: 'Fritz Fenster, MD, Chairman of the Breakfast Club.'

"Other members included:

Bill Traverso, MD, surgeon

Joe Yon, MD, GYN surgeon

David Zehring, MD, plastic surgeon

David Dail, MD, pathologist

Jennings Borgen, MD, community OB/GYN

Art Zoloth, Pharm D, Pharmacy Director

Marion Watanabe, Assistant Director of Food Service

"Often joining in were Roger Lindeman, MD, and administrators Don Olson and Austin Ross. Over time, the group developed close friendships that remain to this day. We often scheduled events outside the hospital. Dr. Fenster was famous for his waffles, and Bill Traverso once brought his llamas along for a hike on the John Wayne Trail. Being with this group is one of my fondest memories of my 25 years at Virginia Mason."

According to another member, Art Zoloth, "Besides the camaraderie, they acted as a support group for each other during times of stress or loss or conflict."

Other Gatherings

Surgeons, anesthesiologists and self-selected, bold internists drank coffee and ate donuts in the surgeons' lounge in the morning. Others met for coffee at the Tully's in the hospital breezeway, or offsite at the nearest Starbucks. Some walked down to the Convention Center through Freeway Park for an off-campus lunch, especially on Fridays. Virginia Mason also organized a street fair on 9th Avenue, closing off the block for vendors, and on the Lindeman patio. Weather might sometimes interfere, but it rarely deterred the hungry workforce looking for different food options and a time for conversation.

Rumors flew that some male staff docs ate lunch in the dark, smoky back room of Vito's Restaurant at the corner of 9th and Madison, reminiscent of the hangouts in big cities where "big decisions" were made. Others met at the Hunt Club at the Sorrento Hotel after work. Another group that gathered off-campus was the infamous poker group including Drs. Dreis, Gortner, Bender, Quigley and Yasuda.

Another highlight was the Tuesday night housestaff versus attendings pick-up basketball games, which helped to "even the playing field". The basketball court was an equalizer, and long-standing relationships developed there are still in existence. This competition culminated in an annual housestaff-attending game for the coveted Donna Hegstrom Trophy, which was usually won by the much younger and (suspiciously) highly-recruited housestaff team. As the unofficial housemother of the graduate medical education staff, Donna was thought to influence the selection of interns based on their height and basketball pedigree. It was a little too obvious when one new intern, the son of comedian Syd Cesar, checked in at 6'11". Fortunately he was a wonderful intern, proving himself over and over on the hospital floors, but he was way too much for the attendings to handle on the basketball court. Relationships formed playing basketball translated into an uncommon collegiality on the hospital wards and in the operating rooms. The housestaff also participated with attendings in annual tennis nights where ten courts at a local public facility were filled with round robin play, followed by dinner at an attending's home. Sections also formed teams to run in fundraisers for Juvenile Diabetes, Alzheimer's Disease, Leukemia (the Columbia Tower Climb), Arthritis (the Jingle Bell Run) and the Heart Walk. VM Hospital fielded other teams in softball and bowling leagues.

Biannual staff retreats for the physician staff and administrators at Port Ludlow, Alderbrook or Semi-ah-moo provided time to discuss sensitive matters in depth, as well as time to get better acquainted through humorous skits, card games, athletic endeavors and excellent cuisine. An in-town meeting held at a Sea-Tac conference center was fun, but too many decided to work part-time and not attend all the sessions, so subsequent retreats were held OUT OF TOWN.

The Annual Professional Staff Dinner during the holidays, as well as the Dreambuilders' Ball, a fundraiser for specific programs at the medical center, were other opportunities to dress up and gather in a festive setting, and continue to this day.

At the medical center, teaching conferences, grand rounds, CME courses and tumor boards were times when specialists from different sections gathered to discuss the medical aspects of challenging cases. The seemingly endless committee meetings were another time to interact, and "New Docs Rock" was a popular morning coffee hour where providers met and welcomed new recruits. The annual Mason Clinic Day was a chance to invite local and regional physicians for a free day of medical workshops, lectures and lunch. Many VM physicians saw this as a way to teach and learn together, developing both internal and external relationships.

One particular administrator, Keith Lundberg, was a master at relationship building. Keith headed the Regional Hospitals' Consortium, and was instrumental in arranging for our specialists to give lectures in outlying communities from the Olympic peninsula to Alaska. A private pilot himself, Keith never flew our staff to these centers, but he arranged for efficient transport, allowing them to maximize patient care and educational time.

Keith was also instrumental in the early adoption of VM's Telemedicine program. An annual lectureship, as well as the control room of our Volney Richmond Auditorium, is named in his honor. He was also the administrator responsible for VM's international medical services work in Asian countries and the Russian Far East, and led VM's participation as a host of the APEC meeting in Seattle in 1993 (see the chapter on International Medicine in this volume). Keith received a special citation from then Secretary of State Warren Christopher for his APEC efforts.

Humor

Humor also influenced the close-knit and connected culture at VM. Allergist Mike Mullarkey organized the infamous St. Patrick's Day spoof grand rounds, when numerous staff doctors took turns presenting tongue-in-cheek "scholarly" treatises. Urologist George Brannen recited an original poem, and Dick Winterbauer offered an evaluation scale for residents based on Superman qualities: faster than a speeding bullet, more powerful than a locomotive and able to leap tall buildings in a single bound. On Dick's scale some residents were slower than molasses, or functioned at one horsepower, or took several bounds to jump over small obstacles. Gary Kaplan presented "Mason Clinic East", renaming the downtown campus "Mason Clinic West". Bruce Nitsche noted several sequential, but contradictory, notes in the hospital charts and termed them "Chart Wars". Orthopaedists Ray Robinson and Tom Green poked fun at various orthopaedic dilemmas and Bill Steenrod took aim at building projects; Andy Healey took on the medical pre-history form. This was one Friday morning each year in the 80s that everyone looked forward to.

The interns always did a skit on housestaff graduation night, spoofing various attending physicians on-stage as "The Buddha", "Dr. Terminal Euphoria", or for displays of certain behaviors in the operating room. Every year the residents clamored for Ed Morgan's famous "mouse trick" using a cloth napkin, and another favorite was a spoof of a rectal sphincter pressure-measuring device called the "bottomanometer", complete with graphs of the daily pressures of various attendings compared to that of an intern during an actual Code 4.

Each year the April issue of VM's monthly newsletter *Pulse* became the *"Re-Pulse"* as an April Fools' joke. A secret committee worked on the publication for weeks, tackling pertinent and timely issues of the day. Robots replacing humans was a front page story that actually came true a couple years later when a robot was designed to deliver inpatient pharmacy medications to hospital floors. Trades of various physicians to other major medical centers for "another doctor, cash and future considerations" were reported – and later an actual trade of residents did occur between VM and UC San Diego. The editorial committee was secret, but rumors flew that Ted Johnson, Peter Manos, John Kirkpatrick and Mardie Rhodes were somehow involved, although no one ever admitted participation.

Talented in-house humorist Ted Johnson was frequently asked to do gigs. Ted was the featured speaker at SENSE Program retreats, and gave over a hundred presentations on lifestyle and health. He also gave a talk to each hospital shift on the medical center's cumbersome floor numbering system. Leave it to Ted to find the humor in "what's the first floor, and what's the ground floor, and why is the ground floor in the hospital really the 4th floor?" Ted was also asked to explain the medical center's new org chart to similar audiences, and there was much in it to poke fun at!! Then there was KVM radio, hosted by Ted and Kim Pittenger, often narrated by the golden voice of VM, Dick Foley. Over 500 weekly episodes were beamed into voicemails touting new programs, important issues or just new providers. Ted and Kim did a wonderful job, always with balance and humor.

Dick Foley had a special role at the medical center. He was the frequent emcee at large medical center celebrations and gatherings, and his recognizable soothing voice could be heard outlining options for the patient calling the medical center for appointments or information, or narrating promotional videos. His wonderful singing voice (Dick historically performed with the popular recording group, The Brothers Four) led the collective holiday troubadour group through the hospital halls with his guitar-playing delighting patients and staff. No matter what he was tapped to do on behalf of VM Communications, Dick was an upbeat and positive presence, and his work gave a warm professional face to Virginia Mason.

I found myself made fun of at my first partner's meeting in 1976. I was 28 years old, having finished college at 21, medical school at 25 and a Mayo residency at 28. We "associates" (two years and an affirmative vote were required for partnership at that time) sat in the back of the room. Then chief clinic administrator, John Dare, stood at the front and directed the group, "I want you to look around the room now. In the year 2013, there will only be one of us still here, and that's Kirkpatrick." Indeed, 2013 was the year I would turn 65, and the Clinic had a mandatory retirement age of 65, a rule that would later be rescinded. This predated the Doogie Howser TV program, so I was repeatedly asked by patients whether I was old enough to be a doctor. After Doogie Howser debuted, nobody asked me how old I was anymore. When I did retire at age 65, I was the longest-serving partner at that time.

Charity

Many staff physicians participated in charitable efforts. The Sweet Charity Auction with its "Gong Show" theme was a popular noon activity. The production pressure that grew after the early 1990s hadn't started, and lunchtime was a chance to take a break and have some fun for a good cause.

The annual Christmas party for physicians' families featured a Santa initially played by the ever-game Mike Mullarkey, and later at least once by John Ryan, whose own children didn't recognize him in the Santa outfit. John's office nurses wore reindeer costumes. The event was organized by the VM Spouses' Association, which was an integral part of the VM community supporting the physicians and medical center activities. The Professional Staff Holiday Party in a downtown hotel has been a time for physicians, administrators and their spouses to dress up and celebrate the season together, and retirement celebrations were black-tie affairs in the 70s and 80s. Many tired of renting tuxedos and just went ahead and bought a tux to save themselves the trouble. As the years passed, that tradition went away, with more people retiring quietly and moving on to the next stage of life without much fanfare.

In Closing

So what is that "special sauce" that makes Virginia Mason so unique? I believe it is the relationships. As one physician who left VM and later worked both in Seattle at a large competing medical center and in Bellevue told me, "VM had uniformly excellent physicians who were easily approachable and worked incredibly well together." He went on, "Even the crusty old guys were giving good care!" My friend didn't find this at other institutions, and hadn't previously at his excellent training programs.

Virginia Mason physicians work together, teach each other, learn from each other, respect each other and, I believe, genuinely like each other. They financially support and volunteer in worthwhile community organizations. Most of all, many have spent their entire working years at Virginia Mason and retired from their first job!

We owe a tremendous debt of gratitude to the founding fathers and the many who followed in their exceedingly large footsteps. They imagined a place where the integration of clinic and hospital, supported by excellent laboratory and radiologic services, would create a place where excellent medicine could be practiced and set the stage for "team medicine" to flower and grow. The next generation now carries that torch forward into the future and one hopes the next 100 years will be as fruitful.

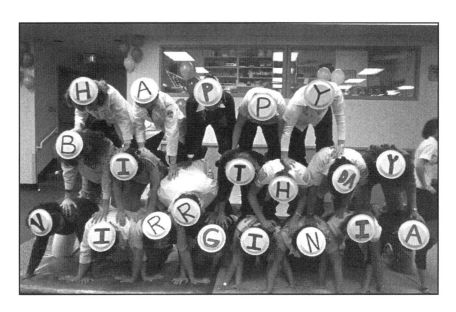

May 1980 - Happy Birthday Virginia! (PH 8996, VMHA)

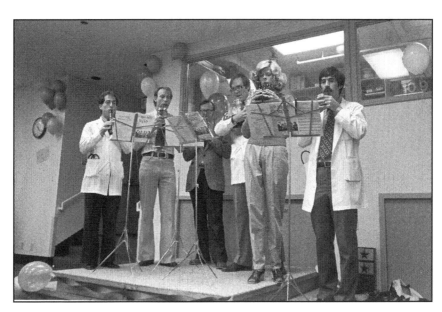

May 1980: Staff Band
L to R:Fred Fox, Dave Gortner, Frank Allen, John Kirkpatrick,
Cori Kirkpatrick, Bob Wilburn (PH 8995, VMHA)

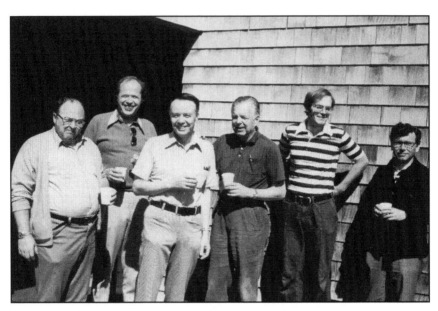

Port Ludlow Retreat 1977
L to R: Jack Houck, Bob Kellum, John Allen, Tate Mason Jr,
John Kirkpatrick, Bob Riggins (PH 2468a, VMHA)

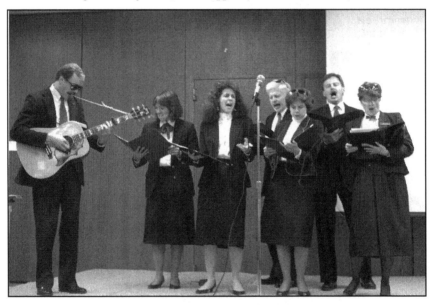

The Administration Singers at the Gong Show 1988
L to R: Mark Secord on guitar, Sarah Patterson, Ann Danford, Don Olson,
Joyce Jackson, Ned Borgstrom, Ingrid Olson (PH 8988, VMHA)

34

Virginia Mason Administration
Perspectives in Management

by Don Olson, George Auld, Sandy Novak, Ruth Anderson,
Mike Rona, Bill Poppy, Craig Goodrich, & John Kirkpatrick, MD

In its 100-year history, VMMC had only seven physicians who served as "Chairman." The original model of a cooperative relationship between physician and the management team started in 1920 and has resulted in a remarkably similar number of Senior Administrators - six: Lewis Dare, his son, John Dare, Austin Ross, Mike Rona, Sarah Patterson and Sue Anderson. These leaders are described below along with their tenures. In addition, there are descriptions and remembrances intermingled from other leaders who significantly impacted Virginia Mason history, included in roughly chronological order.

Lewis Dare (1920 - 1946)
Emeritus Executive Administrator

What would the infant clinic have become without the wise counsel of businessman Lewis Dare? Born in Australia in 1883, at the age of 14 he went to sea with the British Merchant Marine and traveled the world, eventually settling in Winslow, Washington on Bainbridge Island. By 1915 Mr. Dare had moved to

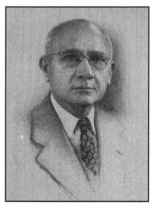

Pendleton, Oregon where he ran the Dare Tire Company, distributing Diamond Tires to the entire eastern half of Oregon. When businesses there suffered from the post-WWI Depression, Lewis sold what remained of the business and returned to Bainbridge Island, where he had maintained his previous home.

A few years earlier, former business associate Mrs. George Dowling had approached him about helping her husband, Dr. George Dowling, and his partners James Tate Mason and John Blackford with the administration of their clinic and a proposed hospital. Upon his return to Bainbridge Island, Lewis finally accepted and helped manage the opening of both the Mason-Blackford-Dowling Clinic, and, two weeks later, the Virginia Mason Hospital on November 1, 1920. Lewis skillfully navigated the clinic through tough financial times that included The Great Depression and after 26 years at the helm, turned the reins over to his son, John Dare, who had been filling multiple roles at the clinic and hospital for about ten years.

John Dare (1936 - 1977)
Emeritus Executive Administrator

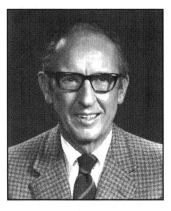

Stories about the capable, dedicated John Dare abound. Born on Bainbridge Island in 1912, John recalled his parents inviting Joel Baker and Louis Edmunds over to their home tennis court, where he and his brother trounced them. After graduation from the University of Washington in accounting, jobs were scarce and he took a position as a night auditor at the Roosevelt Hotel. A year later, Virginia Mason invited him to help out on the business side, and he accepted. One of his jobs was writing payroll checks to the staff. He later recalled that the highest paid employee at the time was the chief cook, a Chinese immigrant named Suey Gim Locke, grandfather of former Washington State Governor Gary Locke. John would write one big check to Locke, who would then divide up the funds and pay his entire kitchen staff, which included many of his own family.

After eleven years John's father stepped down, and John was appointed to the Senior Administrator position in 1946. Exceptionally skilled in financial and system development issues, John was very highly respected by Virginia Mason staff and others in his field. He was founder of the regional Blue Cross, regional hospital associations and many joint services. According to "From the Archives" by Don Low, "John Dare was the President of Washington State Hospital Association, President of the Association of Western Hospitals, President of the Seattle Hospital Council and Chair of the Council on Administration of the American Hospital Association." He was also known for believing that there was too much regulation and paperwork in medicine. In his words, "It's like counting how many times a bird flapped its wings rather than determining if it flew or how far." He also famously said, "Listen to the passengers, but don't let them design the airplane or fly it." [1]

Austin Ross, MPH (1955 - 1991)
Emeritus Executive Administrator

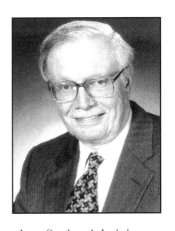

Austin Ross was born in Wisconsin in 1929. He went into the military after graduating from UC Berkeley with a BS in business and later went on to earn his MPH. Austin came to VMH as an administrative resident in 1955 and the next year was hired by John Dare as the Assistant Administrator for the Mason Clinic. He went on to be Associate Administrator of the hospital for twelve years, then Senior Administrator of the clinic for eleven years. He played a significant role in the 1987 clinic restructuring and held the position of Vice President and Executive Administrator for the newly-formed Virginia Mason Medical Center for 4 years. He served as chairman of the College of Healthcare Executives, chair of the Medical Group Managers, president of the Association of Western Hospitals, Washington State Hospital Association, and consultant with the Kellogg Foundation and the Robert Woods Foundation. In 2010, he was inducted into the National Health Care Hall of Fame along with Senator Ted Kennedy. Upon retirement he became Professor in the University of Washington School of Public Health and Community Medicine, where he directed the Capstone projects for MHA students.

Don Olson, BA, MHA (1965 - 1998)
Emeritus Hospital Administrator

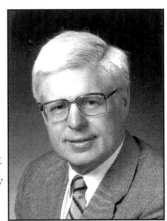

Don was known as an exceptional executive on both the hospital and clinic side of VMMC. He had much to do with the successful relationship with Group Health, and was known as a personal advocate by the entire staff. Don spent nearly 33 years at Virginia Mason and was highly respected by physicians and other employees. His own reflections are included below.

VMMC Reflections: July 1965 - January 1998

In recalling these events, please know that the decisions, actions and outcomes that were undertaken were all with the benefit of an excellent Administrative team, similar to the way the Clinic has always practiced Team Medicine.

I was hired by John Dare and Austin Ross. I came from the M.D. Anderson and Tumor Institute in Houston, Texas, an institution under the auspices of the University of Texas that conducted patient care as well as research devoted to cancer. My arrival at Virginia Mason found four separate organizations that were closely linked – the physician partnerships of The Mason Clinic and the Mason Properties, and the nonprofit Virginia Mason Hospital and Virginia Mason Research Center. At the time of my retirement in 1998, all of these organizations had been joined together to form the Virginia Mason Medical Center with one common Board of Directors providing governance. During my VMMC tenure I served under the leadership of four physician Chairmen: Drs. Baker, Walker, Cleveland

492

and Lindeman and was employed by both the physician partnership and the Virginia Mason Hospital.

There were 55 physicians when I first arrived (total, including the partners and soon-to-be partners). They were all specialists organized within their specialty sections in the Departments of Surgery and Medicine. In 2013 while attending the annual Professional Staff reception and dinner, I was reminded just how much change has taken place as the CEO, Dr Kaplan, read off the names of the 53 newly arriving physicians. Of note, in 1965 there were no Sections of General Internal Medicine or Psychiatric Medicine. The stories of how each of those sections was added makes for interesting tales. Today the Section of General Internal Medicine is the largest section.

Within Administration, the close working relationship between the Hospital and the Clinic had long been established. For financial reasons, the hospital had been created by the physicians but organized as a charitable organization. This close-working relationship and the physical connections made for some interesting operations. Arm's length financial relationships were required to avoid any perception that the charitable hospital was being operated for the benefit of The Mason Clinic. Notwithstanding this operating condition, it was our goal administratively to avoid duplication of services that would unnecessarily add to operating costs – thus we had only one Medical Record Department, one Housekeeping Department, one Food Service, one Maintenance Department, one Laboratory, one Radiology Department, etc. But, of course, we had two distinct business offices that processed all patient accounts.

At the time of my arrival, we had no computers to support patient billing. We had National Cash Register (NCR) posting machines and thousands of pieces of paper that came from physician offices, the laboratory, radiology and any other point-of-patient-care service. It was a paper jungle and nightmare represented by buckets of ledger cards that reflected each patient's account. Soon after my arrival, we began the process of converting to IBM punch cards, guided by our auditing and consulting firm, Arthur Anderson & Co. That began a long relationship as we went from punch cards to the age of computers – in fact, rooms full of computers.

The Campus

Significant changes to the physical campus took place during my tenure. Regretfully, I am not able to include the exact year of these changes.

For example, when I arrived, the first expansion of the original hospital building had already been accomplished, but Terry Avenue was still a thru street connecting Spring Street and Seneca. Additional changes through 1995 are detailed in the excellent book by Austin Ross – *Vision and Vigilance*, and changes beyond that date are left to others to describe.

From: George Auld, CPA (1970 - 1996)
Emeritus Director of Finance
Re: VM Percentage/Compensation
Committee

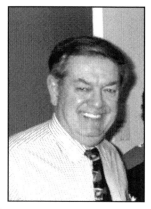

As I look back on my administrative service for the VM Percentage/Compensation Committee, there is no doubt that it was my favorite assignment over the years. The reason is the strong respect I gained working with the type of physicians who were attracted to Virginia Mason.

In the early years, from 1970 to the mid-eighties, it was called the Percentage Committee, since "The Mason Clinic" was a legal partnership, with the seventy partners at that time each owning a certain percentage share.

The Committee was composed of the Chairman of the Clinic, the Chiefs of Medicine and Surgery, plus a Service Chief representative for the Departments of Anesthesiology, Pathology/Laboratory and Radiology. Later on, the Chief of Satellites was added to the committee. In addition, there were three members elected from the rest of the partnership. By design, the "Chairman of the Committee" was always elected from this latter group. The time served was typically four years.

The formula for determining physician compensation when I arrived in March of 1970, was one-third credit for seniority, one-third for productivity and one-third for PAGE (Professional Activities and Group Effort). Don Olson served as the administrative support and I was the number cruncher.

494

After going through the numbers (more on that later) the partners were assigned into ten different groupings, with the same percentage given to each member of the group. A list of the respective percentages was then sent to each partner, so that "all partners" knew where everyone stood. New partners were always added on August 1st of each year.

As an aside, in my first year at VM, after I had sent out the revised percentage list following the August 1970 admission of new partners, I received a phone call from Dr. Birchfield. He said, "GEORGE, why is my new percentage .813, while Nielsen's is .814? We have always had the same number before." I said, "No problem, Dr. Birchfield, the numbers have to add up to 100%, so yours was rounded down." There was silence and then he said, as he slammed down the phone, "Then round it off somewhere else!!!"

That is when I learned that physicians don't always think like accountants. Naturally, I never made that mistake again ☺.

During the seventies, there was a continuing disagreement between Medicine and Surgery, with respect to the one-third credit given for productivity. The surgeons' viewpoint was that since their productivity was considerably higher, they should get more credit and a bigger piece of the pie. The internist's viewpoint was that the surgeons' high productivity was the "direct result" of the many patients that had been sent to them from the Department of Medicine. This was a never-ending battle that took up a great deal of the committee's efforts.

I don't recollect the exact timing, but eventually we did lose several very good surgeons because of salary levels. Accordingly, the formula was changed to eliminate seniority and give greater credit to productivity.

This may be a good place to further elaborate on the professionalism and collegiality of the physicians on the committee. Since it was considered a definite honor to serve, it was a position that was taken very seriously by all. Differences occurred, but did not deteriorate the spirit of "fair play" for all the physicians that would be affected by their decisions. It was definitely NOT a case of the "boys in the back room" making political deals. In addition, as the mix of physicians in the Clinic became more diversified, there were often female physicians on the committee. As new members came on-board, they were welcomed and their input given its proper due. This concept, of making the process one that was determined by "facts not favors", certainly held up over the many years that I served.

In July 1986, when the Medical Center became a non-profit entity, the name was changed to the Compensation Committee. The process of setting the following year's salaries usually started in late September and took anywhere from three to four months.

Productivity: Productivity measurement was based on the charges per MD, through the prior fiscal year ending June 30th. NO CREDIT was given for "ancillary tests ordered". However, there were some added adjustments made for MD, interpretations, such as EKGs, EEGs, etc. and credit was given for Specialty Laboratory supervision and other administrative duties. Disability/sabbatical and other absences were also taken into account.

Since "gross charges" were not the same as collected ones, the concession rate for the period was deducted and productivity was always based on "net charges".

Each year, VM initiated its own "10 Clinic Club member survey" to determine the "ratio" of MD, salary to net charges per specialty, which was then applied to each MD's net charges to arrive at a possible salary figure. For example, if the average salary for a specialty was $175,000 and the average net charges were $350,000, then the "ratio" would be 50%.

An important "MD, Salary Survey" that we participated in was done by the Rochester, Minnesota C.P.A. firm of McGladrey & Pullen. Based on "33 large medical groups", it gave us the 20th percentile, median, mean and 80th percentile for most specialties. Thus, we had a 6,000 physician "reality check" for our initial VM salary figures. Final "grand total comparisons", usually put us modestly above the M & P median.

PAGE: The review of "Professional Activities (PA) and Group Effort (GE)" was done every other year, in order to reduce workload. Fifty (50) points were allotted for PA and (50) points for GE. Each physician was given a Professional Activity form to complete and return. It was then graded by

496

a non-VM employee per grading guidelines, and submitted to the section head for review and adjustments, if needed. In the late eighties, the long-time grader retired and Mike authorized Kay (my wife) to take over the task. In order to be more consistent and save time, she graded five MDs at once on the same question. This worked out quite well and resulted in fewer section head adjustments.

On the GE side, the Committee met with each section head alone and received their input for all MDs in their section concerning "Profession-al Excellence, Relationships, Work Effort and Organizational Growth." Since there was a natural tendency for section heads to grade their mem-bers on the high side ☺, the committee would then discuss the data later and often lower the original evaluations. In this situation, the department chiefs' input was typically given more weight.

While PAGE was not perfect, it was a VM preference that there should be more to salaries than just productivity. The 1996 average for PAGE was 45 points out of 100.

As can be surmised from the above description, the process was very time-consuming. It grew from a ten-key adding machine approach, with penciled spreadsheets for 70 partners, to personal PC-generated data for 275 members. I certainly would not have been able to do it without the invaluable help of Carol Forbes, my primary trusted financial accountant, and secretary Paulette Burrell, who xeroxed dozens of detailed schedules and hand-deliv-ered them weekly in "confidential" envelopes to committee members.

Sandy McMurray Novak, MBA (1978 - 2007)
Retired Administrative Director

A leader in fostering good employee relations and skilled in clinic management, Sandy was a University of Washington graduate with an MBA from City University in Seattle. Winner of the Terin Guinn Award as an outstanding manager, and certified in Lean/Kaizen Lead-ership, she developed and still manages the

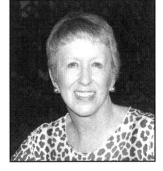

VM Retirees Association. A snapshot photography business keeps her busy in retirement. Sandy contributes her personal thoughts in the following pages.

Joining The Mason Clinic in 1978

In 1978, I was working at the Westin Hotel as the Personnel Director when I got a call from a colleague saying that Dennis Lencioni, the Personnel Director at The Mason Clinic had resigned to take a position at Boeing. He recomended that I apply for his job. I had met Dennis through the Pacific Northwest Personnel Management Association and had a lot of respect for him. So I was intrigued, and decided to apply. A few days later, I got a call from Bob Boyle, who was the Senior Assistant Administrator asking if he could meet me over lunch. We agreed to have lunch at Trader Vic's, which was one of the restaurants in the Westin.

I remember thinking carefully about what I would wear to the lunch, and I settled on a new suit that I had just bought. It was very tailored and well-made and had been expensive although I had found it on sale. I was feeling very professional as I greeted him. He looked at me and one of the first things he said was, "Oh, do you have to wear a uniform here?" Somewhat crushed, I replied something like, "Oh, no, this isn't a uniform."

A couple of weeks later, I was told that I was a finalist for the position and was scheduled for a day of interviews with various physicians and administrators at the clinic and hospital. My competition was the Personnel Director at Cabrini Hospital. I remember being rather amazed at how many people I needed to interview with that day. One of the things that everyone talked about was that the hospital and clinic had just had a big change with all of the key administrators switching organizations. In those days the hospital and clinic had separate sets of administrators and the change had been made in order to shake things up a bit and bring new perspectives to each organization while still retaining the same experienced players.

The next week, I got a phone call from Austin Ross who was the Clinic Administrator, and he offered me the job. In June of 1978, I joined The Mason Clinic as Personnel Director. The department managers greeted

498

me warmly and a number of them took me to lunch. Before long, George Auld, who was the Director of Finance, invited me to lunch. He said we would go out to his favorite restaurant. It turned out to be the International House of Pancakes. As we pulled into the parking lot, he said, "I'll say to you the same thing that I said to Dennis. Dutch Treat." I felt myself panic a little as I wondered, "Shoot, how much money do I have with me?" Once inside, I was able to sneak a peek in my wallet. Only a couple of dollars! When the waitress came, I ordered a small cup of soup and a glass of water. When George questioned me, I just said that I wasn't very hungry and watched him eat a steaming stack of pancakes, eggs and bacon. I tried not to look too envious!

There were a lot of challenges those first couple of years. Prior to my arrival, the laboratory staff had voted in favor of union representation and the clinic was in the middle of contract negotiations. As the contract negotiations went along, the clinic had gone ahead and implemented some of the demands of the union and at the end of it, the laboratory staff looked at the contract and didn't see any substantial gains from what they had, and voted to decertify the union. At that time, there were a lot of new laws relating to discrimination and labor relations. Many of the managers lacked the skills or confidence needed to talk with their staff about performance issues and were under the impression that their hands were completely tied. I did a lot of coaching and role-playing with them to help them gain confidence and realize they could still set goals and expectations for their staff as long as they did it in a fair and consistent way.

The clinic had engaged a wage and salary consultant to review all of the job descriptions and salary levels for staff. This caused a great deal of angst as everyone had their own ideas about the internal value of various positions. Since the structure of the clinic was a for-profit partnership at that time, a lot of the physicians were accustomed to being involved in the governance and were giving their opinions about who should be paid how much. One example I remember was for the position of phlebotomist. One physician confessed that he had always had trouble doing blood draws and I think because it was hard for him, he felt strongly that this was one of the most valuable jobs in the clinic and should be highly compensated - near the level of a nurse.

As the Director of Human Resources, I was considered part of the Administrative team. This was one of the aspects that had appealed to me about the job. Once a week, Austin Ross, Bob Boyle, Paul Friedrich, George Auld and I would meet to brief Fred Cleveland, MD, who was the Chairman of the Clinic. This was a position elected by the physician partnership. I always found these meetings to be very informative and also a chance to observe the various administrative styles. I reported to Austin and I was always very attentive to how he handled things and the writing style that he had. He was a masterful communicator and strategist.

At that time, there were 120 physicians at the clinic and none of them were women. It was even considered quite controversial that the clinic had hired its first internal medicine physician. Some of the physicians regarded this as a step that would diminish the specialty image of the clinic. I was the only woman who worked in clinic administration. Nancy Friedrich was an assistant administrator in the hospital and Jan Dortzbach was a psychologist in the clinic. As a member of administration, I was entitled to eat lunch in the Doctor's Dining Room. The first six months I was there, I found it very intimidating to eat there as I was usually the only woman in a sea of white coats. I have always been a person who sets goals and objectives, so in January of 1979, one of my goals was to eat there once a week. After a few weeks, it became much more comfortable, and then most of the time I did have lunch there. I found that it was a good way to network with the physicians and get to know them on a non-controversial basis, which made it easier to work with them, especially if we had to deal with a tough topic.

About 9 months after I began at The Mason Clinic, Rick Osterhout, an administrative fellow was hired. He had just finished his master's degree in hospital administration and he began attending all of the administrative briefings and doing special projects. It was the custom of the partnership to go to the Rainier Club for dinner after the annual partnership meeting. It began to dawn on me that I was not going to be included in this dinner.

I felt kind of bad, but I decided I would just take it in stride, since I was somewhat new and perhaps not high enough on the totem pole to rate an invite. The afternoon of the event, I happened to be crossing the clinic lobby and I saw a truck pull in and unload a rack of tuxedos. All of the men going to the Rainier Club wore tuxes for this special night. Then I saw Rick come out and select his tux from the rack. The young, male administrative fellow had been invited but I had not. I stood there somewhat stunned.

I went ahead to a meeting that was scheduled that afternoon with Bob Boyle. At the end of it, he said, "Well, I'll see you tonight at the Rainier Club." I just said, "Well, I'm not going." He asked me why not and I replied that I wasn't invited. He was incensed and said he was going to talk to Austin. I told him not to because it was too late in the day and I didn't want to make a big deal out of it.

The next year, I was invited. I knew it was a significant happening for a woman to be included, and I wanted to be as low key about it as possible. I went to Fredrick & Nelson department store and found a black Oscar d' La Renta dress with a white collar and cuffs that was on sale. I was hoping to blend in as much as possible with the tuxes. I was the only woman there but all went well. In the past, the Rainier Club had not even let women attend events and that was just starting to change. They were in the process of adding a women's restroom and while it was useable, it was still roughed in and the plasterboard was unpainted. A few years later, I was even brave enough to take part in a roast at one of these events, which was honoring Louie Hungerford, a volatile but skilled ophthalmologist. I have to admit I asked Diane Clark, who was the manager of the Medical Transcription department, to help me with some of my lines as she had a clever and wicked sense of humor. Fortunately, Louie found my insults hilarious.

At that time, a lot of the physicians had a kind of love-hate relationship with administration. Once in the Doctor's Dining Room, I was at a lunch table with a physician who was a notorious chauvinist, and he started talking about being against letting women in the Doctor's Dining Room as they would probably want to turn all of the conversations into talking about their favorite recipes. I decided to see if I could have a little fun with him and I said, "Well, I kind of admire a man who can cook. I bet that you are a really great cook." Immediately, he took the bait and started telling me how to make his favorite omelet. I listened intently and have wondered many times since if he ever realized what had just transpired.

John Allen, MD, was the Chief of Medicine. He was incredibly effective, but he also had a Machiavellian side to him. His favorite pass time was taunting and testing administrators. Shortly after I arrived, he set up a meeting with me. I went up to the eighth floor where Pulmonary Medicine was located and was told to be seated in the hallway. He was in his office but he kept me waiting for over half an hour. I knew he had done it just to put me in my place, so the next time we had a meeting, I took a bunch of work with me and sat outside doing it while I waited. He came out and saw me doing this, and I could see by the expression on his face that he realized I wasn't going to be intimidated by this tactic. He never kept me waiting again. Another favorite trick of his was to call and leave a message for an administrator if he knew they were out of the building for a personal or professional reason. It was his way of sending them a message that said, "I know you aren't in your office ... why aren't you at work?" Finally, one time as the Christmas holidays were coming up, I sent him a memo listing the days I was going to be taking off and telling him that I was giving him advance notice so that he wouldn't have to bother to see if I was in or not. He stopped calling me when I was gone after that.

Bob Nielsen, MD, an endocrinologist, made no secret of the fact that he thought the Personnel Department was a waste of money and resources. He told me this as well as anyone else who would listen. I started sending him memos and notes every time we implemented a cost-effective policy or program. After doing this for about two years, the day came when I got a note from him saying that I had finally convinced him of the value of the Personnel Department.

One day, I came back from lunch and found him going through some of the personnel files in our office. I was astonished to see him doing this, but at that time, when the physicians were partners, some of them felt like they could do whatever they wanted. After that, we always locked our files.

I mentioned that there were no female physicians in the clinic. Over the years, a few female physicians had been hired, but none of them made it to partnership.

In 1980, a pathologist named Susan Detweiler joined the clinic. She was bright and feisty and ended up being the first woman to become a partner in the practice. I remember that night very clearly. In 1983, after the partnership voted her in, everyone went to the Rainier Club for dinner and there was a little celebration for her where she was recognized and presented with a dozen roses. She gave a short but eloquent acceptance speech and then she broke off one of the roses into a boutonniere, and presented it to Fritz Fenster, who had adamantly opposed her admission. She did it in a humorous way, creating a good deal of laughter, and I admired her for the way she took everything in stride. At the end of that evening, Bob Nielsen came up to me where I was sitting at a table, bent over and said, "If you were a doctor, you would have been the first female partner." I was incredibly touched, considering that one of the greatest compliments I had ever had, and especially coming from him.

In about 1981, there was an opening for an assistant administrator in the clinic. I had been thinking that I would like to get into operations and I decided to apply for the position. One obstacle that I knew I would face was that the administrative fellow, Rick Osterhout, had been groomed for the position. I went to Austin and told him I wanted to throw my hat in the ring. Initially, he wasn't very keen on the idea. But I said that I knew Rick had been groomed for it and I understood my chances were slim; nonetheless, I still wanted to try for it. So Austin agreed to let me. As it turned out, several of the physician leaders voted in support of me and I was promoted. As a compromise, the Executive Committee approved a one-year assistant administrator position for Rick too, and when he left after that year, he had no trouble finding a job. After about three years, he was the administrator of a small hospital in Oregon.

After I was promoted to Assistant administrator, Bob Boyle told me that Roger Lindeman MD, who was then Chairman, was supportive of me being in the position but that he did have one concern. Part of the job duties involved overseeing the construction projects in the clinic. Apparently, Roger had remarked that he wondered what I would do if I needed to get on the roof, for instance, and look at some faulty equipment or oversee a repair (in those days, women wore dresses and heels). So I had an idea about how to reassure him and also have a little fun. I went to JC Penney and bought a set of overalls like mechanics wear to work on cars. Then I had my name embroidered on the front, to mimic how the physicians always had their names on their lab coats. At the first weekly administrative meeting in my new role, I said, "Dr. Lindeman, I understand you might have some concerns about how I would handle situations where I would have to climb on up on the roof or up and down ladders at a construction project. I want to show you my plan." Then I quickly went into my office across the way and slipped into the overalls. I came back and struck a pose. He laughed heartily and that was the last I ever heard of any concerns about me overseeing the construction and engineering projects.

In truth, I didn't know that much about construction and I had seen some of the engineers let an administrator go down the wrong path, much to their amusement, and make a decision that was not well founded. I wanted to avoid this, so right away, I sat down with the key players in the engineering department and told them that this was a new area for me and that I trusted and respected them as professionals. I said that if I was headed on a course they knew was not the best that I expected them to let me know rather than letting me get out on a limb and then watching me saw it off. I had the same conversation with the architects and construction workers. This turned out to be a good approach and we forged solid working relationships.

One slow Christmas holiday, Mike Rona, who was the administrator on call, decided on the spur of the moment not to come in to work that Saturday. My office was just across the way from his, and I noticed it was dark. I was afraid that John Allen would come by, so I opened up Mike's office and turned on the lights. Sure enough, about an hour later, he called for Mike. I answered his telephone, and when John asked if Mike was in, I answered, "Well, I haven't actually seen him yet, but his office is open and the lights are on." Then, I called Mike at home. He said tiredly, "I suppose I'd better come in." This was before caller ID and I said, "Call John from home and he'll never know the difference. But, you'll need to go somewhere very quiet in your house. Go up to the den, close the door, and make sure there are no kids crying or dogs barking in the background." So, he did, and John was never the wiser.

A few years later, we began venturing into satellite clinics, which stirred up a lot of controversy among the physicians. Austin asked me to oversee the Mountlake Terrace clinic, and my career turned in that direction. Eventually, I was overseeing all of them.

Another area that I was responsible for was negotiating the leases for the buildings that we rented to house the satellite clinics that we didn't own. At one point, we were leasing the clinic we had in North Bend from the physician who had practiced there, Dr. Jennings Borgen, who was retired and lived in a condominium just a few blocks away from VM. He usually came in to the hospital cafeteria every morning to have breakfast with a VM group that called themselves the Breakfast Club. He frequently ran into Roger Lindeman there and would complain to him that I was a demanding and tough negotiator. Roger would seemingly empathize with him and say that he would talk to me about it. Then he would come to me, and laughing all the while, tell me the story and end by saying, "Don't give Borgy an inch!" This went on for a couple of years, and I never did capitulate to Dr. Borgen.

The satellites were probably my most rewarding administrative assignment although I went on to have a number of role changes before I retired in 2007. I was fortunate to have a stimulating career full of challenges, but as they say, rarely a dull moment.

Ruth Anderson, MT(ASCP), MBA
Emeritus Senior Vice-President
The change agent in modernizing the lab, Ruth was promoted to an administrative role in order to maximize her exceptional management skills. Ruth retired after a highly

varied and successful career at VMMC. She shares her personal reflections below.

Memories of an Administrator (1981 - 2004)

It snowed the first day I came to work at Virginia Mason – it was known as The Mason Clinic then. January 4, 1981. I didn't know if that portended gloom, givenhow much I dislike snow, or something as wondrous as the view of the snow swirling around when my husband and I went up to the Camlin Hotel Cloud Room for a martini to celebrate my new job. Somehow that is when I knew it would be ok.

I never intended to come to Virginia Mason. I "visited" with Stan Sumida, PhD, out of respect for him. He had invited me to come down and just talk with him about the open position in the Laboratory. I was very clear that I had no intention of interviewing ... but when I got there I learned I was scheduled for 14 interviews! It was enough to make me leave then and there, but somehow I made it through and grew to like the people I met and respect their love for VM. My final interview was with Austin Ross.

Because I was "not interested" in the job, I was totally honest about the situation in the Virginia Mason laboratory at that time – the previous laboratory manager hadn't had a background in the laboratory and didn't stay long. As a result, the departments were running themselves with a lot of dissension. Of course, Austin drew me out, and the discussion was interesting and, dare I say, even promising. However, I started worrying that I'd actually be taken seriously and offered the position. There was a call left for me in Austin's office when I finished, asking me to come back and see Dr. Ed Barron again. At the time he was officially the Director of the Clinical Laboratory. The absolute kindness of that man, who sensed where I might be in my thinking process, made all the difference. He said, "They are going to offer you this job you know." I left after spending that time with him thinking maybe I could do this. However, I still had no intention of changing jobs. I sent a letter to Stan Sumida saying, "Thanks, but no thanks." Stan claims he never received it. We always laugh about that. Ultimately, a set of circumstances (and a whole lot of calls from them) convinced me to come to The Mason Clinic.

Part of the reason for my success, and something to be learned about going to the outside for a hire rather than promoting from within, was that I had no real knowledge of the power structure within the lab. With the full backing of Don Bauermeister, MD, and Ed Barron, PhD, I was given full authority to recommend and actually make changes. What I found was a group of fiefdoms, with no one but each supervisor in charge. Even in the sizeable storeroom, all the supplies were sectioned off by department – they were never shared – even when one department ran out. Little by little I implemented change.

One stipulation I made on hire was that I answer directly to Don with "dotted line" accountability to Ed. This became critical because it meant the anatomical side was covered by the same expectations as the clinical side – a rather big shock to those working directly for the pathologists who were given quite free rein. Over the next several weeks I was visited by the supervisors, one by one, who came to understand that as a medical technologist (the previous manager had only a business degree) and a laboratory manager, I knew all about the laboratory and how it should be run. Grudging respect grew, and I no longer was considered from "that lab in a hospital in the North". This came to a head at a general laboratory meeting when I was "put on the hot seat" to answer any and all questions. Apparently that went all right because on my six-month anniversary, I was guest of honor at a surprise celebration put on by the supervisors with an "evaluation" giving me five stars.

The next three years saw a growth in workload, a control of hiring, an understanding of expenses, and a wonderful working relationship with Don and Ed. Budgets were developed by me in conjunction with the supervisors. There was a strict accountability. Hiring was no longer simply the call of the supervisors – no ads were placed without my agreement. One of the longest-term supervisors said to me, "I've seen them come, and I've seen them go. The same will happen with you." Little did he know.

Don called our weekly meetings together the ABC meeting: the Anderson-Bauermeister-Conversation. We continued that even after I became an administrator, answering across the organization. He was my most valued mentor.

It didn't take long for the powers-that-be to decide I should take on more responsibility outside the lab. I was reminded of the time that one of the supervisors said, "They'll never let us keep you.

The first was with the cardiology laboratories (including transferring the cardiac catheterization laboratory from radiology to cardiology). This was no easy task because each department wanted ownership. Eventually, I was given more and more departments, and then in 1989 I was asked to become an assistant administrator for the hospital. The departments were largely support areas, and I asked to remain connected to the clinical pieces – otherwise I would lose some of the essence of why I went into a medical field. So it happened that I was the first person from the Clinic to bridge both clinic and hospital departments, with administrative responsibility for the Laboratory and Radiology, which was added to the list. I had all of the operational support systems as well, from Environmental Services and Engineering, to Properties and Facility Planning. I learned about the separate cultures that existed in each department as well as in the hospital. Ultimately, by the time I retired, at one time or another, I had had administrative accountability for every department except nursing, finance and the Clinic. Over time, that too melded into one culture to create the Medical Center we have today.

Memorable Events And Times

Retreats

Social events helped to make a cohesive unit out of these two disparate cultures. Management Retreats presented enormous opportunities for working and playing together. Above all, our sense of humor was key. We could laugh at and about ourselves. The skits were well done and poked fun at nearly all. No one was exempt. Even the Executive Committee was parodied. The Physician Retreats did the same for the physicians as they grew from a group practice of 90 (at the time I came) to over 400 (when I retired). Without that mechanism, it would have been far more difficult for physicians to bond as a group. The memories of those retreats became an opportunity to reminisce and laugh over the years. Early days also saw memorable events like the Gong Show, auctions, and talent shows. Then all of a sudden, we grew too big to manage these any more. I still think it was a loss.

The last Management Retreat came just months before the scheduled merger of Group Health Cooperative (GHC) and VM. It was the most powerful, and saddest, we ever experienced. All were allowed to "mourn" what was being lost; and the skits were biting, satiric, and truly funny. Possibly the most memorable was the skit performed to the theme from *The Lion King*. The songs "It's So Good To Be King" (with its underlying parody of the question of whether Mike Rona or Cheryl Scott would be the executive) and "Hakuna Mutata" pretty much said it all. We all left with a rock on which was written "Hakuna Mutata". I still have mine. It was cathartic for all.

The Group Health Alliance

The Alliance was quite a bombshell (to both institutions) when it was announced. There never could have been two more different organizational cultures in all of health care. GHC saw VM as elitist, catering to the "carriage trade," and total snobs. VM saw Group Health as Birkenstock, plain, interested only in the bottom line. Both views were true – and not true. It took the leadership of Don Olson at VM and Scott Armstrong at GHC to bring the disparate cultures into any kind of working relationship. Committees with representation from both organizations were formed. The prestigious McKinsey Consulting was retained to manage the process, at a hefty price.

I was asked to head up the clinical and operational support systems. The biggest contention, predictably, was who would "own" radiology and the laboratories. It was like "herding cats". No sooner would one big argument end then another would raise its ugly head. I remember a time when I was called in to try to mediate a radiology session. Nearly everyone in the room was either in tears or close to it ... including the sophisticated McKinsey consultant. Ultimately, a dicey agreement was reached that stood the risk of being destroyed at any moment. The laboratory was not quite as contentious, largely because of the sophistication of Don Bauermeister and Ed Barron (when Ed retired at the end of 1989, Katherine Galagan, MD, took his role in negotiating particulars related to the laboratory). The assumption had been made that GHC would simply absorb the VM anatomic and clinical laboratories. When it was clear that this was too big a hurdle to start with, it was decided that anatomic would remain in the sphere of each organization (meaning all of the pathologists would remain in place). The sheer size of the GHC Clinical Laboratory made them feel that any other choice but merging the laboratories at GHC was a fait accompli. They were surprised at how sophisticated our laboratory was, of the volumes we handled with a fraction of the staff, and at the level of testing that was present. As the sessions unfolded, a respectful truce ensued, with some progress made at every level. We worked from a classic model that looked at things that were quick and relatively "easy" to accomplish with large and small cultural and financial impacts; those that had a huge positive impact but were very difficult to implement; and others that fell between. It clarified where the group should begin its efforts.

More difficult, even than the clinical areas, were the support areas. The biggest surprise to GHC was how powerful our purchasing power was. They assumed they would take over; they had no idea how strong our consortium was with its national buying group across the entire country, how many outside institutions were buying through us, and how large was the scope of our ambulatory buying, including representing MGMA (Medical Group Management Association). The foundation laid by Austin Ross, Don Olson, and Ken Freeman, and the trust of the other hospitals and medical groups, had paid off handsomely over time. Both groups presented their studies and options, and it was decided that VM was much more powerful than anticipated.

Facilities Management was another surprise for GHC. Again, given the sheer size of GHC, it was assumed they had it all nailed. Again, they were surprised at the strength of our management team as measured in real numbers.

That isn't to say we were always on the top of the heap. Additionally,

510

there had to be "wins" for both organizations if there was to be any hope of an alliance. Ultimately, when the biggest work was done, McKinsey made the presentation to leadership. Each of the committee chairs was present, and the learning was a prize in itself. The biggest kudos at that point had to be given to Mike Rona and Cheryl Scott as well as physician leaders Roger Lindeman from VM and Jerry Beekman from GHC. All would agree that nothing could have happened without the leadership abilities of Don Olson and Scott Armstrong. McKinsey demonstrated the huge monetary advantages possible with a merger, although the devil (as always) was in the details. We were very close to merging.

Then came a bigger bombshell. Just about two months before the Alliance was to take place, the GHC physicians announced that they were becoming part of the Kaiser Permanente Group based in Portland. That organization had expanded as far north as Longview, with the threat of making a base in Seattle as well. The threat was bigger for GHC than for VM because their practice models were so similar. Additionally, all of the GHC physicians felt they would have a voice that they worried would be lost with the highly respected VM physicians. GHC decided to close their hospital and ER and admit to VM; ambulatory surgery would be located at the Capitol Hill GHC facility. Additionally, VM would no longer have an obstetrics unit in our hospital. In all cases, the physicians would stay with their own organizations, with the delivery of services divided. Essentially we were running two systems in one location. Protocols, patient management, and records stayed as they were. It was an unproductive "non-solution" but was the only one feasible at that time.

The Satellite System

The first expansions beyond the downtown campus were "affiliations" with groups in West Seattle, SeaTac and Mountlake Terrace. The first satellite we build independently was Virginia Mason East, which opened in June 1982. These sites were testing ground for determining how to deal with the issues involved: the standards that satellite physicians would have to meet (they were not all board-certified), and the more contentious money issues in the laboratory and radiology – both generators of sizeable revenue from the work that was largely "farmed out". An argument about naming came into play, with the first decision to name by city location, which eventually turned into naming for an area; e.g. VM Federal Way became VM South. There were many comings and goings: Federal Way into South; Mountlake Terrace and Lynnwood into North. Eventually, they were renamed again by city location.

The first sizeable merger was Issaquah. Al Einstein, MD, and I were given the responsibilities of directing physician relations, setting standards, developing policy, remodeling, staffing, overseeing laboratory and radiology, and creating budgets (operations and capital). Ultimately, it was a real success and became a model for the future. It remains as originally named – VM Issaquah.

Some of the less successful attempts were North Bend, Anacortes, Ninth Avenue, Redmond, and Port Angeles. Eventually, three very large satellites (North, South, and East) emerged with brand new buildings and sizeable staff numbers. Smaller, established satellites continued: Bellevue, Issaquah, and Winslow on Bainbridge Island. (see the separate chapter on Satellite Development in volume 1).

Building

Because of my role in Facilities Planning, I was involved in major building and remodeling projects. The first large project was Lindeman Pavilion. The arguments as to which departments would be located in the new setting were quite vocal. It is amazing how many of the sections felt they HAD to be in the new building (let alone the floor with the sky bridge) to be closer to the hospital – and had to be reminded that physician practices all over the city (and country for that matter) found that even cardiologists and OB physicians managed to drive cars to the hospital without losing patients. Double laboratory? Radiology? Outpatient surgery? Central services? Nothing was easy.

I was involved in finishing the items in the ten-year master plan for the campus, as well as beginning some of the items in the next. Largest in that

512

scenario was the expansion of the Lindeman Pavilion. Steve Rupp and I were asked to head up that planning. Unfortunately, a downturn in revenue along with an upturn in expenses (as was happening in all of health care) brought that effort to an untimely end. The new Research Center was built, however, with wonderful results.

Efforts to develop a new wing for the hospital were fraught with challenges. Community challenges were always there, from apartment and condo dwellers who would lose their view, to our VM-owned low-income housing. Taking down the Hudson Arms involved a series of challenges including city hearings and a failed attempt to have it declared an historic building. I never will forget the start of the demolition – I was given one of the bricks as a keepsake!

We always knew that we had to pay attention to some of the critical services that were in the 1929 building - the catheterization laboratory in particular. Unfortunately, that was delayed, but it ultimately landed in the wonderful new Jones Pavilion, which was built after I left.

The biggest disappointment for me about this hospital addition was the pressure that resulted from not housing Central Services in the new wing. Central Services is located in the oldest building, is too small, and depends on "human elevators" to get supplies across the disparate campus on time. Pressure from the clinical sections won out in claiming the basement where Central Services was to be located. So now we must deal with tunneling under the old hospital to get supplies into the new wing effectively. It will continue to be a huge challenge because of the high cost in my opinion. Time will tell.

A major success for the organization was moving the Hyperbaric Chambers across Seneca, with direct hospital access. Originally, the site was in the basement of Blackford Hall. This meant that any patients from the hospital in need of treatment had to be transported in an ambulance to go across the street! City requirements would not allow any other transportation method such as a wheelchair. The cost was prohibitive, and our volumes were growing. We were asked to do one of the first 3P projects in this area, incorporating what we had learned in VMPS

(Virginia Mason Production System) to develop the most efficient and cost effective service possible. The first surprise was the decision to place it in the Medical Library location in the hospital rather than in the large auditorium that was considered a free space for the new hospital wing. It did "pencil" out and became very successful. Neil Hampson, MD, led this effort and the pride we have in this beautiful project is well-founded. The biggest decision included moving to a two-chamber model, rather than one big one, which allowed many advantages including not having to close all services down if one patient had problems needing immediate attention. Time studies found it more effective for scheduling, especially for emergencies; more efficient for staff; and allowed the implementation of many other Lean ideas.

Other "battles" were harder to overcome. Getting the gastroenterologists (GI) to give up their appointment books and helping them to understand the reasoning behind planning for the "usual" vs. the 5% of the patients that needed more time, gave a 20% improvement in room usage. Other Lean improvements developed by the teams, which included GI doctors: standardizing all rooms so equipment and supplies were the same no matter which room a GI physician was using; and offering consultation rooms in the procedure area so the doctors would not have to leave the unit (a huge time-waster). These changes ensured that an appointment would be complete, including documentation, and meant the doctor never had to return to the case to complete dictation or coding.

Another monumental success was the new ambulatory surgery center in Lindeman Pavilion. It was a one-way flow system. The patient checked in directly to the prep room, where every bit of preparatory work (including changing, inserting IV tubes, any testing necessary) was completed. Stocking the rooms was done via two-way cupboards so this could be done from the back and not interfere with patient care. Additionally, stocking was done with just-in-time inventory so just "what was needed", "when it was needed", and "where it was needed" lowered the storage requirements for local inventory that are costly in duplication of supplies and staff. It also addressed part of the problems associated with Central Services being located far from the site. Once the patients were ready for the procedure, they were moved directly from their prep room to the procedure area, and then directly to the Post-Anesthesia Care Unit. The patients never had to be transferred to another bed or table; IV lines remained attached until recovery was complete. Dictation stations were immediately outside the procedure rooms so the surgeons could complete reports in a timely way. Thus there was no need to return to the case once they left the procedural area, no need to monitor surgeons for missing dictations, and immediate capture of coding and billing.

Lean and VMPS

I cannot leave this "tale" without relating my mixed emotions regarding the implementation of Lean practices at VMMC. Ultimately, because I was asked to head up this effort (which stretched my retirement back three years), it ended as my last "hurrah" at the organization.

When Mike Rona first asked me to be involved in a substantial way, I told him I'd consider it, and in six weeks I'd know if it was snake oil or a real opportunity for health care. To this day, I cannot argue about the wisdom of the method. However, I found the early attempts disheartening because of the expense and free rein given to some of the consultants. I spent hours in my office encouraging doctors and managers to at least "try it." We had any number of early successes, only because Mike and Gary held firm to the method. Frankly, that was the reason they convinced me to delay my retirement for this effort. And, I believed (and still do) that if we did not embrace the need to reform ourselves, the government would to it for us ... in ways we would not like.

Which leads me to the first trip to --

Japan

When it was first decided that all of leadership would travel to Japan to experience Lean production first-hand, I cannot begin to describe the turmoil within the organization, as well as publicly. It hit the front page of *The Seattle Times* for which I had to handle the calls.

When Gary Kaplan was elected Chairman to succeed Roger Lindeman, there was change ahead. The biggest change for the physicians to accept was the Board changing the role of Chairman from one elected by the physicians to one appointed by the Board, without time limitations. This happened because of the combination of the Clinic and the Hospital into the Virginia Mason Medical Center, which left the post of Chairman in the hands of the Board. In the past, this role came up for election by the physicians every four years.

I certainly realize that implementation of Lean would not have succeeded if Gary faced an election. Physician resistance was very strong. As it turned out, the planned trip to Japan to experience the Toyota Production System first-hand was a solidifying effort for his new leadership team, both physician and lay.

It would take a document of its own to tell the tale (I refer you to the excellent chapter by Diane Miller who details this story in the next chapter in this volume). As it turned out, we learned a whole lot (as did Toyota) in the implementation of Lean practices as applied to health care. Yes, they had something to learn from us ... the idea of case carts in surgery, for instance. But we had much more to learn from them – ranging from perceiving value from the patient view as well as our own, to seeing all the waste in our system. I consider the basis for what VMPS has become today, including the establishment of the Virginia Mason Institute, as one of the legacies I left for the organization about which I care so much.

The story of the rest of this journey will be left to others.

J. Michael Rona (1981 - 2007)
President Emeritus, VMMC

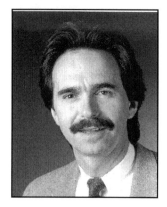

Recruited from Harborview, Mike Rona was the fourth top administrative leader, holding the position of President for nearly 25 years. Mike was a decisive decision-maker, known for his quick and effective use of humor. Paired initially with Roger Lindeman and later Gary Kaplan, he identified the need for change early on, leading to VM's new Production System based on Japan's Toyota Lean Management techniques. After leaving VM, Mike founded a very successful management consulting firm.

Reflections

I joined The Mason Clinic in the Fall of 1981 and left in the Spring of 2007. In those 26 years, admittedly the most challenging and exciting a person could want, the magnitude of change was, to use a very overused expression, unprecedented.

We were a private, for-profit partnership of 125 physicians, related to a hospital, started by physicians in 1920, largely inward-focused, all white, all specialists with one woman partner, pathologist Susan Detweiler. When the partners had their meetings at the Rainier Club, Seattle's oldest business club, the only women's restroom was on the 3rd floor and no one seemed to think that was odd.

Computers were just coming into daily life, largely in finance, with the first desktop being a Wang computer with a green screen. The go-to technology was a 10-key in the office of George Auld, Clinic CFO. Financial and operating data were closely held and, unquestionably, physician partners were number one. While management, early on mostly financial management, was valued, it was largely in the service of the partners.

But in the early 80s, there was a transition happening between management and physician leadership - the beginning of a true partnership and a model of leadership dyads that would set the course for how we would all work together over the next quarter of a century.

My introduction to The Mason Clinic was a seemingly random invitation from Austin Ross, the Executive Administrator of Virginia Mason. I was working in administration at Harborview, the county teaching arm of the University of Washington, and he asked me to come and talk to the administrative team about the structure and function of an academic health system.

I was 27 and knew nothing about The Mason Clinic other than that my grandfather had gone there. I did not realize that the talk was really an interview. Later, Austin asked me to come and learn more about The Mason Clinic and Virginia Mason Hospital. He suggested a Saturday morning, which struck me as odd. He told me that since the physicians saw patients on Saturday mornings, administration worked as well.

We walked the campus, and he told me the history of the place ... his vision for what to do with the old Doctors Hospital and where a research center might go some day ... He took me to the cafeteria to "have a cup of coffee" where "just by accident", the Marcus Welby of specialty care and Austin's physician partner, Roger Lindeman, dropped by.

There were no coincidences for Austin or Roger, as I came to learn over the years ... they were "planful", they had a long view, they were passionate about what they then called "integrated care", and they were interested in me, for a reason, back then, that was unclear to me. I was a hospital guy; they were looking, I thought, for a clinic guy.

At that time, retirement age for physicians at The Mason Clinic was 65 and it was mandatory. It was for that reason that I, as the operations leader at Harborview, was enlisted to help a physician named Tate Mason, Jr., who had reached that momentous age, to start up a urology clinic at Harborview. We met; he was wonderfully humble, but had clear ideas about how his clinic needed to be set up, which was a bit different in those days compared to the battleship green linoleum that was our standard for clinics at Harborview. He even wanted carpet!

We got Dr. Mason settled and later I talked with him about being approached by The Mason Clinic. He was totally against it. He said, "You don't want to go there, you'll be the doctors' handmaiden". He thought it was close to the dumbest thing I could think of.

I loved Harborview and my mentor, the CEO Bob Jetland, but it was clear to me that having an appreciation and understanding of the lives of physicians was a gap for me. We really had not been trained in graduate school about the real lives of physicians; actually we were trained to be wary of them. Many advised me not to do it, that I would be going backwards in my career, but I was enamored with Roger and Austin and I knew I could learn from them. In the 26 years that followed, I learned more from those two men and those they assembled around them than I could ever have imagined.

As I look back at the history of Virginia Mason, it has always been the story of leaders, most frequently in dyads, acknowledging the good of the past and the present and yet knowing that incremental change was not always the right step. While they liked to grow their own leaders, sometimes they would need to go outside. While they liked their specialty niche, they knew they would need to broaden into primary care. While they loved their for-profit partnership, they knew that it was an unsustainable platform to deliver their vision of quality and attract the very best clinicians. While they were fiercely protective of the role and power of physicians, they knew that other clinicians, especially nurses, would need to become part of the team. While they knew that multi-specialty group practice with its own hospital was the best care, it wasn't until the hiring of a marketing executive, Darlene Corkrum (from Group Health, no less), that this vision, what they had always called "integrated care" became "Team Medicine". Team Medicine was the umbrella under which the engagement of all of the people of Virginia Mason became possible.

While they, for the longest time, thought men were best designed for medicine, they leaned heavily into populating the physician staff with the other half of humanity. Women in medicine elevated Virginia Mason and broadened its understanding of both our own staff as well as the patients we were serving.

While they liked fee-for-service medicine, they knew that they needed to incorporate value. Indeed, way before "value in medicine" was the popular term, Austin Ross, in partnership with Fritz Fenster, hematologist and head of our first Practice Patterns Task Force, invented the Value Equation:

$$\text{Value} = \frac{\text{Appropriateness X (Outcomes + Service)}}{\text{Cost}}$$

While they thought they were the best in quality, they acknowledged that safety was not always first. Later, as we truly tackled quality and safety, we would modify Austin's equation by substituting Quality for Value.

While they thought all patients should be treated with equal access, they realized that they would need to be sensitive to an evolving society that did not think that way - thus the Women's Center, Bailey-Boushay House, Mason House and the Dare Center, all controversial but most having a large community impact.

While they loved their organizational independence, they realized that they would need to create significant partnerships, some with heretofore unimaginable partners - like Group Health. And, while they were hailed nationally as being the best in so many areas, the ability to have consistent excellence without some learning from outside of healthcare would be necessary - thus Toyota and the Virginia Mason Production System.

The story of those years is really, in many respects, that of senior leaders encouraging and allowing experimentation with seismic changes. It was always the top leaders enabling those around them to experiment and shift the trajectory of the organization.

Whether it was the then Chief of Radiology thinking in the 70s that The Mason Clinic should have an EMI head scanner, or the then Chief of Surgery simply announcing that he had obtained million dollar funding from a donor with no approval for a DaVinci Robot, or a Chief of Medicine driving the birth of primary care or managed care or the women's center, leaders, mostly in pairs, moved The Mason Clinic to the Virginia Mason Health System, frankly undersized in comparison to its reputation and accomplishments and largely still faithful to its vision of striving to be the quality leader.

It was the Lee Burnetts and the John Ryans and the John Allens who drove so much innovation in the early years and later, the Lucy Glenns and Katherine Galagans and Donna Smiths who carried on and accelerated those traditions.

Of course, no one was without their "wrinkles"; while John Allen, Chief of Medicine was fighting smelters in the community and smoking in the clinic, Lee Burnett, Chief of Radiology seemed nonplussed by setting off fire alarms in Radiology as he absentmindedly smoked his pipe under the smoke sensor. There was the time that John Allen reprimanded me for waking him up while he was sleeping in the board meeting … right in front of the board Chair. And the time that one of our esteemed chiefs decided that clipping his fingernails during the executive committee meeting and watching people duck … was somehow the right thing to do.

For 26 years, I served on the Percentage Committee, which later became the Compensation Committee. Their dedication to getting it right for the small group who comprised physicians was really a model in how to commit to people. It had innumerable silly moments and far too often lasted into the wee hours of the morning. There were times when I thought that John Allen and Richard Anderson were going to have a fight! As the compensation committee chairmanship proceeded from chair to chair and eventually to Joyce Lammert, its first woman chair, it too became less silly and better balanced. If all of the thousands of people at Virginia Mason had that level of attention and discussion, there would be virtually no undesired turnover.

Of course, as we evolved from a very closely-held, almost family-run business to more of a true enterprise, some things changed … like smoking in the building, or having ones' pets brought into clinic or sedated patients recovering on chairs outside exam rooms … even moving our events from the Rainier Club.

The addition of women leaders in so many areas changed the culture … the all-men's dorm with all of its strangeness, became more civilized and enlightened. Having women become Chiefs of Service like Lucy Glenn in Radiology and Katherine Galagan in Pathology/Laboratories; having pioneering women lead change for ambulatory nursing like Mary Anne Moore and Rita Kelly; having women executives rise like Sandy Novak and Ruth Anderson and so many more, dramatically moved the organization forward.

Even those whose tenure would be brief dramatically changed the trajectory of our professions. Barbara Brown, the chief nursing officer of the hospital, was a "force of nature" hired by Don Olson, the hospital administrator, to elevate the quality of nursing. She, of national repute, especially by her own admission, completely changed nursing's sense of what it could be. That change enabled the physicians to have an environment in which they could drive clinical innovation in the hospital. Don was brave in hiring Barbara, but no one really understood that well at the time… Don's hair was already as white as it could get!

That decision by Olson led to the hiring of generations of great nurse leaders like Pat Maguire and Charleen Tachibana and Patti Crome. Each of these leaders changed the course for Cardiology and Cancer, for Nursing, and for Ambulatory Care, respectively.

The story of this time period is that of moving from the quiet preeminence of The Mason Clinic to the simple, but powerful statement - Virginia Mason, otherwise called VM.

In the time that I was privileged to serve at VM there were major "pivots". Each one had their champions. I mention them, not in any particular order, but because they were more than normal shifts.

Most of the big innovations of the 80s were planted by Roger and Austin, either directly or by providing "air cover" for one of their colleagues. One of the largest was integrating the Virginia Mason Hospital and The Mason Clinic. This had been pretty much a tightly woven, but legally separate relationship for 60 years, but it was showing its stress fractures. The fierce independence that the for-profit structure gave The Mason Clinic and its physician partners also exposed it to escalating risk. The need to grow and the inability to retain capital meant that it became increasingly difficult to grow the physician group through the old "buy-in" method. The marketplace was changing where physicians could be in control in other practices and not buy-in. Almost as important, the ability to pay out physicians as they retired became more difficult as these funds were needed to grow and fund the clinic. The hospital, a not-for-profit entity, was well run and generated significant margins, much needed for its own improvements, but hundreds of "inter-financial agreements" between the clinic and the hospital had the effect of funneling significant funds to the clinic. I remember an early assignment of taking responsibility for negotiating these with the hospital and my colleagues Don Olson and Mark Secord. The process was designed to have us fight over money and find even more

522

creative ways to shift funds. At the end of the day, the hospital leadership knew that the clinic had to survive, so the money flowed. But the process was hard on everyone, and was inefficient and risky.

When the hospital and the clinic finally integrated into one structure (a process that evolved after the clinic became a not-for-profit entity), there was a period of adjustment for the group, as they were now members and not partners, under the ultimate control of a lay board with fewer degrees of freedom. However, they also gained greater safety and a source of capital to allow them to compete with less risk. While there was trepidation about this whole process and endless meetings to determine all of the fine points of the new structure, the leaders, Roger and Austin, ensured that there was appropriate power sharing and respect for the important reasonable independence required for good medicine.

I think the rise of Primary Care and the Satellite delivery system was probably one of the next most pivotal moments for VM. We had always had a very strong internal medicine section, but it was traditional internal medicine, clearly not the next evolution of internal medicine-driven primary care and certainly not family practice. In later years, as we considered walk-in clinics in downtown Seattle and having our physicians on television, we interviewed a physician named Bill Crounse, boarded in Family Medicine. I heard later that in the inner sanctum of the Doctors' Dining Room, a group of specialists grilled him on the basics of medicine. It was hard for us to change … it was hard for us to adjust our definition of excellence.

The rise of primary care was controversial for a specialty group for both philosophical and financial reasons. Our practice had been to serve as the referral source for primary care physicians, so what were we doing creating competition? And, these primary care physicians did not generate much money, so what would happen to specialty pay?

The community reaction to The Mason Clinic expanding into primary care was quick and intense. They told Roger that they did not like him or The Mason Clinic being in Kirkland and they would be happy to have him leave. As I heard the story, Roger was crestfallen, as he hated dissension, but he and Austin and John Allen all stayed the course.

The actual execution of the satellite strategy was left to the team of leaders below Roger and Austin. Leaders like Sandy Novak and Bob Webb and Gary Kaplan were instrumental in getting this started. The first clinic started in Kirkland with the acquisition of Del Morris' practice. We learned quickly that having spouses run the front office of our clinics in such acquisitions was probably not the best idea, but we were one of the first in the country to build satellites; there were no models from which to learn.

Good acquisitions and growth fueled the delivery system so essential to the expansion and success of the larger organization, but it was not without its failures. We grew a system very quickly to 16 satellites and eventually shrank that to 9. We hired and then had to let go of groups when we found that we could not really manage practices 100+ miles away. We found that having the largest pediatric practice tied to adult medicine was not as easy as we had thought it would be and we came to understand that while we could do outpatient pediatric care, we weren't as successful on the inpatient side. We learned that "referral leakage", as we came to call it, related to access issues that we had always had and that our satellite system would hold the downtown Seattle delivery system accountable for that as well as for quality.

And, we found that the magical arguments of "downstream revenue" to justify any number of growth scenarios and compensation arguments often had elusive results. As Dr. Winterbauer, Section Head of Pulmonary Medicine and head of the finance committee once said, "I've never met a proforma that we could not fall in love with". He also would lament how infrequently they turned out as advertised.

I remember Austin once telling me that one of the reasons that he wanted me on his team is that I liked numbers and he did not. I think, actually, he knew numbers at least as well as I did, he just preferred me pushing the implications of the numbers rather than himself. In the early years when I was younger and making the 17th pitch to the partners at their regular all partners' meetings to consider "if we could just see one more patient per day per physician"... I was sort of the designated hitter for bad financial messages. Austin and the partners hated those talks … but they also hated drops in partner income … Later I had others make those pitches.☺

When I first started that pitch, we were seeing 10 patients per day in internal medicine. Over many years of changing leadership and the implementation of process improvement, primary care eventually exceeded 25+ per day … of course, that took almost 30 years and new leaders like Jim Bender and Kim Pittenger and Marnee Iseman.

I also remember Roger asking me, as we became the senior dyad in 1991, why I could not ever seem to bring him good news. He often said, "Why can't you bring me a good surprise?" While Roger did not like bad news, he never separated himself from accountability and responsibility. Roger was always about having his partner's back, no matter what. He was selfless and humble. He taught me the code he lived by – his Four F's: Be Fair, Be Firm, Be Frank and Be Friendly. He was, as I reflect on the best teachers in my career, deeply committed to teamwork and team members, regardless of mistakes made along the way. Austin was like this too.

There were many pivotal moments during the time that I worked directly with Roger after Austin retired. We had great fun together and we struggled with some of the most difficult challenges we had ever faced. We had coffee together almost every day as we sorted out the issues of the time. I would bring a tray of styrofoam coffee cups to our meetings and fake trip, sending the cups flying at him. He would jump almost completely out of his chair thinking that a scalding was coming … of course the cups were empty … we did that routine countless times over the years, in front of others attending the meeting, and would just giggle with laughter.

As we were touring clinics and visiting staff in the system, I remember once walking into the Fourth Avenue Walk-in Clinic, when he asked me to remind him who the manager was … I told him Debbie Farnsworth and pointed her out in the white sweater … following which he walked up to her as he entered the clinic and said, "Hi Debbie, I'm Roger Lindeman". She replied, "Great to meet you, but that's Debbie over there." She, too, had a white sweater. From then on, Roger would ask me to be sure to introduce him to Debbie in the white sweater, if I would not mind.

As we became more diverse as an organization (granted this took a long time), Roger would ask how he should announce new physicians who were gay. How should he introduce the couple? He had the Dr. and Mrs. introduction pretty well down ... the others were initially challenging and it was amusing to watch him learn.

We had our more complicated times, including the Group Health Alliance. I think the last thing that Roger ever thought he would be doing in his career was creating an alliance between The Mason Clinic and Group Health. He had always felt there was such a divide between the two institutions. But, we needed their referrals, especially cardiac surgery, and they needed our Obstetrics – a service that we provided, but did not have the numbers for. They really didn't want to be in the hospital business, excepting OB, and all of our money came from being in the hospital business.

Of course, Roger Lindeman and Phil Nudelman were not an instant match ... Roger always led with humility and Phil, not so much. But, Roger exuded class and integrity and soon he and Phil found their cadence; I think they actually liked each other. We had many matching dyads, Cheryl Scott and I; Don Olson and Scott Armstrong; each physician leader with their counterpart; each side managed by bright fellows – Lynda Weatherby on our side and Andrea Voytko on theirs - and McKinsey ... the million-dollar-a-month advisor ... Little ol' VM was in the big leagues, trying to pull off what the UW and others had not been able to. We were trying to execute an alliance during the Clinton healthcare reform years that no one, including Stanford & UCSF, had been able to sustainably do ... but we did ...

At one point, we were close to merging with Group Health, but at the last moment, Nudelman was intrigued by discussions with Kaiser; his physicians enamored by the power of Kaiser's Permanente Group. We were left at the altar, but we were ok ... we had accomplished much of what we wanted to do and decades later, Kaiser would end up acquiring Group Health.

An anchoring decision in Roger's time was the construction of the Benaroya Research Institute. He and Austin had always felt that research was the third leg of the value proposition for physicians at Virginia Mason. While not all participated, there was a core group that needed clinical innovation and exploration as part of their professional lives. Frankly, the reputation of Virginia Mason started first with its core competency of diagnosing and treating complicated medical problems; this created the foundation for the rest of the medical group as well as a role for research and innovation.

To ensure that research did not get swept away in the storms of healthcare change, Jerry Nepom was hired to truly advance the Research Center. He succeeded John Rasmussen, a wonderfully amicable researcher, but added a drive that had never been seen in the Research Center before. While a friendly character, Jerry was totally committed to building a world-class research team. He needed the clinical "bedside" to accompany his "bench" work. We needed his drive and tenacity. Rather than invest in other capital priorities, Roger decided to work with the Benaroyas to get the Research Institute a new building. His long relationship with Jack and Becky Benaroya and their interest in Jerry's research led to the building of the Benaroya Reseach Institute. This decision ensured that while we would innovate on many fronts and evolve, we would also ensure that our core foundational beliefs would carry forward.

A ridiculously hard time together was when, unbeknownst to most, we almost went bankrupt in 1998 and 1999. It was related to pursuing an old strategy that did not work the first time, but that we resurrected during the alliance conversations with Group Health – starting a Health Plan. We had previously done a joint venture, under Austin's leadership, with Blue Cross, called Health Plus ... it had eventually closed down because we didn't know how to manage care.

With the alliance, we formed the Virginia Mason Health Plan, led by our fearless John Allen, and we did reasonably well. But, in the 90s, we were tight on dollars and getting tighter. What we did not understand was that we were incurring out-of-plan costs in the health plan that were not being reported. Called "Incurred But Not Reported", this IBNR represented a $50 million cost to us and came as a complete surprise. It almost sank us and if ever Roger felt like he was getting tired of bad news, it was then. I think it was my fault, largely because I did not listen to people trying to tell me the bad news. Later, when I asked them about it, they said they were afraid to bring it to me because they thought I would get angry. I never thought that I expressed anger all that much, but it does not take much, as I came to appreciate, to have people fear you. I will never forget Julie Sylvester, a manager in the plan, telling me that she had tried to tell me, but that I just refused to accept it. Unfortunately, the bad news was true. Fortunately, with the help of our outside accounting firm and a brilliant young consultant named Sue Anderson, we were able to spread the costs over two accounting periods, sell the health plan to Aetna, not go bankrupt and show a small profit for 2000, the year in which Roger would retire.

Roger decided to retire in 2000 after having been chairman for 20 years and re-elected to his role 5 times. It is telling that throughout those two decades, he was re-elected by huge margins, in spite of the turbulence of those years.

His replacement was Gary Kaplan, an internist, who had progressed up the leadership ladder and who was always interested in leading. He was groomed, in many ways, by his first champion, John Allen, and then later by Roger. Gary was smart and a capable partner. He formed and solidified relationships in his many years at Virginia Mason and was ready to lead when he was elected. He was completely different from Roger - not a specialist, not renowned clinically - but respected in management circles with a long list of accomplishments. If Roger was a leader of "firsts", Gary was more of a "fast follower". Again, not one better than the other, just different.

We were partners for 7 years. In retrospect, I think of those years as transition years. Gary's ascendance to the chairmanship took the senior leadership dyad back to the John Walker/Austin Ross time, where the power was largely with the physician partner … not good or bad … just not the more equal partnership that had existed in the prior 20 years.

The difficulty of the late 90s led to the development of a new strategic plan in 2000, a reset of strategy to re-energize the organization and to create a vision worth pursuing. It was out of this effort that the crisper vision statement emerged and from this strategic planning effort that we became open to the likelihood that without a different way of managing and leading, we were not likely to succeed. It was out of this work that we became more focused.

Our introduction to Toyota happened in late 2000. We decided that we liked pursuing perfection, we liked creating wealth by eliminating waste, we liked the engagement of our people and we liked being more focused on the process than on the individual. The Virginia Mason Production System, while controversial at first, catalyzed the core values of the people of Virginia Mason into a way for leaders to behave. It called us to be accountable and have urgency around things that mattered. It caused us to seriously question our commitment to quality and safety.

Toyota made it possible to be public about the death of Mrs. McClinton - a completely preventable death had we followed our standard work. Her death made us realize how critical leadership discipline and accountability were for patients and staff. Some were fearful about being public, which is completely understandable, but others felt that we must lead.

In addition to the above, with the change in leadership came a restructuring of the leadership appointing process - the election of leaders was eliminated by the board. I led this change, which I see now as one of my greatest errors. While I was concerned that chiefs and the Chairman would be too politically beholden to the physicians as elections approached, I came to understand many years later that the loss of the election process removed the accountability of physician leaders to the physicians. I was too worried that physician leaders would not be able to make the right decisions because of their desire to be re-elected - I had forgotten that Roger had been re-elected 5 times … as had so many of the chiefs, such as John Ryan and Lucy Glenn, just to name a few.

The years of our partnership were a time when strategy was reset, a management system was adopted, quality and safety began to rise to the top and the company started to stabilize into what would be years of stronger performance. Those years also saw the rise of the entire team that would be core to the success of the Virginia Mason Medical Center as it approached its 100-year anniversary. From Jackie at the front desk to Mark Hutchison at the board level, all were critical.

There were three reasons I came to The Mason Clinic – I needed to learn about physicians, I wanted to learn from Austin and I wanted to learn from Roger. I can check all of those boxes. What I did not anticipate were the innumerable friendships that I would make and how much I would learn from each one. There are hundreds of stories that could be told and hundreds of wonderful people who have not been named in this brief piece ... and to whom I am truly beholden.

William Poppy (1984 - present)
Senior Vice-President, Information Technology and Payer Contracting

Some thoughts and reflections regarding my tenure at Virginia Mason

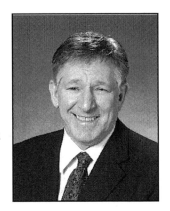

I joined Virginia Mason in 1984 coming from the University of Washington where I had been responsible for all the Information Technology (IT) staff, software and equipment resources supporting the University and their two Hospitals. Mike Rona recruited me and following interviews with Austin Ross and Roger Lindeman, MD, I was hired as an Associate Administrator of the Mason Clinic.

Our first challenge was to address the current status of the IT resources that Virginia Mason Hospital and The Mason Clinic were using to support hospital, clinic and ancillary activities. At that time, the Pharmacy, Laboratory, and Radiology were all supported by software applications designed to run on early generation Digital Corporation equipment (DEC) provided by multiple vendors. The Hospital also had an older generation Honeywell mainframe that was used for inpatient billing. Arthur Anderson consulting was working with the organization to address physician billing and planned to move The Mason Clinic's physician billing to the Honeywell. Mike and Roger wanted a more comprehensive IT Plan and asked for a market scan to insure we were on the correct path. The priority was to determine if there were better multi-specialty physician billing systems that other large clinics were using, that might address Virginia Mason's needs.

We conducted a market review, and found a physician billing system developed by IDX, a company located in Boston, that seemed to be gaining market acceptance with large clinics (Geisinger, Dartmouth Hitchcock and others). Mike asked John Allen, MD, Lee Burnett, MD, Richard Anderson, MD, and myself to visit Geisinger and Dartmouth Hitchcock in order to learn about their experiences with the product, review the overall functionality of the system, and determine its viability for The Mason Clinic. Our trip was extremely promising, and after long days visiting these institutions, we would finish up with a good dinner and refreshments, followed by lots of discussion about what we had experienced, and heated arguments between these physician leaders about other topics that ran well into the night long after I had retired for the evening.

In 1985, we signed an agreement with IDX and began preparations for moving this product into The Mason Clinic environment. In 1992, the Hospital billing system was also moved into the IDX environment and as of today, both the VM physician and hospital patient billing are still provided utilizing the IDX-developed applications. IDX sold the company to General Electric in the 1990s with several buyers thereafter; Athena Health currently owns these products.

As a side note, in 1985 we also elected to move our IT equipment and staff resources to the Metropolitan Park building on Olive Way, approximately 7 blocks from the medical center. At the time, the IT department was located on Madison between 9th and 10th adjacent to the Virginia Mason Sports Medicine clinic. Mike Rona and Don Olson also asked us to include moving the Hospital and Clinic accounting, payroll and billing staffs in order to free up space for the expansion of clinic and hospital services. I had the unique challenge of negotiating a lease agreement with Martin Selig, who owned the building, and was one of the larger commercial office developers in the Seattle community. There was lots of back and forth before we were able to land at a good place financially and as of today, these departments still reside in that same space.

2

Following the selection of IDX for billing and accounts receivable management, we turned our attention to clinic appointments, which at that time were maintained individually by each section and physician utilizing a paper scheduling book. John Allen, MD, had asked if we could possibly find a computerized patient scheduling system for the clinic and its providers to facilitate appointment scheduling across all the medicine and surgery sections. Again a market survey was done, but not much was available to accommodate our diverse specialties and volumes. After much research we landed on a product developed by Control Data and owned by a company named Dynamic Sciences that operated on a large IBM mainframe. We acquired the source code and equipment, and implemented our first computerized patient appointment scheduling system for all sections, which was used throughout the 1990s and eventually replaced in the 2000s by the IDX patient-scheduling application that nicely integrated with the clinic billing system.

During my initial tenure at VM, I was given lots of additional responsibilities, which were both challenging and gratifying as I reflect on those early years. I worked collaboratively with the physician leaders and my colleagues in Occupational Medicine, PM&R, Radiology, Pathology and the Laboratory, Surgery, Sports Medicine, and several of our satellite clinics. One of the more successful accomplishments was the purchase of the land on Gillman Boulevard, which is now the home of our Issaquah Regional Medical Center. Mark Secord, one of the Associate Administrators of the Hospital, and I were tasked with facilitating the construction of the Lindeman Pavilion, which led to the hiring of our first facility director, Scott Anderson, who came to us from Harborview. Our role was to negotiate the initial agreements with Sellen Construction and NBBJ, which was both challenging and beneficial, and to provide continuous oversight. Our goal was to have these firms work collaboratively on the initial design rather than sequentially, which brought real economies to both the design and construction of this facility.

I departed VM for 10 years beginning in January 1990 and therefore was not present for the many challenges Virginia Mason faced during the 1990s with the introduction of Managed Care Capitated insurance plans.

3

Returning to Virginia Mason ...

I returned to VM in 2000 following a call from Roger Lindeman and Mike Rona. Initially, there were two areas of focus: one was to move the Medical center out of capitated insurance arrangements with the third party payers and back to a negotiated fee-for-service payment model; and the second was to develop a long-range IT plan.

We drafted an IT plan, which was presented and approved by the Board in 2001. This plan outlined a strategy of using 3 vendors for our overall enterprise applications. Specifically, Cerner would be used for an electronic health record for both the Hospital and Clinic; Oracle for ERP products (payroll, accounting, HR and supply chain) and IDX (GE) would continue to be used for both the Hospital and Clinic patient billing and accounts receivable management. Radiology would also continue to utilize the IDX product, now owned by GE and interfaced directly to Cerner, and the Laboratory, which was already using the Cerner Lab product, would continue on that platform.

By 2010, most of what was projected in this plan had been addressed and we continued to roll out changes and upgrades across the entire enterprise. There were many successes along the way and a long list of contributors both within the IT department and throughout the medical center. It does "take a village" as I reflect on the many challenges and successes. In early 2015 - 2016, after much lobbying with Cerner, we helped them design the Patient Portal framework (My Virginia Mason), which offers patients ready access to their health information, appointment scheduling, provider information, and secure provider messaging. VM currently has over 250,000 patients utilizing the patient portal. We all are very proud of this success.

Today, the IT department has grown significantly in size and now supports both our hospital and physician practices at Virginia Mason Seattle and Virginia Mason Memorial in Yakima, Washington. We have literally hundreds of software applications supporting patient, clinical, financial, HR, and supply chain, as well as many individual department applications designed to support particular unique requirements outside of our enterprise platforms.

On the payer/reimbursement side, the era of managed care that was spawned during the nineties was ending, with most healthcare organizations in Washington reeling from financial losses. VM had its struggles and our primary focus when I returned was changing the payment models for our services to something more predictable. This was a very challenging time for VM and other Healthcare organizations and time was not on our side as we needed to move quickly to improve the overall financial picture. The insurance carriers were difficult, to say the least, and there were numerous challenges, but in the end we did prevail, ending all of our capitated payment models. This had a huge positive impact on the organization's financials and fortunately we began to see steady profitability and growth from this good work, beginning in 2002 - 2003 and continuing forward. I would be remiss to not mention two colleagues, Julie Sylvester, who worked with me in Contracting, and Craig Goodrich, our CFO, who was previously at Arthur Andersen. Both of these individuals made substantial contributions that indeed changed the course of the organization's financials. Today's payment model for both physician and hospital services is still primarily based on a negotiated fee-for-service pricing model. The market is attempting to recognize quality, and quality metrics with financial incentives are beginning to surface.

As we all have heard and read, there is significant downside pressure from employers to contain the cost of health care or reverse the growth trend, which makes it difficult for health care organizations to negotiate sustainable price increases. The increase in our labor and drug costs year over year are significant expenses that we cannot totally control. Insurance companies now think they are managing health care and have created an overhead in people and processes that are also huge contributors to the healthcare spending in this country. Hopefully we will move closer to a single payer model sooner than later.

4

Closing thoughts …

When I reflect on my career at Virginia Mason over two time periods and now as it starts to wind down, there are so many individuals I truly miss when I walk the halls each day. When I started here in the early 1980s, I had the privilege of working with Don Olson and Mike Rona, the administrators of the hospital and clinic respectively, and Austin Ross, our fearless Executive Administrator who constantly nudged us in the right direction. These men were all incredibly talented individuals who taught me so much along the way. The supporting cast of Mark Secord, Ray Raines, George Auld, Pat McGuire, Bob Boyle and Ruth Anderson were nothing but the best on so many different fronts and I still keep in touch with most of them. Ruth Anderson taught me so much about the Laboratory that perhaps I should have rethought my career! And Bob Boyle and that infamous laugh and his contributions in building the Regional Services and Referral Program were immense. And to Pat who helped me through a difficult medical chapter of my life, I will be forever indebted.

Then there were the physician leaders who really made things work and who helped inspire and drive some of the many advancements over the years. Roger Lindeman, one of the primary reasons I am here, was truly an inspiration to all of us on so many different levels. John Allen, the Chief of Medicine when I started, was visionary, especially around the need to push forward with technology. His efforts helped move us forward in our adoption of IDX for physician billing and the initial IBM computerized appointment system; Lee Burnett, the Chief of Radiology, also recognized the benefits of computerized technologies for Radiology. He was also among the first leaders in Radiology to agree to participate with the Digital Equipment Company as a pilot organization, while they built the first radiology application model referred to as Dec Rad. There are so many more outstanding colleagues I could mention, but unfortunately I would run out of the space afforded.

I cannot close without mentioning my fond memories around a couple events of the past. The annual Sweet Charity auctions, especially the one where Jim Bender, MD, bought a day of Mike Rona's and my time to weed his yard. It was truly hard work and he enjoyed every minute of it, watching the two of us toiling in his gardens. The leadership retreats at Port Ludlow and Fort Casey were annual occurrences that somehow got left behind over the years, but contributed immensely to the VM leadership fabric. These were events driven by our leaders at that time to help bring us together off campus to discuss future challenges, intermingled with lots of laughs, games and some outrageous skits!

For me, it truly has been a journey that has had many challenges along the way. As I walk down the halls of Virginia Mason, I am still reminded of the many individuals I have had the opportunity to work with who have contributed in so many different ways. Virginia Mason has evolved, as do most organizations - it's the people and their contributions at so many levels who make organizations special, and it is these people and memories that I will always treasure.

Sarah Patterson, MHA (1983 - present)
Executive Director, VMI

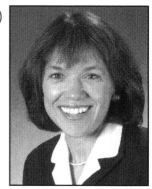

Sarah was the fifth senior administrator, taking the position of Executive Vice-President and Chief Operating Officer in 2007. In 2016, she transitioned to executive sensei at the Virginia Mason Institute and was named Executive Director of the Institute in January 2018. Sarah first came to Virginia Mason for a summer internship in 1983 as part of her master's in health administration program, which led to a fellowship and eventually a full-time position. Equipped with strong management skills, Sarah served in multiple roles in the administration, and was the administrative partner of Gary Ka-plan when he served as Chief of Satellites. Sarah was always flexible and willing to take on key systems and change management practices, and was admired for her ability to foster effective interpersonal relationships. She was instrumental in the acquisition and development of Virginia Mason Memorial Hospital in Yakima and the implementation of VMPS, a role which continues to the present time.

Craig Goodrich (2000 - present)
Senior Vice-President/
Chief Financial Officer

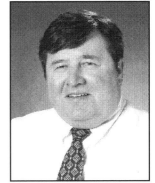

A Brief History of the Virginia Mason Health System Finance

Prior to 1987

Prior to 1987, The Mason Clinic (a for-profit partnership) and the Virginia Mason Hospital (not-for-profit) were closely affiliated but not part of the same controlled group.

In the early 1980s, discussions were held and the conversations evolved into making The Mason Clinic and the hospital into one entity, which would be not-for-profit. This entity would provide certain benefits such as tax-exempt financing for the entire system. This event happened in 1987 when The Mason Clinic was rolled up into the new non-profit corporate entity. According to Roger Lindeman, the physician vote was nearly unan-imous except for one vote that was done "in memory of the partnership." So, in 1987, a significant $100 million of bond was issued, which allowed for the acquisition of Mason Clinic assets and also provided funds for fu-ture building projects.

One of these projects was the new Lindeman Pavilion. In the early 1980s, the hospital had acquired the previous Doctors' Hospital, which provided the facility now renamed the HRB building, as well as the site for the future Lindeman Pavilion building. Real estate acquisition has been an important part of the VMMC downtown campus development. With the growth in property values, these acquisitions have added to the growing asset base of the Medical Center. In addition, the clinic had been developing primary care in some selected satellite locations over the early 1980s, leading up to the 1987 bond issue, which provided funds for the Federal Way and Issaquah construction.

1990s

Having completed the merger into one corporate entity, plans could now be put into place to have a finance function that would cover all entities. By the early 1990s, accounting and finance for the hospital and clinic were combined. This allowed for an overall picture of the financial health of the entity. Also, in the 1990s, a health plan was established but was ultimately sold for various reasons prior to the end of the 1990s.

In 1997, the Research Institute (now a controlled entity under the Virginia Mason Health System) was ready to move from Blackford Hall and acquire much-needed space to grow. A tax-exempt bond was issued to pay for construction of a new research building to be located on the VM parking lot at 9th and Seneca. With a generous donation from the Benaroya family, the Benaroya Research Institute was built. Additional funding would come from cost reimbursement under research grants.

One theme that was always present at VMMC was the need for additional capital and space. In 1997, another bond was issued for hospital campus building development as well as information technology needs.

2000s

As 2000 approached, the healthcare market was moving toward risk contracting models. Virginia Mason did participate but ultimately these contracts were not viable and had to be ended. By 2005, discussions also had started on building a replacement hospital on the east end of the current Central Pavilion. With a significant gift from a generous donor to motivate the Medical Center to move forward, plans for the new hospital were started. In 2007, a bond was issued to provide much of the funds for the new hospital. A lot of learning ensued about construction planning and cost estimates, but finally, the initial phase of construction was completed and the new hospital was occupied. In 2013, an additional bond was issued to further build out several floors in the Jones Pavilion.

We end this brief history with the observation that there are always opportunities and challenges in healthcare finance, but that it is an important and necessary component for providing excellent patient care.

Sue Anderson, MBA (2007 - present)
President, VMMC

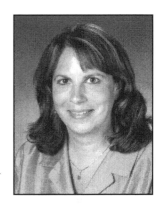

The current senior administrator, Sue Anderson has a background in finance and data processing, and is well known as a health system developer with an appreciation for the complexity of the merging of systems. A graduate of Notre Dame, Sue earned a master of business administration degree from Vanderbilt University's Owen Graduate School of Management, and had a long career in management consulting, including work at Virginia Mason before joining the organization as as senior vice president, chief information officer, and chief financial officer of the medical center in 2007. She was named president of Virginia Mason Medical Center and the executive vice president of Virginia Mason Health System in 2016.

And a few others:

It is impossible to recognize all of the amazing administrators who have served at Virginia Mason over the past 100 years. The following lists a few of these people and their contributions to Virginia Mason. We apologize to all of those we have unintentionally overlooked.

Bob Boyle, MHA (1969 - 1988)
Former Assistant Administrator & Director of Regional Services

The very creative Bob Boyle came to Virginia Mason with an MHA from

UC Berkeley. He was key in the early development of the satellite clinic system and the growth of the Health Sciences Consortium. Bob left VM to assume a position as a top administrator at the Palo Alto Clinic and has had a long career as a health care consultant.

Mark Secord, MPH (1976 - 1993)
Former Senior Associate Administrator

Mark's major contributions were in the area of social and community affairs. He was the lead in developing relationships involving Bailey Boushay House, then left to join Seattle Community Clinic Systems where he served as CEO of Neighborcare Health from 1998 to 2019.

Keith Lundberg (1978 - 1998)
Former Associate Administrator and Executive Director of the Health Care Consortium

Keith, a Seattle Pacific University graduate, was instrumental in the development and leadership of the Health Sciences Consortium, and led the study and initial application of telemedicine technology and international outreach programs before his untimely death at age 55 from acute leukemia. The Media Center within Volney Richmond Auditorium is named in his honor, as is an endowed lectureship.

Joyce Jackson, MHA (1982 - 1997)
Former Associate Administrator

An expert systems problem solver, Joyce was skilled in assessment and tactical approaches to administrative issues. A graduate of Penn State with masters' degrees from Vanderbilt and the University of Washington, Joyce left VM in 1997 to become the CEO of the Northwest Kidney Center and led it through a period of significant expansion before she retired in 2019.

References:
1. Low D. "John A. Dare: Part of Virginia Mason's Administrative Dynasty." *The Virginia Mason Bulletin.* Spring 2017; vol 71(1): 44.

35

The Virginia Mason Institute

by Diane K. Miller, MBA, Executive Director 2008 - 2016

The following chapter describes the events leading to the creation of the Virginia Mason Institute (VMI) in 2008, my personal journey to becoming its first executive director (ED) and the accomplishments achieved there during the first eight years of its existence.

Although VMI was not begun until 2008, there were many events and initiatives that paved the way for the board of directors of Virginia Mason Medical Center to decide to create a wholly owned subsidiary of the medical center that would provide education and training in the methods of the Toyota Production System (TPS). Since I had been involved in many of these initiatives, it was not surprising when Sarah Patterson contacted me while I was employed by a Lean consulting firm to discuss the possibility of me returning to Virginia Mason to lead this new company. I had left Virginia Mason in July of 2004 to work full-time with the Institute for Health care Improvement (IHI), where I served as faculty leading work as a Lean expert. In 2007, at the conclusion of the IHI grant work with Robert Wood Johnson, I then took a position with a consulting firm as a sensei for Lean, working with health care organizations that were adopting Lean management methods. Both positions provided me with invaluable knowledge and continued development in coaching and consulting with health care executives who were learning how to lead improvements specific to Lean, or the Toyota Production System.

Before deciding to return to lead such an organization I asked for assurance from Dr. Kaplan and Sarah Patterson that they were committed to continuing the Virginia Mason Production System (VMPS) journey. The Institute would only be successful if they were honest and transparent leading the transformation. If it was just talk or we lost our focus, the potential clients for the work would not be there. They both, without reservation, agreed that they were fully on the journey and committed to their continued learning for the adoption of VMPS.

Upon returning to Virginia Mason, in addition to being the ED for the Institute, I was also made a vice-president (VP) for the medical center with responsibilities and involvement similar to those of the other executives. This role within the medical center allowed me to experience first-hand the full responsibilities and accountabilities of executives leading a cultural change based on the Toyota Production System. Understanding how policies and the behaviors of executives either supported or were barriers to the full adoption of TPS in health care (beyond the initial changes) was critical to the success of the Institute in this industry.

I led the Institute from the time of formation and incorporation with six staff members and one contract with the Northeast United Kingdom until December of 2016 when I chose to step away from the ED and VP roles and finish my tenure as an executive sensei working with clients. I did so through May of 2017, when I retired fully from VM. The Institute's annual contribution to VM at the time of my retirement was approximately $1M annually with 35 staff members serving many health care organizations throughout the US and the world.

I could never have imagined this journey when I first began working at VM in 1980 as the Director of the on-site child care center. I led this work until 1983 when I was approached by an executive to apply for the admitting manager position. I declined initially as I was not familiar with this work - I wanted to work in child care where I had expertise. After numerous requests from several leaders (whose children were in the day care at

542

the time and knew me) I agreed to meet with Joyce Jackson to understand why I should apply for the position. She persuaded me to consider it so I weighed my options. I had been thinking of going back to graduate school in child and family counseling, since I spent so much of my time doing counseling in the current position; now I was being offered the challenge of the admitting manager position where, candidly, I would earn twice the income rather than spending money for graduate school. I was newly married and wanted to start a family so I decided to give it a try - if it didn't work out I could always go back to school.

I applied for and got the position, and then obtained my admitting manager's accreditation; within three years I was asked to take on the Utilization Review Department and then shortly after to take on the Quality Assurance Department. None of these roles were familiar to me when I was asked to take them on. They required that I learn the strategy for the work but left the technical knowledge to those on the front line.

During these years I was also Chair of the Safety Committee at a time in the mid-80s when smoking was allowed everywhere in the hospital. I, along with committee members, took on the leadership for implementing the no-smoking policy, which to this day is probably the most significant leadership challenge I was involved in other than the leadership for VMPS.

While serving in my role as Utilization Review director and staff to the Utilization Review Committee chaired by Dr. Fritz Fenster, we focused our work on implementing the "managing physician" role. This designation moved the organization to declare "a" physician to be in charge of the care of the patient. In a multispecialty group practice serving patients with many co-morbidities, there were often many physicians involved in their care, but when decisions needed to be made, it was not clear who was in charge. Dr. Fenster led this work with passion and as the years went by, he founded the Office of Value Assessment and helped us define "Value" long before it became a part of the quality equation that we reference today.

While in my role as Quality director in the early 90s, I became frustrated with the study of quality without action to improve. When I learned of Dr. Berwick's course on quality improvement, we took a group of eight to

543

Boston, led by Dr. Susan Detweiler who at the time was Chair of the Quality Assurance Committee. The group included Dr. Lindeman, Mike Rona, Ruth Anderson and Jackie Meurk, who was a member of the board at the time. After the course, we began working with Don Berwick and Paul Plsek to help us provide CQI (continuous quality improvement) training to many managers and physicians. We offered a 4-day workshop entitled "Methods and Tools" for quality improvement for many years. I was invited shortly after to join the IHI faculty for a national course on "Methods and Tools", co-teaching with several including Paul Plsek. Dr. Detweiler led our early work in CQI/TQM (total quality management), which I supported as Director for Quality, providing training and infrastructure. My role as faculty with IHI continued through 2015 with the added benefits of my expertise in Lean and health care leadership that I acquired subsequently.

In 1993 Virginia Mason leaders downsized and reorganized the management team. I took on the role of Education Director with the Departments of Continuing Medical Education, Continuing Nursing Education, the Sense program, our health and fitness program at the time, and staff and management development. I continued to lead this work until my departure in 2004. My title changed to Organizational Development Director as I divested my leadership as admitting manager, and later my work in utilization management and quality assurance. As the Organizational development leader we developed a 6-day leadership course for chiefs and executives - the first joint training for physician and administrative leaders. We began this series of 3 two-day development sessions in 2001. These training sessions provided the platform for introducing Lean to the executive leaders as we began to work with John Black. I also believe it established trust between the executives and physicians by creating shared learning, which then supported the more difficult learning that was about to take place: learning leadership for a Lean culture.

In 2001, Dr. Kaplan and Mike Rona decided to engage John Black to deeply learn this method, which had worked for Boeing and other industries, so I raised my hand to participate. I wanted to be involved in TPS (VMPS) due to my prior role as faculty for quality improvement with Virginia Mason and now as Organizational Development Director. I wanted to be sure we learned from past experiences - what had worked and what had failed. I didn't want to see what we had been doing thoughtlessly tossed out, but rather whether we could add skills to what we were already doing. Adopting a "management method of the day" was a risk and as the Organizational Development Director at the time, I wanted to build, not throw out. I also wanted to understand if it was different or simply the same concepts with a new title.

When we began working with John Black in early 2001, we spent the first 18 months exposing the executive leaders to the work of a Lean organization, the role of executives in this work, and the potential results that could be achieved. Lean had been successfully implemented in other industries but not in health care. In addition to a series of educational sessions integrated into the existing executive learning sessions mentioned above, we took trips to other organizations to speak with their leaders and staff about their experiences. Nemawashi is a word we now understand, "preparing the soil", for the big step of traveling to Japan for an intense learning experience before we decided to step fully into the adoption of TPS as our management method.

The Japan trip was preceded by a series of learning sessions called "Japan Prep". The executive team resisted the strict requirements for attendance, extensive reading assignments and homework. Gary and Mike, with the guidance of John Black, did not waiver on the requirements to both do the work and travel to Japan.

This two-week group trip was an exhausting, exhilarating, challenging and culture-changing first step. More executives began to see the power that this management method could have for health care, where higher quality, safety at lower cost and higher customer and staff engagement were desperately needed. Each evening Gary, Mike, Ruth and I met with John Black to discuss the success and challenges of the day and prepare for the next day. These two weeks were some of the most difficult of my career, but little did I know just how difficult the next three years would be.

On the last day of our journey to Japan, the entire executive team met to debrief the experience and help determine Virginia Mason's continued work to adopt this method. Gary asked each member of the team to state their support for taking on this challenge as an institution, as well as their personal commitment to lead in a new way. It was a moving culmination of two weeks together.

I recall another very significant decision by Gary and Mike while still in Japan, although the formal work had ended. While Gary, Mike, Ruth and I debriefed, we discussed what we would call TPS for health care and Virginia Mason. The decision was made to call it the Virginia Mason Production System, a very controversial name for sure! I was thrilled with this decision, since I had worked in CQI, TQM and many other "naming conventions". This was a signal to me, and more importantly to others, that this was not just more of the same but a significant change in our method for ensuring better quality and safer care at lower cost.

We began with four leaders being certified to lead rapid process improvement workshops (RPIWs), which was an important method to demonstrate the potential of this methodology in health care. I reported to Ruth Anderson, VP for Quality, who was taking the lead for this work at that time. Two of the individuals were operating room (OR) nurses in leadership roles, Susie Creger and Rosemary King, who were pulled out of their roles for 6 months to support the demonstration work in the OR, an area for improvement chosen by Dr. Kaplan and Mike Rona on the recommendation of consultant John Black. Danielle Smith, a Pennington Fellow, and I were the other two leaders certified in Lean initially.

For the next three years I led OVA, the Office of Value Assessment (which became the KPO – Kaizen Production Office - in 2004 following my departure). Between 2001 - 2008, Virginia Mason leaders studied and applied the methods and also became certified leaders, resulting in true cultural transformation. The book *Transforming Health Care: Virginia Mason Medical Center's Pursuit of the Perfect Patient Experience* by Charles Kenney describes those early years of developing the infrastructure for VMPS. [1]

Creation of the Institute

In 2008, I began the work of creating the Institute. My background experience leading OVA at VM, and the additional expertise I acquired at IHI from 2004 - 2007 and as a consultant in Lean with several other health care organizations gave me the tools to set up the Institute effectively.

Incorporation as a not-for-profit educational company with 501c3 designation was our first challenge and one that philosophically was important to us. We did not want to be just another consulting firm but rather be able to share our experiences to support the transformation of health care. We also needed to ensure we could cover the costs associated with the continuous flow of health care leaders who wanted to visit and learn from us, while at the same time assisting us to reinvest in our own learning of the Lean methodology. The leap-of-faith journey we began in 2001 had shown substantial evidence of improved safety and higher quality, and we were ready to share with others who had been asking for some time to learn from us.

A Board of Directors was formed from VMMC board members with Dr. Kaplan as President. We transferred several individuals who had been working with outside organizations, to the Institute; two event specialists, Wendy Barsaloux and Diana Thordarson, who had been managing the visitors we had monthly; two full-time KPO VMPS-certified leaders, Susie Creger and Chris Backous, who had been doing work with the United Kingdom (UK) group and other organizations; one part-time certified leader, Val Ferris, who was interested in working in the Institute; and finally, one physician, Henry Otero, MD, who wanted to work half-time in the Institute while remaining in a clinical role in oncology. Henry later chose to work full-time with the Institute as it became more difficult to balance the clinical demands of patient care with the schedules needed for the Institute.

The Institute also included the Center for Health Care solutions led by Robert Mecklenburg, MD, as Medical Director. This was formed to look at opportunities to decrease waste in medicine by collaborating with the marketplace and streamlining various care value streams. Their first at-

547

tempt, looking at the value stream for back pain management, resulted in a marked improvement in waiting time for patients from 31 days to same day, with 94% of patients returning to work the same day or one day later. Costs were also reduced, and Virginia Mason nearly doubled its back pain care volume in a single year. [1]

During our first year, we offered one-day overview seminars for individuals and organizations, and put considerable effort into the UK contract and the contract with Aetna for clinical value streams. While few other organizations were interested in purchasing our established and proven value streams for key primary care conditions, we were successful in securing a contract with Intel to support their employees in achieving better, safer and less costly care. This story is documented in a chapter of the book, *Pursuing the Triple Aim* by IHI [2]. Throughout the years we routinely had inquiries about how we had accomplished our high level of cooperation with our clinical staff but the power of this work was ideal for an organization that was adopting Lean. Any organization could implement in the short term the changes needed to create the clinical value streams but it was only those organizations that were truly working to change their culture to lead through Lean that could continuously improve and sustain the type of dramatic results we had achieved.

Speaking Engagements and More

Prior to the Institute, all staff, executives and physicians were contacted individually to speak about our Lean work. With the establishment of the Institute, we hoped to prioritize those engagements that were important to VM or to the growth of the Institute.

As the requests to learn, visit, and book speaking engagements continued to grow, it was imperative that the staff (executives and management) remain focused on VM issues using Lean tools, and also experience continued learning. It was equally important to ensure funding for continued work inside and outside of the organization. This took some time and to this day remains a difficult challenge for many. It was with great pride that everyone wanted to share our successes and welcome visitors to their departments. However, historically health care institutions share what they are learning for free, so the concept of the Institute charging for those services or the notion of intellectual property (IP) was quite foreign to many. IP was well accepted for "things" but a difficult concept when applied to the knowledge and processes we had developed within the area of VMPS.

Expanding beyond visits, speaking engagements and one contract for certification with the UK group was the focus in years 2 to 4. We wanted to ensure that organizations and individuals could experience us at a level for which they were ready. Most didn't understand what we were doing and how something that worked at a car company could be appropriate for health care, so the visits were a big portion of our activity. However once they realized that it did have applicability, we needed to be able to offer the next step in their learning. Thus, we developed introductory services such as webinars, articles, and one-day visits, as well as more in-depth coaching for the entire organization, with training and development of their own KPOs.

We saw an increase in requests for custom visits for a single organization's leadership team. This allowed the entire leadership team to have a common experience and talk about what was most important to them. These one-day executive visits became the most common means by which we progressed to contracting with the organizations to support the development of their cultural transformation using the TPS.

The transformation services model we developed was based on what had worked in the past and was critical to success, as well as what hadn't worked and wasn't critical. In addition to the technical component of teaching TPS methodology, we were well known for having a successful approach to working with physician leaders, which set us apart from other organizations offering these types of training services.

One of our most successful training offerings early on was "Flow in the Ambulatory Clinic". The work we had done with primary care was so compelling that we decided to develop a workshop for primary-care teams on the topic of flow. Dr. Otero led the work with the assistance of Drs. Ingrid Gerbino and Kim Pittenger. The first offering was so successful that an organization in Boston contracted with us to train their physician care teams. While we are always reluctant to teach "solutions", this work was so transformative that we shared specific changes needed for results similar to those our primary-care teams experienced. This training in turn led to full transformational services, which included work with the hospital associated with the physician group. Many of the attendees of these workshops over the years also went on to contract with us for transformational services for their executive teams.

Another significant opportunity for the Institute was our contract with John Black and Associates. John had been our consultant in the first 4-5 years and as he worked with other organizations, he contracted with us to provide some services he knew we could provide. Our first contract with him was for the Institute to provide one-day overview visits and create a course for his clients on "Mistake Proofing".

As a commitment from my Japan journey, I agreed to develop a "Gemba Kaizen" experience at VM. Individuals who were becoming certified leaders under contract with John would lead and sub-team lead a Rapid Process Improvement Workshop (RPIW) at VM. One certified leader from VMI would oversee the workshop to ensure the process was followed and was successful for our executive sponsors and departments within the medical center. These RPIWs were very successful but the market for this type of training was limited. We did, however, often use RPIWs to provide hands-on experiences for outside individuals as participants in these VM events.

We also provided week-long shadowing in KPO services for KPO leaders from other organizations to help them understand the role of a KPO within an organization that has decided to embark on the Lean journey.

An important milestone was reached when we were approached by Japanese hospitals to provide them with a multiday visit as part of a study tour. The hospitals were so impressed that we have provided them with two-day visit services every year since. In addition, we began co-sponsoring a conference in Japan once a year to share our current knowledge and assist in the showcasing of the work in Japan.

In 2014 we secured a 3-year contract with 3 hospitals in Denmark and in 2016, they added two additional hospitals. In 2016 we secured a 5-year contract with the UK to work with underperforming Trusts. We also worked in Scotland for several years supporting work they had begun years earlier. Each of these international engagements secured our name as a leader in Lean training beyond the US. At the same time we continued to grow our contracts for transformation services with durations of 3 - 5 years within the US.

While Lean is still looked upon with suspicion as to its value and importance to health care, there is a steady stream of executives looking for ways to support everyone's goals for better, safer and less costly care. What we continued to see was executive leaders struggling to learn and be accountable for new ways of leading.

Lean is a life-long journey for health care organizations; it is not a static learned process. It is not "we're done", and it is not delegated work. These truths mean few leaders have the will needed to take the steps to lead a cultural transformation.

Today we have national and international clients for stand-alone services as well as multi-year services. We continue to have visitors who wish to see and hear from our staff about what a transformed culture looks like. All of this work has also led to the publication of 3 books detailing our journey.

In 2008, when I joined, the organization had begun writing a book regarding their Lean journey. While we had good intentions and a great story to tell, the work was stalled. We decided to commission a writer to help us tell the story and Charles Kenney was commissioned. The book, *Transforming Health Care: Virginia Mason Medical Center's Pursuit of the Perfect Patient Experience*, was very successful and expanded health care's knowledge of what we were doing. [1] We then commissioned a book on Innovation and Lean through Paul Plsek to share how we had been successful in integrating these important concepts and principles into our work, which was published in 2014 (*Accelerating Health Care Transformation with Lean and Innovation: The Virginia Mason Experience*). [2] A third book on the role of executive leadership leading the cultural transformation was again commissioned with Charles Kenney and published in 2015 (*A Leadership Journey in Health Care: Virginia Mason's Story*). [3]

As our success continued, the need to grow staff as well as expanding our strategies to grow the business was critical. We enlarged and assigned dedicated individuals to the marketing and sales team and began attending specific conferences as an exhibitor to expand public awareness of our successes. We offered light touch experiences such as webinars or one-day visits, as well as in-depth engagements with organizations. In addition, as staff expanded, we started looking for new space.

At the beginning in 2008, our staff included six individuals plus the Center for Health Care Solutions staff, and we had a small space in the Health Resources Building (HRB). Our visitors participated in our offerings within our conference room space. This became increasingly challenging as the demands for space over multiple days increased. Since space was at a premium on main campus, we decided to move the Institute staff off main campus to the Metro building and created a new learning space for our visitors. We began with office and training room space on the 5th floor. We quickly outgrew the space, so we expanded and created a complete training and conferencing space on the first floor of Metro.

I'm thrilled VM continues to lead the way over these 18 years and into the future. I know the health care industry's greatest struggle in fully adopting this powerful approach to quality and safety is our willingness to hold ourselves accountable for standard work. I believe health care is riddled with waste that in turn creates higher costs in producing care. A relentless pursuit of how we best implement, improve and sustain standard work is a challenge I know Virginia Mason leaders will overcome if they stay focused on continuous learning. I'm extremely proud of the work I was fortunate to be a part of, before, during and after the adoption of VMPS. I look forward to benefiting from the work as a patient.

References:

1. Kenney C. *Transforming Health Care: Virginia Mason Medical Center's Pursuit of the Perfect Patient Experience*. Boca Raton: FL, CRC Press; 2011.

2. Plsek P. *Accelerating Health Care Transformation with Lean and Innovation: The Virginia Mason Experience*. Boca Raton: FL, CRC Press; 2014.

3. Kenney C. *A Leadership Journey in Health Care: Virginia Mason's Story*. Boca Raton, FL: CRC Press; 2015.

36

The Center for Health Care Improvement Science (CHCIS)

by C. Craig Blackmore, MD, MPH

Virginia Mason's vision is to be the Quality Leader and Transform Health Care. However, transforming health care requires sharing the work at Virginia Mason with others throughout the world. The Center for Health Care Improvement Science (CHCIS) was conceived in 2012 by Craige Blackmore, MD, MPH, and Gary Kaplan, MD, as a vehicle to rigorously evaluate and share Virginia Mason's quality improvement and other Virginia Mason Production System (VMPS) efforts. The Center operates by partnering with quality improvement teams, physicians, nurses, and other leaders throughout the institution, analyzing the ongoing work, and publishing the results in the peer-reviewed academic literature. As of 2019, the Center has supported over 70 published papers on diverse topics including: medication administration safety, experience-based care redesign, inpatient stroke and sepsis care, use of the electronic patient portal, and comprehensive patient care pathways. Our team members have presented this work to academic, provider, and policy audiences throughout the US and in Europe. The Center also has an annual faculty fellowship program, and partners with Graduate Medical Education to encourage resident scholarly work in quality improvement research.

An update from June 2018 gives a representative sampling of activity in CHCIS:

Research Focus Areas

<u>Patient safety</u>

The Institute of Medicine 1999 report "To err is human: Building a safer health system," heightened awareness of the extensive quality challenges in health care. At Virginia Mason, patient safety has been a major focus for more than a decade. At CHCIS, we have multiple research projects studying successful VMPS interventions to improve medication and surgical safety.

Selected publications:

• Ching JM, Long C, Williams BL, Blackmore CC. "Using Lean to Improve Medication Administration Safety: In search of the perfect dose." *Jt Comm J Qual Saf* 2013; 39:199-204.

• Blackmore CC, Bishop R, Luker S, Williams BL. "Applying Lean methods to improve quality and safety in surgical sterile instrument processing." *Jt Comm J Qual Saf* 2013; 39:99-105.

• Idemoto LM, Williams BL, Ching JM, Blackmore CC. "Mistake-proofing to prevent medication timing errors induced by computerized provider order entry." *Am J Hosp Pharm* 2015; 72:1481-1488.

• Kaplan GS, Gandhi TK, Bowen DJ, Stokes CD. "Partnering to lead a culture of safety." *J Healthc Manag* 2017; 62:234-237.

<u>Quality of care</u>

At Virginia Mason, we have implemented standardized clinical value streams across a range of health conditions, designed to prevent unnecessary care while supporting delivery of evidence based, appropriate care. Quality of care also encompasses developing tools to measure quality from the perspective of the patient and health care system. CHCIS research has demonstrated improved outcomes and efficiency from Virginia Mason care improvements.

Selected publications:

• Blackmore CC, Edwards JW, Searles C, Wechter D, Mecklenburg

RS, Kaplan GS. "Nurse practitioner-staffed clinic at Virginia Mason improves care and lowers costs for women with benign breast conditions." *Health Affairs (Millwood)* 2013; 32:20-26.

• Pittenger K, Williams BL, Mecklenburg RS, Blackmore CC. "Improving acute respiratory infection care through nurse phone care and academic detailing," J Am Board Fam Med 2015; 28:195-204.

• Bradywood A, Farrokhi F, Williams B, Kowalczyk M, Blackmore CC. "Reduction of hospital length of stay in lumbar fusion patients with implementation of an evidence based clinical care pathway." *Spine* 2016; 42:169-176.

• Blackmore CC, Watt D, Sicuro PL. "The success and failure of a radiology quality metric: The case of OP-10". *JACR* 2016; 13:630-637.

Patient-centeredness

Health care exists to serve patients. Too often, however, the needs of the patient can get overwhelmed by the health care system itself. At Virginia Mason, we have pioneered Experience-Based Design methods to understand and incorporate the patient care experience while redesigning the health care enterprise. CHCIS is engaged in validating and studying the application of Experience-Based Design.

Selected publications:

• Russ LR, Phillips J, Brzozowicz K, Chafetz LA, Plsek PE, Blackmore CC, Kaplan GS. "Experience-based design for integrating the patient care experience into health care improvement." *Healthcare* 2013; 1:91-99.

• Kaplan GS. "Pursuing the perfect patient experience." *Front Health Serv Manage* 2013; 29:16-27.

• Blackmore CC, Kaplan GS. "Lean and the perfect patient experience." *BMJ Qual Safe* 2017; 26:85-86.

• Hagensen A, London AE, Phillips JJ, Helton WS, Picozzi VJ, Blackmore CC. "Using experience-based design to improve the care experience for patients with pancreatic cancer." *J Onc Practice* 2016;

12:1035-41.

- Kamo N, Bender AJ, Kalmady K, Blackmore CC. "Meaningful use of the electronic patient portal-Virginia Mason's journey to create the perfect online patient experience." *Healthcare* 2017; 5:221-226.

Health care policy

The Virginia Mason vision is to be the quality leader and transform health care. Sharing our success with the broader health care world to inform policy makers is a critical component of transforming health care.

Selected publications:

- Blackmore CC, Mecklenburg RS, Kaplan GS. "At Virginia Mason, collaboration among providers, employers, and health plans to transform care cut costs and improved quality." *Health Affairs (Millwood)* 2011; 30:1680-1687.
- McDonald PA, Mecklenburg RS, Martin LA. "The employer-led health care revolution." *Harvard Business Review* 2015, July-August; 39-50.
- Kaplan GS, Lopez MH, McGinnis JM, eds. *Transforming health care scheduling and access: Getting to now.* 2015: Institute of Medicine. National Academies Press, Bethesda, MD,
- Kaplan GS, Blackmore CC. "The irrational physician defense of fee for service medicine." *NEJM Catalyst*, epub: 3.27.2018.

Organizational Transformation

Adoption of VMPS at Virginia Mason and other institutions is neither simple, nor linear. Understanding Lean organizational transformation is the newest research focus area for the Center. We are engaged in emerging research focused on understanding the process and outcomes of institutional Lean transformation.

Selected publications:

- Kaplan GS, Patterson SH, Ching JM, Blackmore CC. "Why Lean doesn't work for everyone." *BMJ Qual Saf* 2014; 23:970-973.
- Blackmore CC, Kaplan GS. "Lean and the perfect patient experi-

ence." *BMJ Qual Safe* 2017; 26:85-86.

C. Craig Blackmore, MD, MPH, FASER (2007 - present)

Craig Blackmore is Director of the Center for Health Care Improvement Science and a radiologist at Virginia Mason Medical Center in Seattle, WA. Dr. Blackmore underwent radiology training at Dartmouth Medical School, emergency radiology fellowship at Harborview Medical Center, and earned a Master's of Public Health degree from the University of Washington, through the Robert Wood Johnson Clinical Scholars Program. He has authored over 100 journal articles and book chapters, has edited 3 textbooks on evidence-based imaging, and has lectured extensively on emergency radiology, quality improvement, and evidence-based care throughout the Americas and Europe. Blackmore is former chair of the Washington State Healthcare Technology Clinical Committee, responsible for implementing evidence-based medicine in the care of patients covered by Washington state health plans. He is also an Affiliate Professor at the University of Washington. Through the Center for Health Care Improvement Science, Dr. Blackmore's current research focuses on improving health care quality and efficiency through the use of the Virginia Mason Production System, with specific focus on patient safety, evidence-based appropriate care, patient-centeredness, Lean transformation, and health care policy (for additional information, see previous VMI chapter and Radiology chapter in volume 2).

37

Materials Management

by Neeta Moonka, MD and Ken Freeman

Ken Freeman has worked at Virginia Mason for over 45 years and created the Purchasing Department in the 1970s. He went on to develop the Virginia Mason-owned group purchasing corporations, Health Resource Services (HRS) and National Purchasing Partners (NPP).

Ken, born and raised in Seattle, has deep roots in the area, much like Virginia Mason itself. He is a graduate of the University of Washington and was recruited as the pharmacy business manager in 1972 by Art Zoloth, PharmD, following four years of active duty in the U.S. Air Force Medical Service. He was hired to "save the pharmacy from the nurses and doctors" (see notes in the pharmacy history in volume 2), who at the time had keys to the pharmacy and took medications and samples for their families and friends. Austin Ross later revealed a memo from two of the anesthesiologists, which stated: "Fire this guy! We can't get into the pharmacy!" Ken proceeded undeterred and succeeded in his mission, establishing VM's first procurement system.

In 1974, Assistant Administrator Larry Anthony hired Ken as Director of Purchasing, which then was essentially a warehouse and distribution center. Ken envisioned a centralized service center and in 1978, created the Materials Management Department, which integrated central supply, transportation, sterilization and laundry and linen. From 1983 to 1985, the

Transportation Department was further expanded to coordinate movement of equipment, messages and people through the system. This strategy improved efficiency and reduced conflict between departments.

Concurrently, Austin Ross, executive vice-president, created the Rural Hospital Health Services Consortium. The consortium, administered by Keith Lundberg, supplied much-needed physician education to its 18 member hospitals, as well as education in transcription, medical records, pharmacy and supply chain operations.

In 1980 at the Association of Western Hospitals meeting, Austin Ross introduced Ken to Dave Jepson and Bob Walker of Intermountain Healthcare, established five years prior. VM accepted their invitation to join the 13-member, nonprofit, hospital group purchasing organization (GPO): American Healthcare Systems (AmHS). In 1986, AmHS changed its name to Premier, and the new company decided to exclude for-profit members, as well as clinics. Ken joined Bob Walker in forming a new GPO, which would allow clinics to be members. Intermountain, Western Penn, Vector and Healthcare Supply Chain Association (HSCA) formed AmeriNet in 1986 and VM joined as a marketing affiliate and investor. The new GPO enacted the first ever Medical Group Management Association contract.

Significant purchases over the years were the first CT Scanner (EMI) in the Northwest in 1979, the first lithotripter in the early 1980s, and now includes everything from tongue blades to MRI scanners.

VM was administering its buying group, Affiliated Purchase Services (APS), under the supply chain, but in 1993, APS became Health Resource Services, LLC. Ken left operations to serve as President and CEO.

In 2018, Ken started two new companies under the VM banner - Networx Health and Georgetown Specialty Pharmacy. Networx Health provides health care facilities with expert consulting services as well as interim C-suite personnel. The specialty pharmacy supplies patients with more difficult-to-acquire medications contributing to the continuum of care.

Ken's entrepreneurial spirit and dedication to Virginia Mason has and will continue to help make Virginia Mason successful.

560

38

The Virginia Mason Foundation

by Debbie Gordon and Jeanne Jachim

The first gift from a member of the community to the hospital was in 1923 when a donor—kept anonymous—funded the tiny diabetes store in the pharmacy. Other gifts over the years supported the summer camps for kids with diabetes. When the Research and Medical Education Foundation was formed in 1955, it accepted gifts from the clinic partners and a few other friends, but there was little effort to solicit support until the 1960s.

In 1972, the hospital and the research center established an Office of Development to invite gifts as part of the fifteen-year strategic plan. The office was successful in increasing donations, but a study by a committee chaired by Chairman Emeritus Joel Baker found "a need for an incorporated 'umbrella' foundation authorized to receive and allocate funds for both research center and hospital and to coordinate such efforts in the two organizations," and that the office as currently configured "would not allow for possible unforeseen developments, or possible accelerated requirements." [1]

In June 1976, the Virginia Mason Medical Foundation was formed to receive and distribute donations to the hospital and the research center and to provide direction for public relations and fundraising activities. One third of the board came from the hospital board of directors, one

561

third from the research center board of directors, and one third from the community.

In 1980, the Foundation began the Associates Program, not as a fund-raising effort, but as an educational forum on health care policy. Health care delivery and its costs had become a political issue and citizens need-ed to be kept informed. In 1983, the Planned Giving Program began to promote gifts through newsletters, promotional mailings, seminars, and personal contact by volunteers and staff members. In 1984, the first major capital campaign was launched to raise money for the Diabetes and Im-munology Program in the hospital and research center.

In 1986, as part of a system-wide change in governance, the Virgin-ia Mason Medical Foundation was folded in under the Virginia Mason Medical Center. In 1991 the Medical Foundation became the Office of Development. The Medical Foundation board of advisers became the Vir-ginia Mason Board of Governors, conducting outreach on behalf of the Medical Center. In 1994, the Office of Development became the Virginia Mason Foundation with its own board of directors.

The Foundation solicits and receives gifts from the Medical Center's many grateful donors. These gifts may take the form of tributes and me-morials; annual gifts, which result from annual fund solicitations; major gifts (which purchase equipment to support basic clinical and research pro-grams or which take care of special needs at the Medical Center); stocks and bonds; real and personal property; trusts; and estate, insurance, or pension plan distributions. The Foundation donors are patients and pa-tients' families, corporations, foundations, businesses, and friends in the community. [2].

On May 6, 1992, the first Dreambuilders' Ball raised funds for wom-en's health care issues. Every year thereafter, the ball supported a specif-ic program at the Medical Center. Also in 1992, the Foundation began managing the community support for Bailey-Boushay House as part of the Medical Center's care of AIDS patients. In 1994, Volunteer Services joined the Foundation's operations and volunteers were offered formal training as part of their work.

In 2011, the Foundation successfully achieved its goal of raising over $100 million for the Transforming Healthcare Campaign to support Virginia Mason, including the building of the Floyd and Delores Jones Pavilion.

Staff leadership of Virginia Mason's philanthropic efforts began with **Raymond W. Brown** in 1974, followed by **David T. McKee, PhD**, (1978); **Judy Biondi** (1985); **Steven D. Harrison, PhD**, (1989); **Constance J. Winberry** (1994); **Michael K. VanDerhoef** (2002); and **Jeanne E. Jachim** (2014), who continues to serve as President of the Foundation.

Through the years Virginia Mason has benefited from the generosity of thousands of individuals. Some of its most significant individual donors include Hiram Patterson, Jack and Becky Benaroya, Delmer and Mary Buse, Jacki and Carl Meurk, Barbara and Bob Buck, Howard S. Wright, Travis and Suzanne Keeler, Joshua and Pamela Green, George and Wendy Weyerhaeuser, Ann Wyckoff, Floyd and Delores Jones, and Leonard and Norma Klorfine.

Today the Foundation continues to be the philanthropic arm of all charitable activities for the Virginia Mason Health System including the Hospital and Regional Medical Centers, Bailey-Boushay House and Benaroya Research Institute.

References:
1. Baker JW. "Why The Virginia Mason Medical Foundation?" September 23, 1976, VMMC Archives.
2. "What Is the Virginia Mason Medical Foundation?," *ForeSight*, newsletter circa 1989, p. 4, VMMC Archives.

39

The Bailey–Boushay House:
The Healing Power of Compassion and Community

by Ellie David and Brian Knowles

$\mathbf{B}$ailey-Boushay House was built to care for people in the Seattle community who had nowhere else to go.

In 1992, when Bailey-Boushay opened its doors, the epidemic of Acquired Immune Deficiency Syndrome (AIDS) was a decade old. The new disease had already killed 139,000 people in the United States. And by then it had become the number one cause of death in this country for men between the ages of 25 and 44.

With few treatments available and no cure in sight, an AIDS diagnosis was a death sentence.

As the epidemic grew, widespread fear of AIDS and gay people swept the country. People disabled by full-blown AIDS had nowhere to live out their last days in safety and with dignity. Many were estranged from family. Partners and friends were dead, sick, or overwhelmed. Hospitals were too expensive for long-term care. Nursing homes were understaffed for specialized care.

It was in this setting that the Seattle community came together to create the first facility in the nation designed and built from the ground up to provide care for people living with AIDS.

Seattle turned toward, not away from, those most in need.

"It's a beautiful story of people stepping forward to do the right thing," says Betsy Lieberman, one of Bailey-Boushay's founders.

One of the boldest moves came from Virginia Mason Medical Center. At the eleventh hour, Virginia Mason stepped up by volunteering to operate the just-finished facility for the community.

Because of Virginia Mason's "unbelievably fearless and continuing commitment to Bailey-Boushay House," Lieberman explains, the 35-bed nursing home with day health center was able to open on time—and to stay open to serve the community every day since June 24, 1992.

1988-1991:
Building It So They Can Come

A tiny nonprofit named AIDS Housing of Washington (later called Building Changes) built Bailey-Boushay House with a staff of four—and the help of thousands of friends.

Six thousand people, organizations, and community leaders donated $6.2 million to provide cost-effective and compassionate end-of-life care to their coworkers, neighbors, friends, and, increasingly, their own loved ones living with AIDS.

"It was a groundswell of emotion in the community," says Betsy Lieberman, executive director of AIDS Housing of Washington. "It was the right time, the right place, and the right idea."

The need was clear

The still-growing number of people in Seattle with AIDS needed round-the-clock skilled nursing at the end of life. But the beds in Seattle–King County's traditional nursing homes were already full and had long waiting lists.

Even if a bed were available, traditional nursing homes had neither the training nor headcount to give specialized 24-hour AIDS care.

Cultural fit was also a concern. No nursing home specialized in caring for gay men and intravenous drug users, who at that time were numerically the most likely residents for long-term AIDS care.

The window of opportunity was short

Newly announced federal construction funds (leftover from the hospital construction budget) were available for long-term AIDS care.

A compassionate and cost-effective proposal for residential long-term AIDS care was already in hand, thanks to a recent continuum-of-care planning grant from the Robert Wood Johnson Foundation to the Seattle–King County Public Health Department.

And a group from the AIDS Long-Term Care Advisory Committee that wrote that planning report volunteered to help put their research and vision into practice by serving on the new nonprofit's board of directors.

The community was energized

The AIDS Housing staff was small: executive director Betsy Lieberman, fund developer Michele Hasson, accountant and office manager Mark Miller, and administrative assistant Jeff Crandall.

But the paid staff was guided, challenged, and inspired by a power-house board of directors and a prominent advisory committee. Their voices and expertise reached far into the community. They were activists, health care professionals, business and civic leaders, people living with AIDS and people who'd lost a loved one to the disease, philanthropists, communications experts, front-line providers of AIDS services, lawyers, educators, and leaders of faith-based groups—all of whom volunteered their time, talent, and treasure to the cause.

AIDS Housing of Washington hit the ground running in May 1988. First priority: start-up funding.

A $2,000 loan from the Northwest AIDS Foundation was the first bank deposit. A still anonymous (and still thrilling) $100,000 gift was delivered through the Catholic Archdiocese of Seattle—soon followed by an equally encouraging $100,000 pledge from the Archdiocese itself. By September the first federal grant came through: $500,000 from the Human Resources and Services Administration (HRSA). And by year's end a $1,500 donation from employees at Swedish Hospital marked the first gift in a community-wide fundraising campaign.

The ground-breaking celebration on October 10, 1990, was an emotional high point. ("I thought we'd reached the top of Mt. Everest," Betsy Lieberman says.) Just a year later W.G. Clark Construction Company turned over the completed building to AIDS Housing of Washington. In June 1992, four years after AIDS Housing went to work, Bailey-Boushay admitted its first residents and clients.

There were, as on every big project, plenty of problems to solve along the way. Two stand out because each would have delayed—and even shuttered—the desperately needed new facility.

Controversy slowed building permits

When the building site at 2720 East Madison Street was announced in fall 1988, the Madison Valley neighborhood expressed concern. And people kept talking for two years. Was an AIDS care facility appropriate for their small business district? The neighborhood was divided—strongly for, strongly against, and not-sure-but-concerned.

Objections ranged from familiar urban-density worries (added traffic and parking problems, the look and scale of the building, the size and location of the parking lot) to indications of Not In My Back Yard (NIMBY) flat-out resistance. The fear of lowered property values was a much-discussed topic.

The stigma of AIDS as a gay-related disease unsettled nerves, stirred misunderstandings, and polarized discussion.

"It was very hard, and I was very naïve," Betsy Lieberman says. "If I'd known what I was getting into, I would have been too scared to do it."

The debate spread throughout the city when four Madison Valley property owners lodged a last-minute legal appeal to deny the master building permit for the proposed health care facility.

In a memorable letter, the challengers wrote: "Like it or not, most people do not wish to be around ill people often, and here we may be adding the sorts of behavior sometimes associated with AIDS—overt homosexuality, dementia, and drug abuse."

When their first appeal lost, they filed another.

As a delaying tactic, the legal challenges were powerful. Waiting for permits meant costly construction delays that could put both the budget and the facility opening date in jeopardy.

Social pressure helped resolve the conflict. Supporters of the new facility took action to change minds:

- Radical Faeries dressed up in attention-getting outfits for a "terrorist shopping spree," cheerfully handing out pro-AIDS Housing fliers to Madison Valley merchants while overtly spending money in the shops.
- Community activists staged support rallies at the building site. News articles, editorials, and letters to the editor widened the community discussion.
- ACT-UP Seattle (local chapter of AIDS Coalition to Unleash Power) scheduled a protest against the permit challengers.

Just before the protest, the legal challenge was dropped. ACT-UP joyfully held a party instead of a confrontation. The scheduled ground-breaking was no longer at risk.

Turnout for that milestone event underlined the broad community support galvanized by the permitting controversy.

Seattle mayor Norman Rice and King County executive Tim Hill joined the AIDS Housing of Washington board and a crowd of 400 for the ceremony. Looking back 20 years later, Mayor Rice remembered: "I was proud of Seattle at that moment. I was proud to be mayor."

The search for a new operating partner

A less visible, but equally project-threatening situation arose in 1991.

AIDS Housing of Washington needed an established health care partner to run the completed AIDS care facility. AIDS Housing would retain ownership of the building; the medical partner would lease and operate it.

Early on they found a respected partner in the Sisters of Providence Health Care Corporation, a longtime Seattle provider of nursing home care.

Sisters of Providence guided financial planning for a skilled nursing home with higher than usual operating costs (AIDS care requires more

568

nursing hours per resident). They also navigated the state regulatory process for new health care facilities: a Certificate of Need was in hand by August 1989 and a timeline for licensing the new health care facility was in place.

The partnership hit a roadblock in early 1991. The Providence group opposed the presence of birth control products in the facility and the partnership was ended.

Finding a new operating partner became a fast-track priority. After talks with several top health care organizations, AIDS Housing offered the operating partnership to Virginia Mason.

Saying Yes to Great Need

Leaders of Virginia Mason's board, administration, and physicians faced two formidable questions.

One: *Do we belong in this field?* Virginia Mason had no experience running nursing homes. And while it had provided AIDS care in the hospital, it was not known (in the way Swedish Hospital and Harborview Medical Center were) as a place for patients with HIV.

Two: *Is the financial risk justifiable?* The state had yet to approve the higher Medicare reimbursement rates needed for labor-intensive AIDS care. The new facility couldn't open without them: standard daily nursing home rates fell far below expected operating costs.

"We took months to carefully vet the idea," says Mark Secord, the Virginia Mason administrator who carried AIDS Housing's message to decision-makers.

Working with a long-term care consultant assured due diligence on Virginia Mason's part. And open meetings throughout the medical center assured all concerns could be voiced.

Facing doubts, choosing commitment

Executive administrator Mike Rona and the hospital board advisor Austin Ross made a forceful case for Virginia Mason's opportunity and obligation to meet the community's need for AIDS care.

As in the wider community, energetic discussion raised awareness of fear and latent homophobia even within the health care setting.

"Those against were greatly outnumbered," Mark Secord recalls. "The whole program called to Virginia Mason's better angels."

The board of Virginia Mason voted unanimously for the operating agreement in April 1991.

That courageous act, says Betsy Lieberman "moved Virginia Mason way outside their comfort zone. And there was no financial case for it. They did it just to do good in health care."

Naming the new facility

AIDS Housing of Washington chose the completed building's name before turning it over to Virginia Mason in November 1991. Bailey-Boushay House honors Thatcher Bailey, a publisher who grew up in Seattle, and his life partner Frank Boushay, who died of AIDS in 1989.

Thatcher Bailey joined the board of AIDS Housing soon after Frank's death. As co-chair of the capital campaign, Bailey was a tireless fundraiser (he single-handedly raised $200,000 for the new facility). But it was his personal ties to the Madison Valley neighborhood and his personal story that inspired the AIDS Housing board to unanimously choose to use his and Frank's names.

"It was a time when AIDS was stigmatized as a gay-related disease," Thatcher Bailey later said. "It meant a lot for the board to name this facility after an openly gay couple who were directly affected by the epidemic."

Engaging the community in AIDS care

Once Bailey-Boushay House was staffed, equipped and furnished, licensed, granted higher Medicaid reimbursement rates, and caring for patients, Virginia Mason told its story to the community. The Fall 1992 issue of Virginia Mason's *Review* magazine featured a compelling photographic essay called "Images of Compassion: Caring for people with AIDS at Bailey-Boushay House."

Those 14 pages put a new face on the AIDS epidemic in Seattle.

The cover story presents intimate, intense, and respectful portraits of a dozen fragile patients, taken by photojournalists Saul Bromberger and Sandy Hoover during Bailey-Boushay's first 30 days. The unforgettable black-and-white images convey both the burden of having AIDS and the healing power of compassionate care in a homelike setting. In the article Virginia Mason explained its new role and commitment:

> "In this issue we invite you to experience the opening of Bailey-Boushay House ... [It is] a national trendsetter [and] a living legacy to the vision, compassion and leadership of this community.
>
> "Virginia Mason Medical Center was asked to manage and provide care at Bailey-Boushay. From a purely financial standpoint, the decision could have been difficult. The cost of caring for a person with AIDS is far greater than the reimbursement, but Virginia Mason responded with its heart.
>
> "We found it impossible to say no. The need was so great.
>
> "As you look at the pictures, we hope you'll agree that we made the right decision."

June 24, 1992:
Bailey-Boushay House Opens

For people living with AIDS in 1992, daily life was a roller coaster. Their loved ones and the Bailey-Boushay staff were on the same ride with them.

It was a time of "immense suffering and loss and trauma and stress," says Chris Hurley, Bailey-Boushay's first executive director. "The emotional intensity level was beyond volatile. Patients and their families suffered intense grief and outbursts of joy."

The unstoppable pace of an epidemic

People were so sick when they moved into the nursing home that average length of stay in 1992 was counted in days and weeks, not months. Chris Hurley remembers: "It took us six months to have one 'full house' day because people kept dying."

In the day health program 8 to 12 frail clients died each month.

Volunteer Matthew Behrle remembers the shocking number of losses: "Two or three people passed [away] my first two or three days," he says. "We were at the front lines of the battle with AIDS."

The complexities of comfort care

Patients' needs changed often and unpredictably. Comfort care spanned a wide range of clinical needs: respiratory infections, wasting syndrome, debilitating and disfiguring opportunistic infections, depression and anxiety, blindness, and dementia.

Managing their pain was complicated. And it was even more complex for patients with a history of addiction, because they required higher doses of pain medication for relief.

Upstairs in the nursing home patients had more choices than they would in a hospice setting. Some battled to stay alive long enough for a cure, choosing to join clinical trials or experiment with treatments for symptom relief. Others chose comfort care alone. All were subject to a swirl of emotions—anger, relief, grief, acceptance, despair, determination, and fear. And all had the right to change their minds at any time.

The roller coaster for clients downstairs in the day health program was, if slower, no less frightening. Still well enough to stay home at night with caregivers, they were too frail to be alone during the day. Many were tethered for hours to poles dispensing IV therapies. And though they found comfort, companionship, and encouragement in Bailey-Boushay's safe haven, the shorthand phrase "going upstairs" triggered dread. In 1992 those who moved from the outpatient program up to the nursing home didn't come back down.

Bailey-Boushay House promised to stay with all residents and clients on the AIDS roller coaster. That commitment, by building trust, offered stability to people in the maelstrom of an epidemic.

Brian Knowles, the first director of outpatient services at Bailey-Boushay, described the essence of the comfort care that staff and volunteers provided to patients: "Our job is to meet them wherever they are, at that moment, and to love them."

572

Inside the House: Two Constants

Without examples of long-term AIDS care to study, "Bailey-Boushay was a blank slate," says former executive director, Chris Hurley. "We had to make it all up, but we understood the problem."

Since June 24, 1992, two things have remained constant at Bailey-Boushay House: the compassionate mission and the building's welcoming embrace. Both make possible experiences of calm, joy, connection, and meaning even in people dealing with a terrifying and isolating illness.

A clear and effective mission

Bailey-Boushay House provides cost-effective and compassionate care to people living with HIV/AIDS, with the goal of improving their quality of life and helping them remain as independent as possible, for as long as possible.

The strength of Bailey-Boushay's mission is that it makes good sense: it's the right thing to do for all the best reasons.

Whenever it's safe for patients, staying out of the hospital saves money. And focusing on independence helps people retain the power and dignity of self-direction. Each resident and client at Bailey-Boushay has a broad choice of options in how to live and a nonjudgmental community to support their decisions.

Two core beliefs underlie the mission and guide staff and volunteers in their work. First, that everyone deserves to live and die with dignity. And, second, that those who provide care can learn from the people they serve and always find ways to do better.

A welcoming home: The physical setting

By design, the physical environment contributes to compassionate care and quality of life at Bailey-Boushay House. Its architects envisioned a care facility "as comfortable and gracious as a small hotel."

The three-story building's footprint is the same today as in 1992. Nursing home residents live in 35 private rooms on the top two floors; clients receive outpatient services on the ground floor. Everyone on site uses the shorthand "upstairs" and "downstairs" to distinguish inpatient and outpatient care.

Downstairs. The home for outpatient services is the Big Room: a large, light-filled gathering space just off the lobby. Clients who live independently—on their own or with caregivers—can safely and comfortably spend the day in a supportive community.

A nursing team is on duty all day. Restrooms, showers, laundry, and a nap room are down the hall. Hot meals and snacks come fresh from the in-house kitchen. A wall-size board lists the day's activities (open to all, but not required). A TV and music alcove is located next to doors that lead out to a large, lushly planted fenced patio.

Upstairs. In the nursing home, large single rooms give residents privacy. Common spaces—dining rooms, solaria, a greenhouse, an art room—encourage mobility, independence, and social connection through shared meals, group activities, and conversation.

Private rooms provide homelike comfort: a wooden frame for the hospital bed, a large view window, a private bathroom, and comfortable seating for visitors. In-room controls for environment (lighting and temperature) and entertainment (TV, DVD, stereo) reinforce individual choice. Room decoration is encouraged (as long as it's safe) to express a resident's personality, style, and life experience.

All through the house. Art was a top priority from the earliest stages of AIDS Housing's planning. The whole building is alive with original art that engages, nurtures, and lifts the spirit. Patients can also create their own art projects with Bailey-Boushay's artist in residence.

Shared spaces connect people to nature in the greenhouse and solaria upstairs. Downstairs, gardens edge the building. A meditation room upstairs—open to all patients, loved ones, staff, and volunteers—offers a calm and quiet space for reflection.

All these thoughtful touches impart a gentle influence on everyone inside the house.

Living in comfort, graciousness, and beauty calms the mind, feeds the senses, and enriches the spirit. Even for those at the end of life. And especially for those who are isolated by fear, pain, loneliness, despair, and social stigma.

A welcoming embrace: Staff and volunteers

The staffing model at Bailey-Boushay House takes advantage of interdisciplinary teams to treat the whole person. Patient-centered care includes medical and nursing services, complementary therapies, counseling, and spiritual support.

Everyone on the care team—from doctor, nurse, and nursing assistant to social worker, physical and occupational therapists, psychiatrist, dietitian, chaplain, artist in residence, and music and recreational therapists—works together to understand what each patient wants and needs. The shared goal: to promote well-being and independence.

The team upstairs also supports everyone the resident loves. Birth family or chosen family, partners and spouses, friends and children—all are made welcome, given comfort, and enabled to step away from the burdens of caregiving to spend their time renewing the personal connection that sustains both patient and loved one.

It's no exaggeration to say that Bailey-Boushay House couldn't run without volunteers. The combined dollar value of their unpaid hours places the group at the top of every year's donor recognition list.

Their service is both cost-effective and compassionate. Volunteers handle traditional tasks (helping in the office, at the reception desk, and with events). They also directly assist patients by serving meals, giving rides, running errands, and keeping people company—all of which frees staff members to spend more time in direct care. Certified professionals also volunteer their skills to enrich daily life for patients through acupuncture, haircuts, massage, Reiki therapy, spiritual support, and therapy pet visits.

Through their gentle and genuine connections with clients and residents, volunteers help create the supportive community within Bailey-Boushay. Their presence also connects patients to a wider community that has not forgotten them.

The Third Constant: Change

AIDS Housing of Washington envisioned re-inventing the traditional nursing home to provide hospital-level nursing in a homelike setting until medical science could end the AIDS epidemic.

"We really thought there'd be a cure," recalls Betsy Lieberman, "and that we'd turn over the building to serve another health care crisis."

But AIDS kept changing. The virus changed, the treatments changed, the needs of patients changed, and the people in most need of care changed.

"I've never seen a greater frequency of change and response," Chris Hurley says of Bailey-Boushay's nearly three decades of evolution.

The history of Bailey-Boushay House has been shaped by the need to repeatedly reinvent programs and services to fit the changing needs of people living with HIV/AIDS.

1992 - 1999:
Life-Changing Care at End of Life

Half the people who have died of AIDS in King County spent their final days at Bailey-Boushay House.

In Bailey-Boushay's early years, waiting lists written by hand on a yellow legal notepad grew ever longer for both inpatient and outpatient care.

With no cure in sight (1992-1995)

In 1993, just a year after opening, the Adult Day Health program had blown past enrollment projections by 50 percent. Originally designed to serve 35 clients a day (from a total roster of 70), it was now serving 50 people a day. To better meet frail clients' daytime needs, Bailey-Boushay added weekend care to its weekday services.

The expansion was "a huge and scary change for a small program," recalls director Brian Knowles, citing the increased responsibilities to recruit and manage more staff and volunteers, transport more patients, and coordinate increased facility use. "But that's what people needed, so we found ways to stay open longer."

The 35-bed capacity upstairs wasn't expandable. But the expertise of interdisciplinary care teams and high staff-to-patient ratio enabled Bailey-Boushay to provide life-changing care for people with AIDS at the end of life. Even without hope of a cure, many experienced healing of the heart, mind, and spirit before they died.

Stories of end-of-life healing

Upstairs: Two residents moved into the Bailey-Boushay nursing home shortly before their deaths in early 1995.

Gus, an artist in his early fifties, suffered from deep bouts of depression. The stigma of being gay and a recovering alcoholic added to his isolation and turmoil.

His wife describes the healing he experienced: "Gus thrived here," she says. "This place let him be exactly who he was and wanted to be. He was free. Everybody loved him. He could do his artwork. He could just be Gus. And not have any of that outside stigma to deal with."

Stephen, at 39, was angry about dying young. He didn't want to give up his future with the man he loved. And like everyone in his large family, Stephen was haunted by the neglect and indignities his older brother Gary suffered when he died of AIDS in 1990 in a New York City hospital.

A third brother describes Stephen's very different experience: "The contrast between New York City and [Bailey-Boushay] was night and day. From the very first day it was clear what a wonderful place it was. Stephen had resisted coming, but he knew it was the right place to come in the end. He was treated ... the way we all want to be treated: with dignity and respect for our humanity."

Downstairs: Steve was one of Bailey-Boushay's first outpatients. A few months before he died in early 1993, he said: "This place saved my life. The year before I came here I was just sitting home waiting to die."

The power of community support surprised Steve: "Being here is like family, without the arguing. Before I came here I was *definitely* against group things, but now it feels good to fit in. I don't know what it is about this place, but my entire outlook changed. I've had inside healing growth here."

Life-Saving Drugs Give New Hope

Two dates stand out in the history of AIDS. In 1981 the first AIDS diagnosis in the United States was made. After fifteen harrowing years of the epidemic, reports at the 1996 International AIDS Conference raised hope for the first time that new drugs were successfully controlling HIV, the virus that causes AIDS.

HAART (highly active antiretroviral therapy)—often called "the AIDS cocktail" because it combined three or more drugs—didn't claim to cure HIV/AIDS. But for many patients the new medication could slow the disease. Depleted immune systems showed signs of recovery: T-cell counts moved above 200 (the accepted marker of full-blown AIDS), and the amount of virus in the blood dropped to undetectable levels.

Many people—though, sadly, not all stopped dying and started getting better. For the first time since 1981, death rates began to fall. Nationwide deaths from AIDS dropped 47 percent in one year (1997-98).

Bailey-Boushay House was no exception. Before 1996, only 5 percent of all residents had returned to their homes. By 1997 Bailey-Boushay's fifth anniversary the year's discharge rate jumped to 30 percent.

Milestones in Meeting Changing Needs: 1992 - 1999

AIDS wasn't over with the introduction of the new AIDS medications, but the lives of many clients and residents at Bailey-Boushay House changed dramatically in the early years from 1996 to 1999. As health, energy, and hope returned, patients' growing independence required more flexible levels of care, both upstairs and downstairs.

Adding shorter-stay respite care (1996)

The word tune-up entered the Bailey-Boushay House vocabulary. "Going for a tune-up" gave people the option of moving into the nursing home for a few weeks or months of 24-hour care. The goal: to rest, heal, and re-charge after a medical crisis. It's a chance to fine-tune medication, rebuild strength, re-establish healthy eating and habits, and get support for other health concerns.

578

Offering medication management (1997)

The new AIDS drugs were incredibly difficult to take as directed. Dosing requirements were rigid and taxing. Toxic side effects were severe. Outpatients took 10 to 30 different medications every day—dozens and dozens of pills in 24 hours. Missed pills let the virus mutate and become drug-resistant, creating both the personal suffering of treatment failure and increased public health risk of passing the resistant virus on to others.

Bailey-Boushay recognized the new need—and the opportunity—to help clients take their pills every day, as directed, without fail. Effective medication management became a key goal in outpatient services.

"Taking 20 pills five or six times a day had become the life-saving part of HIV/AIDS care," says Brian Knowles. "It's not dramatic or glamorous, but after 1997 that became our work."

Widening the circle of care (1998)

In 1998 for the first time, the nursing home regularly had unused beds. With no waiting list, people seeking AIDS care upstairs were admitted without delay. But empty beds put the operating budget at risk, and underused resources were going to waste.

Bailey-Boushay began accepting residents without AIDS but who needed expert care that traditional nursing homes couldn't provide. They needed skilled nursing and end-of life care for complex conditions including trauma, cancer, large wounds, and stabilization before and after transplant surgery.

By 1999 half the residents upstairs did not have AIDS. Serving them ensured the doors stayed open to serve people with AIDS during uncertain financial times.

Helping clients graduate from care (1999)

In 1999 eligibility criteria for outpatient care changed. To make sure that the most vulnerable of those disabled by HIV—the physically frail, the homeless, the addicted, and the mentally ill—could get medical services, Bailey-Boushay asked 32 clients who no longer needed medical support to return to full independence.

Staff spent four months helping them plan for life beyond Bailey-Bou-shay House. It was a bittersweet turning point: they were alive and well, but leaving the supportive community that saved their lives.

And like everyone on HIV medication, they worried how long and how well the new pills would work. Bailey-Boushay reassured them: any-one who got sick could be readmitted within a week.

The remaining clients, the staff, and volunteers celebrated the depart-ing survivors as the community's first graduating class.

2000 - 2005:
In Transition, Facing Uncertainty with Flexibility

The new AIDS treatments approved for humanitarian reasons on a fast-track basis without long-term studies—brought both great hope and many unknowns.

Early in 1998 executive director Chris Hurley wrote: "Our crystal ball for the future is on the fritz these days. We do not know where the needs of people with AIDS will go in the next years. One thing is certain; we will be there with them."

From 2000 to 2005, as the inpatient and outpatient census fluctuated and as cuts continued in state and federal Medicaid funding, staff frequent-ly reevaluated changing patient needs. Three trends became clear:

• The powerful protease inhibitors didn't work for everyone. End-of-life care must remain a core Bailey-Boushay specialty.

• Residents and clients who were living longer, thanks to the life-sav-ing drugs, had more complex—not simpler—needs.

• Not all people taking HIV drugs had an equal chance of success. The risk of treatment failure was higher for those whose lives were also complicated by mental illness, chemical dependency, and home-lessness.

The Changing Face of HIV/AIDS

Even greater diversity had become a hallmark of the Bailey-Boushay com-munity by its 10th anniversary in 2002.

People receiving care were male and female, gay and straight and transgender, poor and not poor. They spoke English and half a dozen other languages (including American Sign Language), with ethnic heritages ranging from European and Latino to Middle Eastern and African. They were Christian, Muslim, Buddhist, Jewish, and not believers. They had been diagnosed with HIV/AIDS as long ago as 15 years and as recently as the last year.

In 2002 the mix of residents in the nursing home held steady at half with AIDS and half with other life-threatening conditions. Of the 110 clients in the outpatient program, 65 percent had a dual or triple diagnosis (HIV/AIDS plus chemical dependency and/or mental illness).

A Full House (Again) in 2005

The demand for services changed again. The outpatient program grew by an astounding 30 percent in one year. Inpatient care refocused exclusively on AIDS care and end-of-life care: 95 percent of nursing home admissions in 2005 were people with AIDS.

Medical director Dr. Wayne McCormick explained the need for more AIDS care upstairs: "It's not because we're seeing a steep increase in new infection or because we've run out of gas with HIV meds—it's because people with AIDS are living longer."

With steady medication, stable lives, and good luck, many people living with AIDS had few medical crises. For others, being on long-term HIV treatment added severe health complications that triggered a cycling from one level of care to another. They moved from hospital to Bailey-Boushay to ICU to Bailey-Boushay to home and back again.

"We're helping manage their struggle with medications and the in-out cycle of hospitalization," said Brian Knowles (who succeeded Chris Hurley as executive director in 2005). "They need us because they're alone, there's no one else to help, and they're too sick to be at home."

Milestones in Meeting Changing Needs: 2000 - 2005

Faced with increased demand for services in 2005, Bailey-Boushay staff used the Virginia Mason Production System to create efficiencies, adopted cost-effective new technology for patient safety, and reinvented the flow of services to ensure peace of mind for both inpatients and outpatients.

Streamlining the admission process

Using LEAN tools to reduce housekeeping room-turnover time and to streamline paperwork and procedures, the lead time for admitting a new resident, start to finish, dropped from seven days to three hours.

More people were served in the nursing home on a daily basis than ever before: the occupancy rate jumped from 75 to 98 percent.

Mistake-proofing medication delivery

Bailey-Boushay became the first skilled nursing facility in Washington State to adopt automated, single-dose packaging of medication. Working with Seattle pharmacy partner Kelley-Ross, Bailey-Boushay chose the new technology to avoid errors, save time for nursing staff, reduce waste in unused pills, and increase ease-of-use for patients. The machine-created, continuous perforated rolls of customized, single-dose medication packets are called medistrips.

Helping patients move easily between levels of care during health changes

Before effective HIV treatment, the flow from outpatient to inpatient care was a one-way, one-time event; staffing was separate in the two programs. With the advent of more cyclical care—moving back and forth between outpatient care and nursing home to resolve acute medical crises—Bailey-Boushay moved to an All for One staffing plan. Now the same social work and rehabilitation team follows the patient during health changes, emphasizing the patient's peace of mind and consistency of care over program convenience.

2006 - 2017:
Managing Chronic Illness

It seems a fitting marker that the first once-daily HIV pill was introduced in 2006. Twenty-five years after the first case was diagnosed in the United

States, AIDS had evolved, for most patients in this country, from an imminent death sentence to a treatable chronic illness.

A disclaimer is always necessary: HIV treatments don't work for everyone, and everyone on HIV medication has unique needs and medical experiences. Most outpatients at Bailey-Boushay House take an average of 11 different drugs every day (as many as 15-30 pills in 24 hours).

Though serving the most vulnerable people with HIV/AIDS—those who also live in the turmoil of chemical addiction, mental illness, and homelessness—Bailey-Boushay House has had notable success helping outpatients take life-saving pills correctly.

On average, Bailey-Boushay clients who live independently take their medication correctly 97 percent of the time. In most programs for chronically ill people with mental health and chemical dependency issues, pill-taking success is at best 50 percent.

With patients ranging in age from 18 to 80 and new treatments in development (and one day a vaccine), chronic care management at Bailey-Boushay will require continued reinvention to meet changing patient needs.

The building blocks of success

Lessons learned from the early years of giving comfort care to the dying continue to inform Bailey-Boushay life-saving services today.

- Build trust first.
- Approach all with respect and dignity.
- Ask patients what they need and want.
- Honor their choices.
- Provide the safety of a nonjudgmental community.
- Repeat every day.

"Food has always been our gateway to care," Brian Knowles says. Drawn to Bailey-Boushay for nutritious food, supportive nursing services, comfortable surroundings, and hassle-free medication management, clients—if and when they choose—also have the opportunity to participate in support groups, to work individually with mental health and addiction counselors, and to build skills to get and keep housing.

"We work first to build trust," Brian says, "so clients can move on to greater independence when they feel safe and supported."

Once clients are taking their medications as prescribed, Bailey-Boushay's ultimate goal for outpatient care is to provide every person with HIV equal access to positive outcomes (defined as undetectable HIV viral load), optimum physical and psychological health, a stable living situation, adequate nutrition, and supportive social connections.

It's a lot to accomplish, and it takes patience and persistence. But it's what everyone deserves.

"Good things happen when clients and residents take HIV medication successfully," Brian Knowles says. "The better they feel, the more hope they have. And hope can mobilize people to take courageous steps forward."

Bailey-Boushay is committed to develop tools and services that work for patients who are ready to use them.

Extending Healing at End of Life

Bailey-Boushay always has and always will give end-of-life care to nursing home residents with AIDS. We continue to encourage maximum independence—whether it's going on outings, dressing up for parties, learning how to golf, getting a pedicure, making music and art, or recording a StoryCorps interview for loved ones.

When people with AIDS do not need an available nursing home bed, Bailey-Boushay House now offers end-of-life care to people with degenerative nerve disease.

The care needs for people with amyotrophic lateral sclerosis (ALS) and Huntington's disease are complex and labor-intensive. Traditional nursing homes are unprepared and reluctant to care for them.

"These patients are in exactly the same position as people with AIDS were back in the early years," says Brian Knowles. "Their families are overwhelmed. And no one else can or wants to take care of them. We knew Bailey-Boushay was where they belong for dignified and respectful care. It is our honor and privilege to help them."

Bailey-Boushay is the only nursing home in the state of Washington that offers specialized care for these patients.

Because Housing Is a Health Issue

Mental health and addiction problems can trigger homelessness, and housing instability has long been a problem for a number of our clients trying to rebuild their lives after successfully taking HIV medication. But after 2012 (Bailey-Boushay House's 20th anniversary), homelessness has become a major health care crisis for outpatients living with HIV/AIDS.

In late 2013 and early 2014," reports Brian Knowles, "we saw a big change. More homeless clients were coming in—especially younger men in their twenties—and with a much higher level of desperation. The outpatient program hadn't been this full since 1998."

By 2015 a third of our outpatients were homeless and another third were at high risk of losing the housing they had.

Taking HIV medication correctly is hard enough when you have a safe place to store medication and reliable access to water, food, a refrigerator, and a toilet. Living in a shelter or on the streets provides none of those necessities.

After asking clients what they wanted and needed, Bailey-Boushay began devising and reinventing unique services to provide both immediate and longer-term help.

The Housing Stability Project (HSP) took shape in 2015 when four dedicated Bailey-Boushay team members began mapping ways to help clients acquire and maintain permanent housing.

This is work Bailey-Boushay cannot do alone. And we cannot predict where it will take us. But we are committed to ensuring that outpatients have the tools to take HIV medication, regain their health, and rebuild their lives.

Milestones in Meeting Changing Needs: 2006 - 2017
Transferring ownership to Virginia Mason

In 2007, the year of Bailey-Boushay's 15th anniversary, AIDS Housing of Washington (by then renamed Building Changes) transferred ownership of

Bailey-Boushay House, confident of Virginia Mason's unflagging commitment to AIDS care. The building-transfer plan ensured a sustainable future for Bailey-Boushay House within the larger Virginia Mason Health System.

Promoting independence for the most disabled

In 2008 Bailey-Boushay was the first nursing home in the state to install safer, more efficient equipment to lift patients.

One staff member can quickly and easily lift from bed to wheelchair any resident who can no longer control his or her own body. Mobility greatly improves quality of life. Our residents with Huntington's disease and ALS can more fully engage in the Bailey-Boushay community.

Improving communication on care teams

In 2010 Bailey-Boushay was the first nursing home in the state to convert fully from paper to electronic medical records.

Nursing staff and social workers on site, doctors in their offices, and our offsite pharmacy partner all have ready access to the latest information on each resident's care. Sharing real-time information promotes coordinated care, better decision-making, and patient safety.

Respecting patient rights

Bailey-Boushay is the only nursing home in the state to support a patient's legal right to choose when to die.

Most terminally ill patients do not exercise their legal right to physician-assisted suicide. If they do, Bailey-Boushay respects the decision to stop treatment and to end their lives with dignity, in the presence of people who will miss and remember them.

Opening a renovated kitchen

In 2014 Bailey-Boushay renovated its original 1992 kitchen (which started out with used appliances). The improved workspace promotes Bailey-Boushay's increased emphasis on making healthier food choices for self-care.

Living at the Winter Motel

In the winter of 2014-15, 45 homeless clients each got a motel room to call their own. The respite from life in shelters and on the street came through the "Winter Motel," a pilot project with Lifelong AIDS Alliance, to safely house the most vulnerable and hardest-to-house Bailey-Boushay clients. The goal was to keep frail people out of the hospital during Seattle's coldest, darkest, and wettest months.

Fighting hunger for better health

In 2017 (its 25th anniversary year), Bailey-Boushay opened an on-site food bank for homeless outpatients. Shelves were stocked to meet the special needs of people without cooking facilities, refrigerators, access to water faucets or even can openers (pop-top canned goods solve that problem). Clients fill their own bags only with what they want and know they will eat.

2017 and Beyond:
The Need to Change Never Changes

Bailey-Boushay started execution of its new five-year strategic plan in 2017. Developed over two years by Bailey-Boushay's all-volunteer, community-based board of directors, it's an ambitious, detailed attempt to improve Bailey-Boushay House's services, develop wider partnerships, and seek funding for future projects.

All of it is aimed in the same direction: to enhance the lives of people with HIV.

"Every year we've been open," says Brian Knowles, "we've never known what the future would hold. What we're good at is taking what we've learned from the people we take care of, and using that knowledge to reinvent ways to give them what they need and want next."

The Future of Bailey-Boushay House

Bailey-Boushay House embraced two brand-new opportunities in 2018 to meet the changing needs of its homeless outpatients.

Opening the world's first emergency homeless shelter for HIV-positive people

Funded as part of Mayor Jenny Durkan's initiative to add 500 shelter beds in the city of Seattle, Bailey-Boushay opened a safe and accessible overnight emergency shelter for up to 50 of its most vulnerable HIV-positive clients who are homeless.

All were medically fragile and already sleeping on the street. They avoided existing shelter services for fear of personal harm or having their medication stolen.

Opened on November 1, from 4 pm to 6:30 am the emergency shelter occupies the first-floor space used in the daytime for Bailey-Boushay's Chronic Care Management outpatient program.

"We're not set up for shelter," said Bailey-Boushay executive director Brian Knowles, "but who else would do it? We already provide other services to them as outpatients, and we know them so well. It just makes sense to have them sleeping inside instead of dying of the cold. "

Administering a rental assistance project to house homeless HIV-positive adults and their families

The City of Seattle in 2018 also asked Bailey-Boushay House to partner with and lead six local nonprofits that find housing for homeless clients. Focusing first on people of color and women, the project used federally funded vouchers to supplement rent on market-rate apartments in King and Snohomish counties.

"We're excited to share what we've learned in our 25-plus years of working with HIV-positive clients," Brian Knowles said. "And to learn from our six partners' extensive expertise in finding housing for the homeless."

Bailey-Boushay collaborated with Babes, POCAAN, Center for Multicultural Health, Entre Hermanos, WA State Dept. of Corrections, and Seattle Indian Health Board.

"It's such a great period we're in now," Brian Knowles said in 2018. "Bailey-Boushay has respect from government funders for the ground-breaking work that we do."

It's a wonderful context for looking back at 25 years of serving this community, he said.

"And it's only because of Virginia Mason that we're here. Virginia Mason is so wonderful to us. And they're all so proud of Bailey-Boushay House."

40

Dentistry at Virginia Mason

by John Kirkpatrick, MD

Although a dentist has never been under VMMC's governance, from the very beginning a dentist has been on-site and included in professional staff events. **O.T. Dean, DDS**, was one of the original investors. From the Archives, Lewis Dare wrote, "The Western half of Floor A had been specially divided into operating rooms, office and patient rooms for use as a dental suite by Dr. O.T. Dean, oral surgeon and stockholder in the hospital". [1] Dr. Dean had originally opened an office for tooth extraction and oral surgery in the Cobb Building in 1914, and presumably moved his practice to Virginial Mason Hospital shortly after 1920. He was the first oral surgeon in the state of Washington. A notice from 1934 announced a speech to the Seattle Council of the Parent-Teacher Association on "Effects of Cigarettes on the teeth and gums". Preventive dental care started with this – it's not clear when fluoride in toothpaste, sugarless gum and flossing became other important recommendations.

Roy Correa, Sr., DDS, joined the dental practice in 1928 and had his office on the VM Campus until his retirement over 40 years later. Locations included a small building between the Buck Pavilion and VM Hospital, and another on the west side of Terry Avenue next to the pharmacy, before the hospital expansion closed off that block of Terry Avenue where the current main entrance to the hospital is located today. The office moved to its most recent location across the hall from the hospital cafeteria on the 4th floor in 1975. Another oral surgeon, **E. Ulin Schreiner, DDS**, was listed on the staff in 1939. It's not clear how long he stayed.

Dr. Correa had met new UW Dental School graduate **Art Snyder, DDS**, in a downtown study group in 1961. When Dr. Correa had a heart attack in 1963, Dr. Snyder took over his practice. After his recovery, Dr. Correa and Dr. Snyder worked together for 10 years until Dr. Snyder bought the practice at the time of Dr. Correa's retirement in 1973.

After the move to the space across from the hospital cafeteria, several dentists joined Dr. Snyder for brief periods. The first was **Bruce Rothwell, DMD, MSD**, from 1975-1978, an aspiring academician who went back to the UW Dental School where he had a distinguished career as the longtime director of the Graduate Practice Residency Program and chair of Restorative Dentistry. He won national recognition for spurring creation of a computer program that used dental records to identify victims of Seattle's infamous Green River killer. He also won acclaim for creating a painkilling mouthwash for oral cancer patients undergoing radiation and chemotherapy, The Bruce R. Rothwell Distinguished Teaching Awards are given annually at UW. Dr. Rothwell died at age 52 in 2000. [2]

Others who shared the dental suite with Dr. Snyder included **Chester Woodside, DDS** (1982-1985), **Eric Opsvig, DDS** (1985-1988), and **Carrie York, DDS** (1992-1994). Each of them apparently wanted to buy into the practice but according to his wife, Dr. Snyder wanted to keep ownership of the practice until he was ready to retire, which he felt would make that final transition easier. **Ken Burnett, DDS**, the son of longtime Mason Clinic radiologist Lee Burnett, MD, joined Dr. Snyder in 1998. A year later, when it was time for Dr. Snyder to retire, Ken bought the practice, which he kept until his retirement in 2019. Ken's wife, also a dentist, joined his office in 2015 as a very friendly practice manager and scheduler. The Burnett team provided convenient, highly capable, and wonderful dental care ranging from routine preventive cleanings to hospital consults, and from tooth extractions and crowns to restorative and cosmetic dentistry. Dr. Burnett retired due to health concerns in 2019.

References:

1.Remembrances from Lewis Dare. VM Archives.

2. "School of Dentistry honors two outstanding teachers." At: https://www.washington.edu/news/2010/06/24/school-of-dentistry-honors-two-outstanding-teachers/; accessed 25 Nov 2019.

Made in the USA
Coppell, TX
20 July 2020